Phospholipids in
Nervous Tissues

Phospholipids in Nervous Tissues

Edited by

JOSEPH EICHBERG

Department of Biochemical and Biophysical Sciences
University of Houston
Houston, Texas

A WILEY-INTERSCIENCE PUBLICATION

JOHN WILEY & SONS

New York • Chichester • Brisbane • Toronto • Singapore

Library of Congress Cataloging in Publication Data:

Main entry under title:
Phospholipids in nervous tissues.

   "A Wiley-Interscience publication."
   Includes bibliographies and index.
   1. Phospholipids.   2. Neurochemistry.   I. Eichberg,
Joseph, 1935–   .   [DNLM: 1. Nerve Tissue—analysis.
2. Phospholipids—physiology.   WL 104 P575]

QP752.P53P47   1985   599'.0188   84-25660
ISBN 0-471-86430-7

Printed in the United States of America

10 9 8 7 6 5 4 3 2 1

*This book is dedicated to
the memories of*

*Jordi Folch-Pi, a neurochemical pioneer
who gave me unstinting encouragement,*

and

*Giuseppe Porcellati, a friend
and talented professional colleague.*

Contributors

BERNARD W. AGRANOFF Neuroscience Laboratory and Department of Biological Chemistry, The University of Michigan, Ann Arbor, Michigan

JOHN CALLAHAN Research Institute, The Hospital for Sick Children, Toronto, Ontario, Canada

R. M. C. DAWSON Department of Biochemistry, ARC Institute of Animal Physiology, Babraham, Cambridge, United Kingdom

STEPHEN K. FISHER Department of CNS Research, Lederle Laboratories, Pearl River, New York

LAURIE L. FOUDIN Sinclair Comparative Medicine Research Farm and Biochemistry Department, University of Missouri, Columbia, Missouri

ROBERT M. GOULD Department of Pathological Biochemistry, Institute for Basic Research in Developmental Disabilities, Staten Island, New York

LLOYD A. HORROCKS Department of Physiological Chemistry, College of Medicine, The Ohio State University, Columbus, Ohio

FIROZE B. JUNGALWALA Department of Biochemistry, Eunice Kennedy Shriver Center, Waltham, Massachusetts; Department of Neurology, Harvard Medical School, Boston, Massachusetts

ROBERT W. LEDEEN Department of Neurology, Albert Einstein College of Medicine, Bronx, New York

GRACE Y. SUN Sinclair Comparative Medicine Research Farm and Biochemistry Department, University of Missouri, Columbia, Missouri

EPHRAIM YAVIN Department of Neurobiology, The Weizmann Institute of Science, Rehovot, Israel

Preface

The accumulation of knowledge concerning phospholipid chemistry, metabolism, and function has been intimately associated with and paralleled our growing understanding of the complexities of nervous tissue at the cellular and molecular level. The presence of phospholipids in brain undoubtedly made it possible for Hensing as early as 1719 to demonstrate the existence of phosphorus in this organ. Pioneering neurochemists, from Thudichum to the late Jordi Folch-Pi, primarily and necessarily concentrated on the isolation, characterization, and quantification of these compounds in nerve and brain. This era in phospholipid research was succeeded by one in which the metabolic pathways involved in the biosynthesis and degradation of these substances were largely elucidated. Most recently attention has focused increasingly on the dynamic role of phospholipids within cellular and subcellular elements of the nervous system.

In the future, advances in this field will rely extensively on improved procedures for cell separation and culture, subcellular fractionation, sophisticated instrumental and microchemical analyses, and immunochemical and cytochemical techniques that will permit progressively more precise studies of defined structural components of the nervous system. Using these methods, numerous investigations are already underway on the distribution and metabolism of individual phospholipid molecular species in neurons, glia, and their subcellular organelles and on the exchange and transport of phosholipids within and among nervous system structures. A further goal will be to pursue tantalizing hints and to fortify existing circumstantial evidence that individual phospholipid classes or molecular species may play important roles in a variety of membrane-mediated phenomena.

To a considerable extent, the properties of phospholipids are utilized to fulfill analogous functions in all tissues. However, it is a reasonable premise that the characteristics of these amphipathic lipids have been adapted in particular ways to serve many of the unique functional requirements of nervous tissue. Indeed a major impetus for preparation of this book is to foster widening appreciation among neuroscientists of the importance of phospholipids in many aspects of nervous system function.

This volume has three principal aims: to bring together and summarize well-established information concerning phospholipids in nervous tissues, to discuss the status of major problems and areas currently being investigated, and to indicate likely future directions of research. The intent is not to be exhaustive or encyclopedic, but rather to identify and interpret important findings and, wherever possible, to set them in a structural and functional context. It is hoped that the book will be of significant and lasting value to experienced and novice phospholipid researchers alike and, in addition, of use to others whose interests may impinge on the phospholipid field.

Each contribution has been written by one or more experienced investigators. The book begins with a chapter that outlines recent advances in analytical methodology pertinent to phospholipids. Then follow chapters on the enzymatic transformations of phospholipids in brain and nerve and on changes in phospholipid distribution and metabolism during development and aging of the nervous system. Attention is next given to the movements of phospholipids in nervous tissue, including exchange and transfer within and between cells and axoplasmic transport of these substances. Because phospholipds are the primary source of free fatty acids that may be released in brain as a consequence of metabolic stress and subsequently exert a variety of effects, a chapter dealing with the generation, fate, and possible physiological significance of fatty acids is included.

The rapidly growing importance of cultured cells of neural origin in studies of phospholipid metabolism and function has reached the point at which a chapter on this subject is timely. This is followed by a chapter on the role of inositol-containing phospholipids in receptor-mediated phenomena in the nervous system, a currently fast-moving and provocative area.

In the last two chapters abnormalities of the nervous system that affect the status of phospholipids are considered. These include experimental models for nervous system disorders, as well as selected diseases involving nervous tissue in which alterations in phospholipid composition, distribution, and metabolism are either well documented or believed to play a significant part.

Throughout this volume a goal has been to demonstrate how information and approaches derived from diverse disciplines, including biochemistry, pharmacology, cell biology, anatomy, and neurology, have added to our knowledge of phospholipids in the nervous system in health and disease. In this way it is intended to impress the reader with the broad impact that continuing investigations of phospholipids will have on neuroscience.

The completion of this book could not have been accomplished without the cooperation and help of many individuals. In particular, I would like to acknowledge the perseverance, not to say forebearance, of the authors. I would also like to thank Dr. Brian Middleditch for valuable suggestions and for reading portions of the manuscript as well and Ms. Cheryl Fisher and Dorothy Smith for invaluable typing assistance. Finally, I owe much to my wife, Kathleen, and family for their encouragement and support.

JOSEPH EICHBERG

Houston, Texas
January 1985

Contents

List of Abbreviations   **xvii**

1. Recent Developments in Techniques for Phospholipid Analysis   **1**

Firoze B. Jungalwala

1.1	Introduction	2
1.2	Phospholipid Extraction	3
1.3	Purification of the Phospholipid Fraction	4
1.4	Phospholipid Analysis by Conventional Methods	4
1.5	Phospholipid Analysis by Newly Developed Methods	11
	References	40

2. Enzymic Pathways of Phospholipid Metabolism in the Nervous System   **45**

R. M. C. Dawson

2.1	Introduction	46
2.2	Biosynthesis of Phospholipids in the Nervous System	48
2.3	Catabolism of Phospholipids in the Nervous system	64
	References	73

3. Phospholipid Composition and Metabolism in the Developing and Aging Nervous System   **79**

Grace Y. Sun and Laurie L. Foudin

3.1	Introduction	81

xiii

3.2   Phospholipid Composition of Brain   82
3.3   Acyl Group Composition of Phospholipids in Brain   93
3.4   Composition of Phospholipids and Their Acyl Group
      Profiles in Spinal Cord   104
3.5   Composition of Phospholipids and Their Acyl Groups
      in Peripheral Nerve   106
3.6   Dietary Effects on Brain Phospholipids   107
3.7   Phospholipid Metabolism in Brain   115
3.8   Conclusions   125
3.9   Summary   128
      References   129

4.   **Transport, Exchange, and Transfer of Phospholipids in the
     Nervous System**   **135**

     Robert W. Ledeen

4.1   Introduction   136
4.2   General Considerations   137
4.3   Axonal Transport   140
4.4   Axon–Myelin Transfer   153
4.5   Intracellular Phospholipid Transfer   161
      References   167

5.   **Metabolism and Function of Fatty Acids in Brain**   **173**

     Lloyd A. Horrocks

5.1   Introduction   174
5.2   Transport   177
5.3   Oxidation   178
5.4   Synthesis   178
5.5   Release of Free Fatty Acids   186
5.6   Utilization of Fatty Acids   191
5.7   Summary   194
      References   195

6. Phospholipids in Cultured Cells of Neural Origin   **201**

Ephraim Yavin

6.1 Introduction: Lipids and the Neural Cell Surface   202
6.2 Methods for Nervous Tissue Culture   204
6.3 Chemically Defined Media, Lipid Constituents, and Neural Cell Growth   212
6.4 Composition and Metabolism of Phospholipids   214
6.5 Phospholipids and Neural Cell Growth and Function   228
6.6 Summary   233
References   234

7. The Biochemical Basis and Functional Significance of Enhanced Phosphatidate and Phosphoinositide Turnover   **241**

Stephen K. Fisher and Bernard W. Agranoff

7.1 Introduction   243
7.2 Pharmacology of Receptors that Elicit Enhanced Phospholipid Turnover   253
7.3 Biochemical Characteristics and Mechanisms   264
7.4 Cellular and Subcellular Localization of Enhanced Phospholipid Turnover   271
7.5 Functional Significance of Enhanced Phospholipid Turnover   277
7.6 Summary   287
References   288

8. Phospholipids in Disorders of the Nervous System   **297**

John Callahan

8.1 Introduction   298
8.2 Sphingomyelin Lipidoses: Primary Defects of Phospholipid Metabolism   299
8.3 Neurological Disorders with Secondary Involvement of Phospholipids   307
8.4 Animal Models of Phospholipid Disorders   313
References   314

9. **Animal Models of Neurological Disorders: Insight Through Studies of Phospholipid Metabolism**   **321**

Robert M. Gould

9.1   Introduction   322
9.2   Phospholipid Metabolism in Neurons and Glia   324
9.3   Approaches for Studying Phospholipid Metabolism in
       Animals   327
9.4   Wallerian Degeneration   328
9.5   Models for Demyelination and Hypomyelination   348
9.6   Experimental Diabetic Neuropathy   361
9.7   Conclusions   367
       References   367

Index   **379**

═══ Abbreviations ═══

Unless otherwise indicated, the following abbreviations are used throughout the book.

Ach	Acetylcholine
CI	Chemical ionization
CNS	Central nervous system
DG	Diacylglycerol
DPG	Diphosphatidylglycerol
EFA	Essential fatty acids
FFA	Free fatty acis
GLC	Gas–liquid chromatography
HPLC	High-performance liquid chromatography
LysoPC	Lysophosphatidylcholine
LysoPE	Lysophosphatidylethanolamine
MS	Mass spectrometry
NGF	Nerve growth factor
PA	Phosphatidic acid
PC	Phosphatidylcholine
PCpl	Choline plasmalogen
PE	Phosphatidylethanolamine
PEpl	Ethanolamine plasmalogen
PG	Phosphatidylglycerol
PI	Phosphatidylinositol
PIP	Phosphatidylinositol-4-phosphate
PIP_2	Phosphatidylinositol-4,5-bisphosphate

PNS	Peripheral nervous system
PS	Phosphatidylserine
QNB	Quinuclidinylbenzilate
SCG	Superior cervical ganglion
TLC	Thin-layer chromatography

Phospholipids in
Nervous Tissues

═ one ═══════════

RECENT DEVELOPMENTS IN TECHNIQUES FOR PHOSPHOLIPID ANALYSIS

FIROZE B. JUNGALWALA

Department of Biochemistry
Eunice Kennedy Shriver Center
Waltham, Massachusetts

Department of Neurology
Harvard Medical School
Boston, Massachusetts

CONTENTS

1.1   INTRODUCTION   2

1.2   PHOSPHOLIPID EXTRACTION   3

1.3   PURIFICATION OF THE PHOSPHOLIPID FRACTION   4

1.4   PHOSPHOLIPID ANALYSIS BY CONVENTIONAL
       METHODS   4

    1.4.1.   Deacylation and Phosphate Determination, 4
    1.4.2   Thin-Layer Chromatography, 6
    1.4.3   Molecular Species Analysis, 10

1.5   PHOSPHOLIPID ANALYSIS BY NEWLY DEVELOPED
       METHODS   11

    1.5.1   Class Separation of Phospholipids by HPLC, 11
    1.5.2   Determination of Molecular Species of Phospholipids
          by HPLC, 16
    1.5.3   HPLC–Mass Spectrometry (MS) of Individual
          Phospholipids, 22
    1.5.4   HPLC–MS of Phospholipid Mixtures, 34

    REFERENCES   40

1.1   INTRODUCTION

Phospholipids are the major lipid components of the nervous system. They make up about 20–25% of the dry weight of neural tissues and are important constituents of all neural membranes. Other complex lipids such as cholesterol and glycosphingolipids (cerebrosides plus sulfatides) are also abundant, each accounting for about 10% of the dry weight of neural tissue. It is therefore desirable that a preliminary class separation of phospholipids from these other lipids be achieved before detailed analysis of phospholipids is attempted. Many methods for the class separation and for individual phospholipid analysis have been described. This chapter will concentrate on procedures that are currently in general use, with emphasis on some of the recent developments in high-performance liquid chromatography (HPLC) and mass spectrometry (MS) techniques developed in the author's laboratory and elsewhere.

1.2   PHOSPHOLIPID EXTRACTION

Extraction of phospholipids from brain and other tissues has been amply discussed by Spanner (1973) and Nelson (1975). The most successful and commonly used solvent is still chloroform–methanol, described by Folch et al. (1957). Different workers have used varying proportions of this solvent mixture for extraction of neural tissues. In the most convenient procedure, the tissue is homogenized with 10 volumes of chloroform–methanol (1:1, v/v) followed by centrifugation at about 800g for 5–10 min to sediment the tissue residue. This extraction step normally removes 95% of the total lipids from the tissue. The residue is reextracted with 5 volumes of the same solvent, followed by 15 volumes of chloroform alone to bring the composition of the final extract to chloroform–methanol (2:1, v/v). Most of the phospholipids are solubilized by this procedure; however, if one is interested in recovering the polyphosphoinositides, special care is necessary due to their metabolic lability and ionic nature. The neural tissue should be frozen as quickly as possible; in the case of small animals the entire head is dropped in liquid N_2 after decapitation. For extraction of polyphosphoinositides, the tissue is first extracted with chloroform–methanol (1:1) containing 60 µmol of calcium chloride. The residue is reextracted twice with chloroform–methanol (2:1). The damp tissue residue from the neutral solvent extraction is then extracted 3 times for 20 min each with 8 volumes of chloroform–methanol (2:1) containing 0.25–0.5% concentrated HCl (Hauser and Eichberg, 1973).

More recently, concern for the toxicity of chloroform and methanol has been expressed. Hara and Radin (1978) have presented evidence that an alternate extraction solvent, namely 18 volumes of hexane–isopropanol (3:2), is nontoxic and efficient.

In all of the above extraction procedures some nonlipid material is solubilized along with lipids, particularly the proteolipid proteins. In the case of chloroform–methanol extraction the lipid extract is washed by solvent partition once with 0.2 volumes of aqueous medium containing 0.4% $CaCl_2$, 0.9% NaCl, or 0.74% KCl, followed by 2–3 washes with 0.2 volumes of methanol–0.9% NaCl–chloroform (48:47:3, by volume). This washing procedure will remove most of the gangliosides and ceramide polyhexosides together with small amounts (about 0.6%) of phosphatidic acid (PA), phosphatidylserine (PS), phosphatidylinositol (PI) and phosphatidylethanolamine (PE), whereas proteolipid protein will still remain in the organic phase. In the case of polyphosphoinositides the lipid extract is washed with 0.2 volumes of 1 N HCl, followed by methanol–1 N HCl–chloroform (48:47:3) and methanol–0.01 N HCl–chloroform (48:47:3) (Hauser and Eichberg, 1973). The alternate procedure for removing non-lipid materials is by Sephadex G25 column chromatography as modified by Nelson (1975). Phillips and Privett (1979) recommended that the washing procedure or the dextran gel chromatography can be avoided if the tissue is preextracted with 5 volumes of 0.25% aqueous acetic acid, pH 4.0–4.4, prior to extraction with organic solvent chloroform–methanol. Lipids are not lost in the aqueous lipid extract and the extracts are free of nonlipid contaminants. Hara and Radin (1978) recommended washing of the hexane–isopropanol extracts with 7% aqueous sodium sulfate to remove nonlipid contaminants.

1.3   PURIFICATION OF THE PHOSPHOLIPID FRACTION

The lipid extracts from neural tissues contain, besides phospholipids, mainly cholesterol, glycosphingolipids, and other nonpolar lipids. These non-phosphorus-containing lipids are removed by column chromatography on a silicic acid column (Vance and Sweeley, 1967). The solvent from the lipid extract is removed under N_2 and the extract is redissolved in a small volume of chloroform and chromatographed on a "Unisil" silicic acid column. The column is packed with adsorbant about 75 times the weight of the lipid. The less polar lipids, namely steroids (mainly cholesterol), free fatty acids, and mono-, di-, and triacylglycerols, are eluted with 20 times the column bed volume of chloroform. The glycosphingolipids are then eluted with 20 bed volumes of acetone–methanol (9:1, v/v) followed by phospholipids with methanol.

1.4   PHOSPHOLIPID ANALYSIS BY CONVENTIONAL METHODS

1.4.1   Deacylation and Phosphate Determination

The procedure of sequential chemical degradation, separation, and analysis of phospholipid hydrolysis products was developed by Dawson (1954). The procedure and various modifications have been described in great detail (Dawson, 1967; Sheltawy, 1975; Dawson, 1976). The basic principle of the method is that various phospholipids are chemically degraded to facilitate selective removal of hydrophobic groups. The initial step of mild alkaline alcoholysis removes the fatty acids linked in the ester form to the glycerol moiety of phosphatides and consequently forms water-soluble glycerophosphoryl derivatives from diacyl and monoacyl phosphoglycerides. Mild alkaline alcoholysis also removes fatty acids esterified in alk-1-enyl, acyl phosphoglycerides (plasmalogens) and alkyl, acyl phosphoglycerides; however, they retain their solubility in lipid solvents as lysophospholipids. The second step is to treat the remaining phospholipids with mild acid hydrolysis in the presence of $HgCl_2$ at 37°C. The alk-1-enyl lysophospholipids are degraded by the acid treatment to form water-soluble glycerophosphoryl derivatives. The last step is to treat the remaining alkyl lysophospholipids and sphingomyelin with strong methanolic acid at 100°C to break down the fatty acid–amide bond of sphingomyelin and predominantly liberate water-soluble phosphorylcholine and some sphingosylphosphorylcholine. The unhydrolyzed alkyl lysophospholipids retain their solubility in organic solvents and are estimated by direct phosphorus assay. The liberated water-soluble glycerophosphoryl derivatives as well as phosphorylcholine and sphingosylphosphorylcholine are separated either by paper chromatography and paper electrophoresis or by ion-exchange chromatography. Clarke and Dawson (1981) have recently introduced further advantageous modifications in the earlier procedure. Quantitative O-deacylation of phospholipids was achieved by incubation at 53°C for 1 h with a reagent containing monomethylamine, methanol, and water instead of alkali metal hydroxides previously used. The advantages are that the reaction is not complicated by secondary decomposition of deacylated phosphorus products and the base is easy to remove from the reaction mixture since it is volatile. This eliminates the need to pass the hydrolysate over an ion-exchange resin to remove the alkali. Furthermore, since fewer deacylated phosphorus-containing products are formed, it is not necessary to perform paper chromatography followed by second-dimensional paper ionophoresis. The water-soluble glycerophosphoryl derivatives are completely separated by single-dimensional paper ionophoresis. The lyso alk-l-enyl-(plasmalogens), lysoalkyl-phospholipids, and sphingomyelin are analyzed by thin-layer chromatography (TLC) before and after catalytic $HgCl_2$ hydrolysis of the alk-l-enyl-lysophospholipids (Clarke and Dawson, 1981).

After ionophoresis, the dried paper is sprayed with 0.25% ninhydrin in acetone and heated at 100°C for 3 min to locate the amino group containing glycerophosphorylethanolamine and glycerophosphorylserine. They can be also detected with greater sensitivity under long-wavelength ultraviolet light after spraying with 0.05% fluorescamine (4-phenyl-spiro[furan-2(3H)-1-phthalan]-3-3 dione) in acetone (Felix and Jiminez, 1974). Other phosphorus-containing compounds are located on the paper as blue spots, after lightly spraying with ammonium molybdate–perchloric acid reagent (Clarke and Dawson, 1981), drying the paper at room temperature and briefly exposing it to ultraviolet light. The phosphorus content in the spots is determined by digesting the phospholipid-containing areas of paper with perchloric acid (Dawson, 1976) and measuring liberated inorganic phosphorus by a modified Bartlett (1959) procedure (Cook and Daughton, 1981).

The lyso alk-1-enyl-, lysoalkyl-phospholipids, and sphingomyelin on thin-layer chromatograms are located with a sensitive phosphorus-detecting reagent (Vaskovsky and Kostetsky, 1968). For quantitative analysis, the spots are scraped off the plates and phosphorus determined as described above.

1.4.2   Thin-Layer Chromatography

A large number of procedures for the separation of phospholipids by TLC has been described (Nelson, 1975; Spanner, 1973; Skipski and Barclay, 1969; Kates, 1972; Renkonen and Luukkonen, 1976). In general, single-dimensional separations have been found inadequate to resolve all of the different classes of phospholipids. Better resolutions have been achieved by two-dimensional TLC methods. In most cases 20 × 20 cm silica gel HR (which has no binder) precoated plates have been used. These commercially available plates are coated with different thicknesses of adsorbant. A variety of solvent mixtures to develop the plates for the separation of phospholipids has been employed (Nelson, 1975; Spanner, 1973; Skipski and Barclay, 1969). One of the commonly used procedures for the separation of phospholipids of the nervous system, including plasmalogens, was developed by Horrocks (1968). Silica gel G, 0.5 mm thick plates are used and developed with chloroform–methanol–15 M NH$_4$OH (65:25:4, by volume) in the first direction. The plates are then dried and exposed to concentrated HCl fumes for 10 min. After dispersal of HCl fumes, development in the second dimension is carried out with chloroform–methanol–15 M NH$_4$OH (100:50:12, by volume). By exposing the plates to HCl fumes, 1-alk-1-enyl, 2-acyl phosphoglycerides present in the mixture are cleaved to form monoacyl phosphoglycerides and a long-chain aldehyde. The latter migrates with the solvent front, whereas the mobility of the former is retarded compared to diacylphosphoglycerides. Other phosphoglycerides are also well resolved in this system. The other commonly used system, which we have used extensively in our laboratory, is the two-dimensional TLC method originally described by Getz et al. (1970) and modified by Eichberg et al. (1973). The separation is achieved on a silica gel HR plates, with chloroform–methanol–acetic acid–water (52:20:7:3, by volume) in the first dimension. The plate is air dried and washed with acetone to remove the first solvent completely and air dried again. The plate is developed in the second dimension with chloroform–methanol–40% methylamine–water (65:31:5:5, by volume). If separation between 1-alk-1-enyl, 2-acylphosphoglyceride, and diacyl-phosphoglyceride is desired, the plate is exposed to HCl fumes after the development in the first dimension, as suggested by Horrocks (1968). Fairly good separation of the major phospholipids is achieved by this system, including the difficult separation of acidic phospholipids, PI and PS. In either of the above methods, however, 1-alkyl-2-acylphosphoglycerides are not resolved from the diacylphosphoglycerides. Unless the thin-layer plates are developed in an atmosphere of low and constant humidity, the separations are not consistent. Recently several other two-dimensional systems, including multiple development, for the separation of lipids and phospholipids of neural and other tissues have been described (Pollet et al., 1978; Hubmann, 1973; Blass et al., 1980; Portoukalian et al., 1978; Poorthuis et al., 1976; Vitiello and Zanetta, 1978).

The major drawback of two-dimensional TLC is that a direct comparison of different phospholipid extracts separated under identical conditions cannot be made in a single run. In recent years interest in one-dimensional TLC of phospholipids has revived, and several systems employing modified adsorbants on the plate have appeared. Thus Althaus and Neuhoff (1973) have described one-dimensional microchromatography of phospholipids on sodium silicate–impregnated silica gel layers with reasonably good separation of the individual phospholipids. Allan and Cockcroft (1982) separated anionic phospholipids such as PS, PI, and PA on an EDTA-impregnated plate developed with chloroform–methanol–acetic acid–water, (75:45:3:1, by volume). However, diphosphatidylglycerol (DPG) and phosphatidylglycerol (PG) were not well resolved from ethanolamine-phosphoglycerides in this system. Fine and Sprecher (1982) have reported good separation of phospholipids, including the anionic phospholipids, on boric acid–impregnated plates with chloroform–methanol–water–ammonium hydroxide (120:75:6:2, by volume) as the solvent in a single dimension. (Fig. 1.1). Recently Gilfillan et al. (1983) have described a single-dimension TLC separation of phospholipids from lung with chloroform–methanol–petroleum ether–acetic acid–boric acid (40:20:30:10:1.8, v/v/v/v/w).

The acidic phospholipids, phosphatidylinositolphosphate (PIP) and phosphatidylinositolbisphosphate (PIP_2), although minor components of neural and other tissue phospholipids, have gained special biochemical interest. Their rapid turnover in response to physiological stimuli in various tissues has suggested that they may have an important biological role

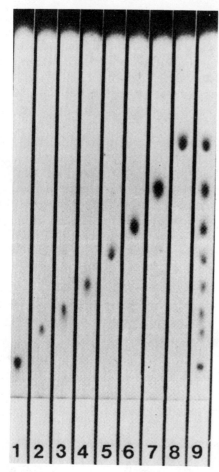

FIGURE 1.1 Single dimensional TLC of phospholipid standards on boric acid–impregnated plates. Whatman precoated LK5 and LK5D TLC plates with a preadsorbent area were impregnated by dipping them upside down into a solution of 1.2% boric acid in absolute ethanol–water (1:1, v/v). The plates were air dried and activated at 100°C for 1 h. Standard phospholipids were applied to the undipped preadsorbent area and developed with chloroform–methanol–water–ammonium hydroxide (120:75:6:2:, by volume). Lane 1, PI; 2, LPC; 3, PS; 4, SP; 5, PG; 6, PC; 7, PE; 8, DPG; and 9, a mixture of 1–8. (Reproduced by courtesy of Fine and Sprecher, 1982, and *J. Lipid Res.*)

in cell membrane function (Michell, 1982). These phospholipids are usually separated on thin-layer plates coated with silica gel H impregnated with potassium oxalate, developed with *n*-propanol–ammonium hydroxide, 4 *N* (2:1, by volume) or with chloroform–methanol–ammonium hydroxide, 4 *N* (9:7:2, by volume) (Gonzalez-Sastre and Folch-Pi, 1968). Polyphosphoinositides have also been resolved on precoated silica gel 60 high-performance TLC plates with either chloroform–methanol–15 *N* NH₄OH–water, 90:90:7:22, by volume (Schacht, 1978), or with chloroform–methanol–20% methylamine, 60:36:10, by volume (Bell et al., 1982). Rapid and quantitative purification of polyphosphoinositides have been achieved on an affinity column of immobilized neomycin coupled to reactive glass-beads (Schacht, 1978). Polyphosphoinositides in acid-washed lipid extracts interact strongly with neomycin and are retained on the column, whereas other lipids are eluted by washing the column with 150 mM ammonium acetate in chloroform–methanol–water (3:6:1, by volume). PIP is eluted with 600 mM ammonium acetate in the same solvent, whereas PIP$_2$ is eluted either with chloroform–methanol–15 M ammonium hydroxide (3:6:1, by volume) or with chloroform–methanol–12 M HCl (3:6:1, by volume). Based on the same principle, Palmer (1981) has reported separation on a neomycin column of other weakly acidic lipids, including PS, PA, DPG, and PI besides the polyphosphoinositides by using different combination of the eluting solvents. Acidic and other phospholipids can also be resolved on alumina columns and quickly eluted with solvents containing ammonium salts to reduce breakdown of the lipids (Luthra and Sheltawy, 1972).

The detection of phospholipids on thin-layer plates is usually done by formation of the phosphomolybdenum blue complex. The composition of several sprays used to generate this complex has been described (Vaskovsky et al., 1975). Ninhydrin and fluroescamine are used to detect amino group–containing phospholipids as discussed above, prior to spraying with other reagents. Various fluorogenic spray reagents, such as rhodamine 6G (Nelson, 1975), 2′, 7′-dichlorofluorescein (Nelson, 1975), 1-anilinonaphthalene-8-sulfonate (Heyneman et al., 1972), N-phenyl-1-naphthylamine (Bernard and Vercauteren, 1976), and 6-p-toluidino-2-naphthalenesulfonic acid (Jones et al., 1982) have been reported. After their application, as little as 1–10 nmol of phospholipids could be detected visually under appropriate ultraviolet light. The fluorogenic reagents are nondestructive, and intact phospholipid can be usually recovered from the thin-layer plates for further analysis, such as radioactivity determination or quantitation by phosphorus analysis (Dawson, 1976; Vaskovsky et al., 1975; Ryu and MacCoss, 1979; Goswami and Frey, 1971; Kundu et al., 1977). The detection limit of phosphorus analysis is generally about 0.5 µg. If greater sensitivity is desired, other methods such as direct measurement of spot intensities on TLC plates using a densitometer (Ryu and MacCoss, 1979) should be used. The lower limit of quantitative analysis reported for this procedure is about 0.05 µg phosphorus. Alternately, Schiefer and Neuhoff (1971) have described a fluorometric microdetermination procedure with rhodamine which claims quantitative analysis with a lower limit in the range of 0.5 ng phosphorus. Harrington et al. (1980) have developed a fluorometric procedure for the analysis of polyunsaturated phospholipids by separating the lipids on high-performance TLC plates, converting the lipids on the plates to a fluorescent derivative and quantifying them by densitometric scanning. The lower limit of quantitation is about 0.5 ng phosphorus, but the formation of the fluorophore requires the presence of at least two double bonds in an acyl chain. Hess and Derr (1975) have published a method for determination of phospholipid phosphorus based on the principle that at a low pH Malachite Green forms a complex with phosphomolybdate with a marked shift in absorption maximum and a higher molar absorption coefficient. The method is sensitive with a lower limit of 1 nmol (0.03 μg) phosphorus for reliable assay.

1.4.3 Molecular Species Analysis

The total fatty acid composition of a phospholipid is analyzed after alkaline or acid hydrolysis followed by the analysis of fatty acid methyl esters by gas–liquid chromatography (GLC) (Kishimoto and Hoshi, 1972). Such a determination provides information on the overall fatty acid species in the phospholid class but not on the molecular species of the lipid. Recently special interest in the analysis of molecular species of phospholipids has been generated since it has been demonstrated that the biological properties of membranes such as transport of small molecules, cell membrane integrity, enzymic activity, action potential, receptor function, and so on, could be manipulated by changing the molecular species of lipids in the membranes. Several methods for the analysis of molecular species of phospholipids have been published (Renkonen, 1971; Kuksis, 1972; Kuksis and Marai, 1967; Myher et al., 1978; Wiegand and Anderson, 1982; Myher and Kuksis, 1982). Basically these methods involve dephosphorylation of the intact phospholipids, resolution of the resulting diacylglycerols by argentation TLC, and GLC of the separated diacylglycerols. The dephosphorylation of the phospholipids is achieved by enzymatic hydrolysis with *Clostridium welchii*, type I phospholipase C (Renkonen, 1965; Park and Thompson, 1973). The diacylglycerols obtained can be analyzed directly by GLC on capillary columns after forming volatile trimethylsilyl derivatives (Myher and Kuksis, 1982). Alternately, they are acetylated with acetic anhydride and the acetyldiacylglycerols formed are first resolved on AgNO$_3$-impregnated silica gel TLC plates, based on degree of unsaturation, and then analyzed by GLC after methanolysis (Wiegand and Anderson, 1982; Aveldano, and Bazán, 1983).

Separation of intact phospholipids based on their degree of unsaturation has been achieved by argentation TLC (Arvidson, 1965, 1968); however, this method is not entirely quantitative and variable recoveries are obtained from the TLC plates. If one is interested in distinguishing between the fatty acids on position 1 or 2 of the diacyl phospholipids, it is necessary to use specific phospholipases A_1 or A_2 for hydrolysis followed by GLC of the released fatty acids.

Analysis of molecular species of phospholipids containing 1-O-alkyl or 1-O-alkenyl group require special consideration. Viswanathan (1974) and Schmid et al. (1975) have reviewed earlier work on the analysis of these phospholipids. For the quantitative analysis of the total and individual alkyl and alkenyl group-containing phospholipids, the lipids are chemically degraded and the alkenyl and alkyl glycerols formed are then derivatized to alkyl-substituted dioxanes or isopropylidene derivatives, respectively, and the species determined by GLC (Su and Schmid, 1974; Schmid et al., 1975). Alternately, alkyl and alkenyl glycerols are formed from the phospholipids by phospholipase C followed by saponification or vitride reduction. The alkyl- and alkenylglycerols are then converted to long-chain fatty aldehydes (formed by acid hydrolysis of the alkenylglycerols) or O-alkyl glycolic aldehydes (formed by periodate oxidation of the alkylglycerols). Colored complexes produced by reacting the aldehydes with fuchsin reagent are measured spectrophotometrically (Blank et al., 1975). The alkyl and alkenylglycerols have also been analyzed by GLC after formation of their trimethylsilyl ethers or their diacetates (Lin et al., 1977; Albro and Dittmer, 1968). Renkonen (1968) has separated alkenylacyl, alkylacyl, and diacyl forms of ethanolamine phosphoglycerides as O-methylated N-dinitrophenyl derivatives by TLC on silica gel G plates. Sundler and Akesson (1973) have resolved molecular species of these ethanolamine phosphoglycerides after conversion to their N-acetyl-O-methyl or N-benzoyl-O-methyl derivatives by argentation or reversed-phase partition TLC followed by GLC analysis.

1.5 PHOSPHOLIPID ANALYSIS BY NEWLY DEVELOPED METHODS

1.5.1 Class Separation of Phospholipids by HPLC

High-performance liquid chromatography (HPLC) is now widely employed for the analysis of substances that are nonvolatile and thus cannot be separated by conventional GLC technique. An HPLC system includes a reusable and efficient column filled with microparticulate (size 3–10 μm diameter) adsorbant, a high-pressure solvent delivery and sample injection device, and a suitable sample detection system. The most commonly used detectors are variable wavelength ultraviolet light monitors with low cell volume (8–10 μl). However, all compounds do not absorb light at a suitable wavelength and therefore a more universal detector such as a mass spectrometer is now increasingly favored.

Several HPLC methods for the class separation of phospholipids have been reported. Jungalwala et al. (1976) first showed that the phospholipids can be separated on a silica column by HPLC with ultraviolet light detection at about 200 nm. The absorption of ultraviolet light at 200 nm and below for phospholipids is mainly due to $\pi \rightarrow \pi^*$ transition of electrons in double bonds in the fatty acid side chains as well as functional groups such as carbonyl, carboxyl, phosphate, and amino groups. The response of the detector varies with the number of functional groups, primarily the number of double bonds in the phospholipid molecules (Jungalwala et al., 1976). Thus, direct quantitation of phospholipids with an unknown degree of unsaturation is not possible with the ultraviolet detection mode. However, separated phospholipids can be easily collected and quantitated by independent micromethods.

An HPLC separation with ultraviolet detection of commonly occurring phospholipids is shown in Figure 1.2 (Jungalwala et al., 1982). The analysis of brain and other tissue phospholipids in the lipid extracts is usually performed after isolation of the phospholipid fraction by silicic acid column chromatography (Vance and Sweeley, 1967). The sensitivity of the detection is dependent on the degree of unsaturation of the phospholipid. Approximately 1 nmol of a phospholipid containing at least one double bond per molecule can be detected.

Geurts van Kessel et al. (1977) reported separation of phospholipids by HPLC on a 10-μm silica (Li Chrosorb Si-60) column using n-hexane-2-propanol-water as the solvent system with detection at 206 nm. With this solvent system PE, PI, PS, and lysoPC were resolved, but sphingomyelin and phosphatidylcholine (PC) were not separable.

Gross and Sobel (1980) described an HPLC procedure with ultraviolet detection at 203 nm for the separation of phospholipids on a column of 10 μm silica with covalently bound benzene sulfonate (Whatman PXS 10/25 SCX) using isocratic solvent acetonitrile–methanol–water (40:10:34, by volume). Although separation of PC, lysoPE, lysoPC, and sphingomyelin was achieved, PE was not resolved from PS.

Hanson et al. (1981) used a column of 10 μm silica bonded to amino groups (Ultrasil-NH$_2$) with a gradient elution of a solvent mixture of hexane–isopropanol–methanol–water. Under this condition, the order of elution was PC, sphingomyelin, lysoPC, PE, and lysoPE. However, acidic phospholipids such as PS and PI were tightly bound to silica coated with amino groups and thus were not eluted.

James et al. (1981) have used silica cartridge with Waters' radial compression module and gradient elution with hexane–isopropanol–

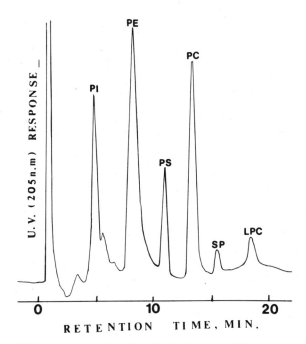

FIGURE 1.2 HPLC separation of pig liver PI, bovine brain PE, bovine brain PS, bovine brain sphingomyelin (SP), and lysophosphatidylcholine (LPC) on a Micropak-Si 5-μm column. The elution was with a 20-min linear gradient of acetonitrile–methanol–water–ammonium hydroxide (15 *M*) from 95:3:2:0.05 to 65:21:14:0.35, pumped at 2 ml/min. The rise in the baseline at 205 nm was corrected by using a Schoffel memory module with the monitor. (From Jungalwala, Sanyal, and LeBaron, in Horrocks, Ansell, and Porcellati, Eds., *Phospholipids in the Nervous System*, Vol. 1, *Metabolism*, 1982. Reproduced by permission of Raven Press, New York.)

water solvent with similar results as described by Guerts van Kessel et al. (1977).

Briand et al. (1981) have reported HPLC separation of phospholipids on a tandem column of (25 cm × 4.6 mm) Li Chrosorb Diol, 10 μm (diol phase chemically bonded to silica gel) along with a short (3 cm × 4.6 mm) 10-μm silica gel column. A gradient elution solvent system of acetonitrile–water was used. The order of elution under this condition was PG, PI, PS, PE, PC, sphingomyelin, and lysoPC. If only the Diol column was used without the silica column, the order of elution was slightly changed; PE was eluted between PC and sphingomyelin.

Yandrasitz et al. (1981) used sulfuric acid in their solvent for ion suppression of ionizable phospholipids in order to resolve them better on a Micro-Pak Si-5 column. However, such a solvent system degraded plasmalogens in the phospholipid mixture.

Chen and Kou (1982) have reported HPLC separation of phospholipids with a Micro-Pak Si-10 (10-μm) column (30 cm × 4 mm) with isocratic elution with acetonitrile–methanol–85% phosphoric acid (130:5:1.5, v/v). The order of elution was PI, PS, PE, LPE, PC, lysoPC, and sphingomyelin in about 30 min. Diphosphatidylglycerol was eluted with the solvent front, whereas PA and PG coeluted with PC. The disadvantages of this method are that the presence of phosphoric acid in the solvent does not allow quantitation of phosphorus after digestion, and the strong acidity may lead to degradation of plasmalogens.

Patton et al. (1982) described separation of phospholipids on a 10-μm Lichrosphere-Si-100 column (25 cm × 4.6 mm) with isocratic elution using a complex solvent system of hexane–isopropanol–25 mM phosphate buffer–ethanol–acetic acid (36.7:49:6.2:10:0.06, by volume). The phospholipids were eluted in the following order, PE, PA, PI, PS, DPG, PC, sphingomyelin, and lysoPC in about 120 min.

Kaduce et al. (1983) have reported an isocratic elution HPLC method for the analysis of phospholipids with acetonitrile–methanol–sulfuric acid (100:3:0.1, by volume) on a Beckman ultrasphere Si, 5-μm column (4.6 × 250 mm). Although PI, PS, PE, PC, lysoPC, and sphingomyelin were resolved, the elution time was almost 50 min and the later-eluting phospholipid peaks were broad. Again due to presence of acid in the solvent, the method is not suitable for plasmalogens.

HPLC detection based on short-wavelength ultraviolet absorption described above is convenient and the injected samples can be entirely recovered after the chromatography for further analysis such as radioactivity, phosphate, or fatty acid species determinations. However, there are certain drawbacks to this mode of detection. The choice of solvents is limited since ultraviolet-transparent solvents at around 200 nm are required for chromatography. Direct quantitation of phospholipids is not possible as discussed previously. Sensitivity of detection for the same molar amount of phospholipid varies with the number of double bonds. Thus disaturated fatty acid–containing phospholipids such as dipalmitoylglycerylphosphorylcholine are detected with rather low sensitivity. Large amounts of ultraviolet-absorbing impurities could interfere with the analysis. For these reasons other modes of detection have been tried for the HPLC analysis of phospholipids. Kiuchi et al. (1977) used a Pye Unicam transport flame ionization detector. Eluate from the column is partially dropped on a continuously moving wire that is heated to evaporate the solvent. The residue is then detected in the flame ionization mode. However, the sensitivity of such a detection mode is low since only a small part of the sample is retained by the moving wire. The detector is no longer commercially available. Kaitaranta and Bessman (1981) described an automatic phosphorus analyzer for quantitative determination of phospholipids after HPLC. The eluate from the column is directed into a rotating table containing 40 silica cups. At 30-s intervals the aliquots are automatically oxidized with nitric acid, dried, and ashed to inorganic phosphorus. The molybdenum blue color reagents are automatically added to each cup, and colored solution is then pumped through a 25-μl flow cell and read at 820 nm. Although reasonable linearity and reproducibility for samples in the range of 1–100 nmol have been reported, the detector is not yet widely used. Blom et al. (1979) have described a flow-through radioactivity monitor for the detection of phospholipids. [^{32}P]orthophosphate is first incorporated into the phospholipids followed by HPLC and radioactivity monitoring. This procedure facilitates detection of minor phospholipids after HPLC, but quantitation cannot be achieved by such a method.

An alternate approach to quantitative analysis of phospholipids is to form ultraviolet-absorbing or fluorescent derivatives and analyze these by HPLC. Most of the phospholipids have functional groups available for such derivatization except for PC. This difficulty precludes simultaneous analysis of all the phospholipids after derivatization. However, many phospholipids have been derivatized and quantitatively analyzed in the picomole range by HPLC. Jungalwala et al. (1975, 1982) reported preparation of biphenylcarbonyl derivatives of amino group-containing phospholipids, such as PE, PS, lysoPE, and lysoPS followed by HPLC with ultraviolet detection at 280 nm. The amino phospholipids containing vinyl ether bonds (plasmalogens) can be determined separately from diacyl and alkylacyl phospholipids by HPLC before and after treatment of the samples with HCl as done with the TLC method (Horrocks, 1968). The lower limit of detection by HPLC of these lipids is about 10–15 pmol or 0.3–0.4 ng of phospholipid phosphorus.

Chen et al. (1981) have described a similar method for the analysis of amino group–containing phospholipids after formation of their fluorescent dimethylamino naphthalene-5-sulfonyl derivatives. The sensitivity of the fluorescent method was similar to that reported for the biphenylcarbonyl group ultraviolet absorbance method.

Sphingomyelin, PG, and PI can be also derivatized with 10% benzoic anhydride in tetrahydrofuran or with dimethylaminopyridine to form benzoyl derivatives of the phospholipids (Jungalwala et al., 1982; Smith et al., 1981). The derivatized phospholipids were then quantitatively analyzed by HPLC (Fig. 1.3 and 1.4). Thus, although derivatization of phospholipids permits sensitive quantitative HPLC analysis of some of these

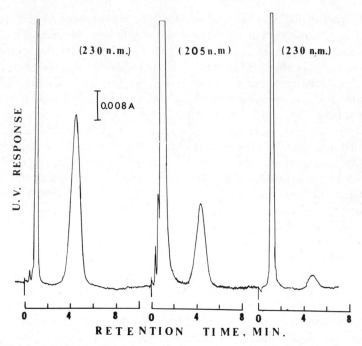

FIGURE 1.3 Quantitative HPLC analysis of sphingomyelin. The phospholipid extract of rat brain subcellular fractions was first resolved by HPLC as shown in Figure 1.2. The sphingomyelin fraction was collected and, if necessary, a possible trace of contaminating PC was removed by mild alkaline hydrolysis. The sphingomyelin fraction was then benzoylated with 0.5 ml of 10% benzoic anhydride in tetrahydrofuran at 70°C for 2 h. The 3-*O*-benzoylated sphingomyelin was isolated and analyzed by HPLC on a Micropak Si-10 column with acetonitrile–methanol–water (75:21:14, by volume) pumped at 1 ml/min. *Left:* 3-*O*-benzoylated sphingomyelin (6.7 nmol, 0.21 μg P) with detection at 230 nm. **Middle:** same amount but with detection at 205 nm. *Right:* 3-*O*-benzoylated sphingomyelin (0.6 nmol, 0.019 μg P). Bar represents ultraviolet absorption response due to 0.008 Å units. (From Jungalwala, Sanyal, and LeBaron, in Horrocks, Ansell, and Porcellati, Eds., *Phospholipids in the Nervous System*, Vol. 1, *Metabolism*, 1982. Reproduced by permission of Raven Press, New York.)

compounds, a general universal method using this approach has not emerged.

1.5.2 Determination of Molecular Species of Phospholipids by HPLC

Recently great interest in the analysis of the molecular species of individual phospholipids has been evident. Reversed-phase HPLC has been generally used to achieve molecular species separation. The important

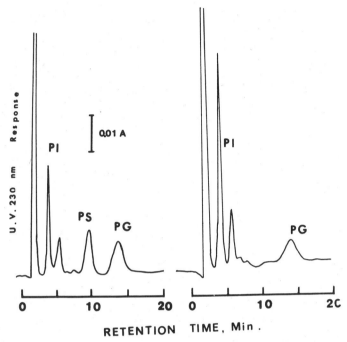

FIGURE 1.4   HPLC separation of benzoylated PI, PS, and PG. The standard phospholipids and the acidic phospholipid fraction of rat lung isolated over a DEAE column was benzoylated with 100 µl of 5% (w/v) benzoic anhydride and 50% saturated 4-dimethylaminopyridine in tetrahydrofuran at 37°C for 30 min. The reaction mixture was partitioned between hexane and methanol/saline (1:1) containing 0.05 N HCl. The hexane phase was collected and injected on a Micropak Si-10 column. *Left:* standard, PI, PS, and PG. *Right:* acidic lipid fraction of rat lung. The elution was with a 20-min linear gradient of hexane–isopropanol–2 N NH$_4$OH from 93:6.9:0.1 to 80:19.7:0.3, by volume, pumped at 1.5 ml/min. Bar represents ultraviolet absorption response due to 0.01 Å units. (From Jungalwala, Sanyal, and LeBaron, in Horrocks, Ansell, and Porcellati, Eds., *Phospholipids in the Nervous System*, Vol. 1, *Metabolism*, 1982. Reproduced by permission of Raven Press, New York.)

feature of the reversed-phase chromatographic process is the magnitude of the hydrophobic interaction determined by the nonpolar contact area between the solute and the ligand of the stationary phase. The actual molecular geometry involved in the binding of the solute to ligand is unknown due to scant knowledge of the topography of the stationary-phase surface and the arrangement of the hydrocarbonaceous ligands. Nevertheless, in practical chromatographic systems it has been determined that the free energy change is minimized when the contact area between the solute and the ligand and the net energy of interaction with the solvent are maximal (Horvath and Melander, 1978).

Jungalwala et al. (1979) reported the separation of molecular species of sphingomyelin by reversed-phase HPLC. Sphingomyelin species from bovine brain, sheep, and pig erythrocytes were resolved into 10–12 separate peaks on a μ-Bonda-Pak C_{18} or Nucleosil-5-C_{18} column with methanol–5 mM potassium phosphate buffer, pH 7.4 (9:1, v/v) as the isocratic solvent and detection at 203–205 nm. The separation was based on the number of carbon atoms and degree of unsaturation in the fatty acid and sphingoid side chains of the various sphingomyelin species.

The HPLC analysis of sphingomyelin species was made quantitative and more sensitive by separating the benzoylated sphingomyelins on a "fatty acid analysis" column from Waters Associates (Smith et al., 1981). About 5 μg of benzoylated sphingomyelin was separated into various molecular species in 30 min with detection at 230 nm (Fig. 1.5). LeBaron et al. (1981) have used this method to determine the turnover rates of molecular species of sphingomyelin in rat brain subcellular fractions. Although good separation was achieved on the reversed-phase column, sphingomyelins having a double bond in the acyl side chain (e.g., 24:1) were not resolved from the lipid having a saturated fatty acid with two less carbon atoms (e.g., 22:0). This difficulty can be overcome by the combined use of argentation HPLC and reversed-phase HPLC (Smith et al., 1981). First, separation based on the degree of unsaturation was achieved with a commercially prepared silica-bonded silver column on which 3-O-benzoylated sphingomyelin was resolved into two peaks. One contained the lipid with only saturated fatty acids, whereas the other contained sphingomyelin with only the monounsaturated fatty acids. The two peaks separated on the silver column were collected and individually reinjected on the reversed-phase column to resolve all the possible molecular species of sphingomyelin (Smith et al., 1981).

Separation of molecular species of other phospholipids has been also achieved by reversed-phase and argentation HPLC. Smith and Jungalwala (1981) have reported the reversed-phase HPLC separation of PC from various sources. Reversed-phase HPLC separation of egg PC is shown in Figure 1.6 and the major fatty acid species separated are listed in Table 1.1. It is also shown that from the chromatographic behavior of each PC species one can determine the relative hydrophobicity of various molecular species. As can be seen from Table 1.1, all molecular species are not resolved on the reversed-phase column. However, separation based on the degree of unsaturation can be achieved on a silver-coated silica gel HPLC column. The separation of rat brain microsomal PC on such a column is shown in Figure 1.7. Peaks 3 and 4 display a partial resolution of molecular species containing 18:0 and 16:0. In the case of hexaenoates (peak 6) the earlier peak was mostly due to PC with 18:0-22:6 whereas

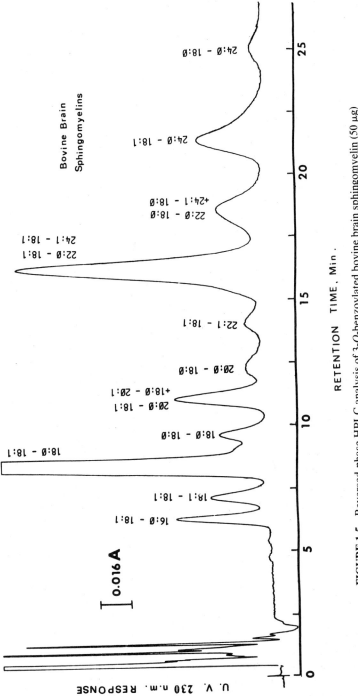

FIGURE 1.5 Reversed-phase HPLC analysis of 3-O-benzoylated bovine brain sphingomyelin (50 μg) on a "fatty acid analysis" column with tetrahydrofuran–acetronitrile–water (25:35:40, by volume) pumped at a flowrate of 2 ml/min. Bar represents ultraviolet absorption response due to 0.016 Å units. The fatty acid (first number) and the sphingoid base (second number) composition of the resolved molecular species is listed near each peak.

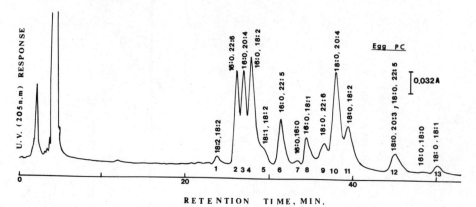

FIGURE 1.6   Reversed-phase HPLC analysis of egg PC on Nucleosil-5-C_{18} column with methanol–1 mM phosphate buffer, pH 7.4 (9.5:0.5, v/v) as a solvent with a flowrate of 1 ml/min. Five hundred micrograms of PC was injected and the PC species eluted were collected as indicated in the figure by numbers and analyzed (see Table 1.1). The major fatty acid composition of the PC in an individual peak is given near the peak. Bar represents ultraviolet absorption response due to 0.032 Å units. (Reproduced by permission of *J. Lipid Res.*)

the later peak was due to PC with 16:0–22:6. The peaks collected from the silver column can be reinjected on the reversed-phase HPLC column in order to completely resolve major molecular species of intact phospholipids.

Patton et al. (1982) also have described similar separation of molecular species of PC, PE, PI, and PS by reversed-phase HPLC with detection at 205 nm. Hsieh et al. (1981a) reported preparation of phosphatidic acid dimethyl esters from PC after enzymatic hydrolysis of PC followed by esterification of the phosphatidic acid with diazomethane. The dimethyl esters of PA were then chromatographed on a reversed-phase column. For some reason the resolution obtained by the HPLC column of these derivatives was not very impressive. Improved resolution using two Partisil-10 ODS columns in tandem was later reported for these derivatives (Hsieh et al., 1981b). Batley et al. (1980) reported separation of diacylglycerol *p*-nitrobenzoates by reversed-phase HPLC. Phospholipids were first degraded by the action of phospholipase C to diacylglycerols, which were then derivatized and quantitatively analyzed. The latter method is based on partial degradation of phospholipids and may not be suitable if phospholipids labeled with radioisotopes in the base or phosphorus moiety are to be analyzed.

HPLC methods for the separation of alkenylacyl, alkylacyl, and diacyl acetylglycerols derived from ethanolamine glycerophospholipids and for

TABLE 1.1 Percentage Composition of Fatty Acid Species of Egg Phosphatidylcholine Fractions Obtained by HPLC

Peak No.	Fatty Acid									Probable Major Molecular Species of PC	Percent Composition of PC
	16:0	18:0	18:1	18:2	18:3	20:3	20:4	22:5	22:6		
1	8		9	70	13					18:2–18:2; 16:0–18:3; 18:1–18:3	0.4
2	40		12						48	16:0–22:6; 18:1–22:6	1.7
3	37		18				45			16:0–20:4; 18:1–20:4	2.8
4	47		2	48			3			16:0–18:2	18.9
5	22		30	48						16:0–18:2; 18:1–18:2	3.2
6	43		8	8		10		31		16:0–22:5, 16:0–20:3, 18:1–18:2	2.0
7	95		5							16:0–16:0	0.5
8	47		53							16:0–18:1	37.0
9	36	6	52						6	16:0–18:1; 18:1–18:1; 18:0–22:6	9.3
10		35	27				38			18:1–18:1; 18:0–20:4	6.3
11		50		50						18:0–18:2	7.3
12		45				25		30		18:0–22:5; 18:0–20:3	0.6
13		49	51							18:0–18:1	10.0

Source: Reproduced by permission of J. Lipid Res.

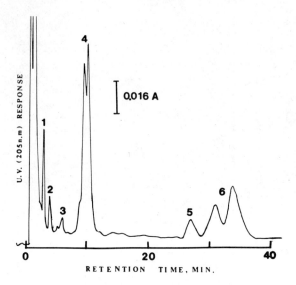

FIGURE 1.7 HPLC analysis of rat brain microsomal PC on a Nucleosil-10 sulfonic acid Ag$^+$ (Chrompak) column with methanol as the eluting solvent pumped at 2 ml/min. The temperature of the column was maintained at 45°C. The number near each peak represents the total number of double bonds in the fatty acids of PC. Bar represents ultraviolet absorption response due to 0.016 Å units.

separation of the individual molecular species from each of the separated classes have been described by Nakagawa and Horrocks (1983).

1.5.3 HPLC–Mass Spectrometry (MS) of Individual Phospholipids

Although significant improvements in the separation of individual phospholipids and molecular species of phospholipids by HPLC have been achieved, facile quantitative detection of these lipids is not quite satisfactory. HPLC–mass spectrometry (MS) in recent years has generated a lot of interest as a means for detection and simultaneous analysis of the resolved compounds (reviews edited by Lederer, 1982). Coupling of MS with HPLC offers an important advance in analytical methodology. The mass spectrometer not only functions as a highly sensitive universal detector but also serves to provide valuable structural information not obtainable otherwise on small quantities of compounds.

In the past few years significant progress has been made in overcoming technical problems associated with the interfacing of HPLC to MS. An "on-line" HPLC–MS system is preferred, which is capable of analyzing compounds eluted as sharp narrow peaks without loss of resolution. A transport type of interface has been found quite suitable for removal of HPLC solvent and introduction of the solute into the mass spectrometer (Alcock et al., 1982). We and others have demonstrated that moving belt–type interface works well for such a purpose and that peak broadening is minimal (Hayes et al., 1983; Jungalwala et al., 1984).

The compounds are then analyzed by the chemical ionization (CI) method in which positive and negative ions are generated with CI reagent gases such as ammonia, methane, or nitrous oxide (Sugnaux and Djerassi, 1982). We have used a commercially available Finnigan HPLC–MS interface. A continuously moving belt made from polyimide collects the HPLC eluant. The solvent is removed by two high-vacuum pumps and a heater located above the moving belt. The sample on the belt is carried directly to the ion source of the quadrupole mass spectrometer. Alternate positive/negative ion spectra are obtained by the system under the control of a Teknivent model 56K MS computer.

Although theoretically any solvent could be used for HPLC analysis in this system, in practice solvents with high volatility are preferred to facilitate evaporation from the belt. Naturally occurring phospholipids are a complex mixture of compounds having similar polarity so that separation of phospholipids on a chromatographic column is difficult. Separation by this means is also hampered by the existence of various salt forms of the same phospholipids or a mixture of salts and free bases. In our experience the HPLC of phospholipids on silica columns is best achieved by the use of solvents containing ammonia and is reproducible provided the solvent is well equilibrated with the column. Most of the commonly occurring phospholipids are well resolved; however, the separation could be improved to achieve the resolution of other minor phospholipids in natural mixtures, such as PA, DPG, and lysophospholipids as well as PS, which tails on such columns.

In previous studies utilizing MS for phospholipid analysis, Klein (1971) reported electron ionization MS of several intact PC molecular species. A few reports have also appeared on the analysis of phospholipids by field desorption and fast-atom bombardment MS (Wood et al., 1977; Sugatani et al., 1982; Lehmann and Kessler, 1983). Isobutane chemical ionization mass spectrometry (CIMS) of dioleoyl-PC has been previously reported by Foltz (1972), whereas positive-ion ammonia CIMS of synthetic PCs has been reported by Crawford and Plattner (1983). We have described positive and negative CIMS of several naturally occurring phospholipids including PC with ammonia and methane as the reagent gases (Evans et al., 1983; Jungalwala et al., 1984).

1.5.3.1 Phosphatidylcholine

Positive and negative CIMS with ammonia and methane as the reagent gas were obtained for various synthetic and naturally occurring phospholipids before HPLC–MS was attempted. The phospholipid, about 5 μg in 10 μl solvent, was directly applied to the moving belt with a microsyringe. The major characteristic ions and ions in high-mass range of each phospholipid are listed in Table 1.2. Based on the study of mass spectra of various synthetic PC, the following ions were recognized in positive-ion ammonia CIMS of PC: $[M + 1]^+$, $M^+ - 41$, $M^+ - 182$ (i.e., $M^+ - $ phosphocholine) and $[M + 35]^+ - 182$. The positive-ion ammonia CIMS of lung PC is shown, as an example, in Figure 1.8 and the ions that provide fatty acid species information are listed in Table 1.3. Nineteen different molecular species of lung PC were identified from this spectrum.

From the relative intensity of these diacylglycerol-related ions, the percentage composition of the molecular species present in each phospholipid can be calculated. The relative percentage compositions of major species of lung PC as calculated from the relative intensity of three different ions in the mass spectrum were very similar (Table 1.3). Good correspondence of results was obtained with $M^+ - 41$ and $M^+ - 182$ ions because they are major ions in the spectrum. The results from $[M + 1]^+$ (not shown) or $M^+ - 147$ ions showed some differences due to their relatively low intensity. The total fatty acid species of the lung PC were also analyzed by GLC and the relative percent distribution is given in Table 1.4. The total fatty acid composition of lung PC was calculated from MS data (Table 1.3) by adding the relative amounts of each fatty acid in various molecular species and then dividing by 2. The percent distribution of fatty acids as analyzed by GLC was very similar to that as calculated from the MS data (Table 1.4). This result indicated that the molecular fatty acid species assignments as determined by MS are mostly correct. A small degree of overlap cannot be ruled out since the molecular weights of different combinations of fatty acids can be the same, for example the molecular weight of 16:0–20:4, 18:2–18:2, and 18:1–18:3 PC. However, generally phospholipids contain one saturated and one unsaturated fatty acid and therefore the assignments are made on this basis. Analysis of monoacylglycerol and free fatty acid ions at the lower end of the MS also helped to eliminate certain possibilities. For more accurate analysis, it is probably desirable to perform reversed-phase and/or argentation HPLC with on-line MS. The position of the fatty acid on the glycerol moiety can also be determined since ions specific for the sn-1 and sn-2 positions have been reported to be produced (Hatch, 1982).

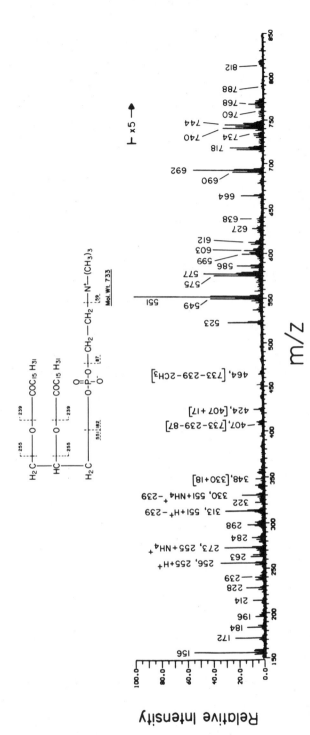

FIGURE 1.8 Ammonia CI mass spectrum of lung PC in positive-ion mode. About 5 μg of PC was applied to the moving belt of the Finnigan model 4500 mass spectrometer interface. MS data were collected from m/z 150–850 in the CI mode with ammonia (0.75 torr) as the reagent gas, every 6 s. The ion source temperature was 150°C. $M^+ + 1$, $M^+ - 41$, $M^+ - 147$, and $M^+ - 182$ ions of various molecular species of PC are listed in Table 1.3. The ordinate scale is expanded fivefold from m/z 725. Fragmentation of dipalmitoylglycerophosphorylcholine is given as an example.

25

TABLE 1.2 Major Characteristic Fragment Ions in the Positive and Negative Ammonia and Methane CIMS of Various Phospholipids

Phospholipid	Ammonia CI		Methane CI	
	Positive	Negative	Positive	Negative
PC	142 [M + 1]$^+$ M$^+$ − 41 M$^+$ − 182 [M + 35]$^+$ − 182	182, 123 [M − 1]$^-$ M$^-$ − 13 M$^-$ − 24 M$^-$ − 33 M$^-$ − 42 M$^-$ − 60 M$^-$ − 184	125, 139, 153 [M + 1]$^+$ M$^+$ − 41 M$^+$ − 182	159, 182 [M − 1]$^-$ M$^-$ − 13 M$^-$ − 24 M$^-$ − 33 M$^-$ − 42 M$^-$ − 60 M$^-$ − 130 M$^-$ − 148 M$^-$ − 184
PE	141 (Ethanolamine phosphate) M$^+$ − 140 [M + 35]$^+$ − 140 [M + 17]$^+$ − 140		124 M$^+$ − 140	191 M$^-$ − 88
PS	105 (Serine) M$^+$ − 184 [M + 35]$^+$ − 184		M$^+$ − 184	139, 173 M$^-$ − 132

PI	180 (Inositol) 198 (Inositol + 18) $M^+ - 259$ $[M + 35]^+ - 259$	$M^+ - 259$	152, 179 $M^- - 207$
SP	142 $M^+ - 182$ $M^+ - 182 - 18$	$M^+ - 182$ $M^+ - 182 - 18$	
LysoPE	141 (Ethanolamine phosphate) $M^+ - 140$ $[M + 35]^- - 140$ $M^+ - 43$ $M^+ - 17$		
LysoPC	142 $M^+ - 182$ $[M + 35]^+ - 182$ $M^+ - 31$ $M^+ - 41$		
PG	172 (Glycerol phosphate) $M^+ - 171$ $[M + 35]^+ - 171$		

Source: Reproduced by permission of *J. Lipid Res.*

27

TABLE 1.3 Molecular Species of Lung Phosphatidylcholine by Ammonia CIMS[a]

Molecular Species	$M^+ + 1$	$M^+ - 41$	$M^+ - 147$	$M^+ - 182$
14:0–16:0	706	664 (9.1)	558 (6.2)	523 (7.6)
15:0–16:0	720	678 (2.0)	572 (2.3)	537 (1.9)
14:0–18:3	728	686 (0.5)	580 (1.1)	545 (1.1)
14:0–18:2	730	688 (2.1)	582 (2.3)	547 (2.2)
16:0–16:1	732	690 (12.8)	584 (9.9)	549 (11.4)
16:0–16:0	734	692 (29.2)	586 (23.0)	551 (28.3)
17:0–18:1	746	704 (0.7)	598 (1.5)	563 (0.9)
16:0–18:3	756	714 (1.4)	608 (3.0)	573 (1.5)
16:0–18:2	758	716 (11.0)	610 (9.9)	575 (10.6)
16:0–18:1	760	718 (13.9)	612 (12.1)	577 (12.8)
16:0–18:0	762	720 (3.6)	614 (5.3)	579 (4.5)
16:0–20:4	—	740 (3.4)	634 (4.5)	599 (4.5)
18:0–18:3	—	742 (2.3)	636 (4.2)	601 (2.8)
18:0–18:2	786	744 (3.4)	638 (5.3)	603 (3.9)
18:0–18:1	788	746 (1.6)	640 (2.6)	605 (1.9)
16:0–22:6	—	764 (0.6)	658 (1.5)	623 (0.9)
16:0–22:5	—	766 (0.6)	660 (1.5)	625 (0.9)
18:0–20:4	—	768 (1.8)	662 (3.8)	627 (2.2)
16:0–22:3	—	770 (0.1)	664 (—)	629 (0.1)

Source: Reproduced by permission of *J. Lipid Res.*

[a] Numbers in parentheses represent the mole percent composition of the fatty acid species of the phospholipid as calculated from the relative intensity of the indicated ion. In the case of $M^+ + 1$ these values are not reported because some of the species did not present the expected $M^+ + 1$ ions. The values are averages of three determinations.

Besides the above-mentioned diacylglycerol related ions, the phospholipid "base"-related ions were identified (Table 1.2). In the case of PC and also sphingomyelin, m/z 142 (100%, not shown in Fig. 1.9), 156, 172, 184, 186, and 196 were identified. The most characteristic ion for choline-containing phospholipids was m/z 142 and was used, as shown later, for monitoring these phospholipids after HPLC.

Fatty acid– and monoacylglycerol-related ions were identified between m/z 200 and 450. For example, m/z 239, 256, 273, 313, 330, 348, 407, and 424 were all related to 16:0 fatty acid (mol. wt. 256), whereas m/z 267, 284, 301, 341, 358, 376, and 452 were related to 18:0 fatty acid (mol. wt.

TABLE 1.4 Percent Fatty Acid Composition of Lung Phosphatidylcholine by GLC and MS[a]

Fatty Acid	GLC	MS		
		$M^+ - 41$	$M^+ - 147$	$M^+ - 182$
14:0	2.1	5.8	4.8	5.4
15:0	0.8	1.0	1.1	1.0
16:0	53.2	58.1	50.6	56.2
16:1	6.2	6.2	5.0	5.7
17:0	0.5	0.3	0.8	0.5
18:0	8.0	7.0	11.3	8.1
18:1	9.8	8.1	8.1	7.7
18:2	9.9	8.2	8.7	8.4
18:3	2.2	2.1	4.1	2.7
22:5	0.5	0.3	0.7	0.5
20:4	5.0	2.6	4.1	3.3
22:3	0.5	0.05	—	0.05
22:6	1.0	0.3	0.7	0.5

Source: Reproduced by permission of *J. Lipid Res.*

[a] The values are average of three separate analysis. The percentage fatty acid composition by MS was calculated from $M^+ - 41$, $M^+ - 147$, and $M^+ - 182$ ions by summation of the percentage of individual fatty acid in different molecular species (Table 1.3) and dividing by 2.

284). The corresponding ions for fatty acid 18:1 and 18:2 were also identified in this spectrum.

1.5.3.2 Ethanolamine Phosphoglycerides

The major ions in the high-mass range were $M^+ - 140$ ($M^+ -$ phosphoethanolamine) and $M^+ - 105$ (i.e., $M^+ + 35 - 140$) and $M^+ - 123$. ($M^+ + 17 - 140$) was also present with low intensity. The characteristic ion for ethanolamine base was at m/z 141, with highest intensity in the spectrum. This was useful in monitoring this phospholipid after HPLC. The positive-ion ammonia CIMS of bovine brain ethanolamine phosphoglycerides is shown in Figure 1.9. Bovine brain PE contains mainly alk-1-enylacylglycerophosphorylethanolamine (GPE), together with both diacyl and alkylacylglycerophosphorylethanolamine. The $M^+ - 140$ and $M^+ - 105$ ions for the alk-1-enylacyl-GPE could be distinguished from the corresponding ions derived from diacyl-GPE; the former

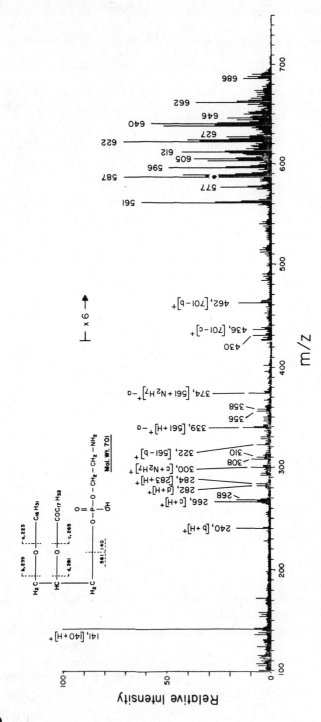

FIGURE 1.9 Ammonia CI mass spectrum of bovine brain ethanolamine phosphoglycerides (5 μg) in the positive-ion mode. The spectrum was obtained as described in the legend of Figure 1.8. The ordinate scale is expanded sixfold from m/z 425. Fragmentation of 16:1 alkyl-18:1 acyl-GPE (plasmalogen) is given as an example. (Reproduced by permission from *J. Lipid Res.*)

30

having 14 units less mass than the latter. They cannot, however, be distinguished from the corresponding odd-chain fatty acid containing diacyl-GPE. Based on the intensity of the $M^+ - 140$ ions (all having odd numbers), the proportion of alkenylacyl plus alkylacyl-GPE was calculated to be 69%, whereas diacyl-GPE was 31% of the total PE. This agreed with the values published in the literature for bovine brain PE (Nakagawa and Horrocks, 1983).

The major diacyl-GPE molecular species tentatively identified were 18:0–18:1 (21.2%, m/z 605 and 640); 18:0–18:2 (16.2%, 603 and 638); 16:0–18:1 (15.3%, m/z 577 and 612); 16:0–22:6 (13.8%, m/z 623 and 658), 18:0–20:4 (13.4%, m/z 627 and 662); 16:0–22:5 (8.3%, m/z 625 and 660); and 16:1–20:4 (7.1%, m/z 597 and 632).

The major alkenylacyl- and alkylacyl-GPE molecular species tentatively identified were 16:1–18:1 (21%, m/z 561 and 596); 18:1–18:2 (20.5%, m/z 587 and 622); 18:1–18:1 (12%, m/z 589 and 624); 18:1–22:3 (11%, m/z 641 and 676); 18:1–20:4 (6%, m/z 611 and 646); and 18:0–20:4 (5%, m/z 613 and 648). About 15 other molecular species of PE in small quantities were identified but are not listed here.

1.5.3.3   Phosphatidylserine

The positive-ion ammonia CIMS of bovine brain PS (Fig. 1.10) exhibited as major ions $M^+ -$ phosphoserine ($M^+ - 184$) and $[M + 35]^+ - 184$ in the high-mass range. The characteristic ion of all serine-containing phospholipids was at m/z 105. The major molecular species were identified as 18:0–18:1 (54%, m/z 605 and 640); 18:0–18:2 (7%, m/z 603 and 638); 18:0–20:1 (17%, m/z 633 and 668); 18:0–20:2 (6.3%, m/z 631 and 666); 18:0–22:2 (2%, m/z 694); and 16:0–18:1 (1%, m/z 577 and 612) with minor amounts of other species. Small amounts of alkenylacyl-PS were also identified as 18:1–22:6 (7%, m/z 607 and 642) and 18:1–18:0 (2%, m/z 591 and 626). The fatty acid composition of PS as determined by GLC was in agreement with that as analyzed by CIMS. Thus, GLC analysis of the same sample of PS showed major fatty acids as 18:0, 40%; 18:1, 30%; and 20:1, 11% whereas calculations from the relative intensity of the $[M^+ + 35] - 184$ ion indicated 18:0, 43%; 18:1, 28%; and 20:1, 9% as the major fatty acids.

1.5.3.4   Phosphatidylinositol

The positive-ion ammonia CIMS of bovine brain PI (Fig. 1.11) revealed $M^+ - 259$ ($M^+ -$ phosphoinositol) and $[M + 35]^+ - 259$ as the major ions in the high-mass range. The characteristic ions of PI were m/z 198 and 180. The major molecular species were identified as 18:0–20:4 (40%,

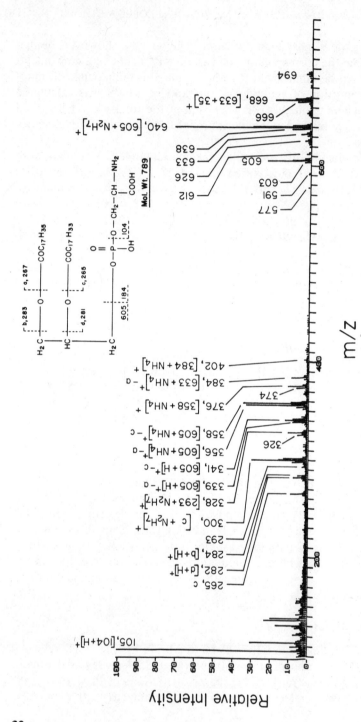

FIGURE 1.10 Ammonia CI mass spectrum of bovine brain phosphatidylserine (5 μg). The spectrum was obtained as described in the legend of Figure 1.8. Fragmentation of 18:0–18:1 glycerophosphorylserine is given as an example. Ions m/z 293, 328, and 402 are from 18:0–20:1 fatty acid–containing PS. (Reproduced by permission from *J. Lipid Res.*)

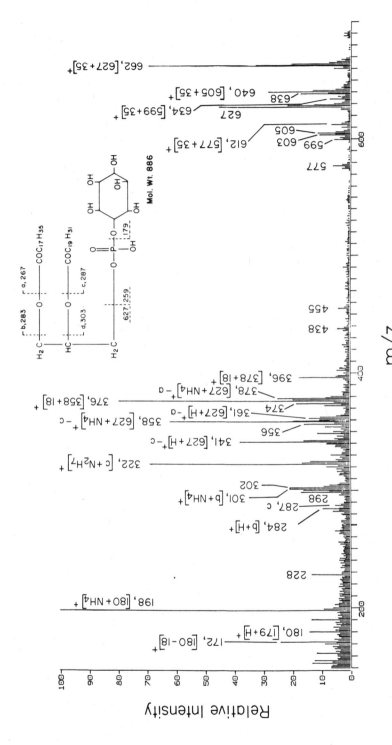

FIGURE 1.11 Ammonia CI mass spectrum of bovine brain phosphatidylinositol (5 μg). The spectrum was obtained as described in the legend of Figure 1.8. Fragmentation of 18:0–20:4 glycerophosphorylinositol is given as an example. (Reproduced by permission from *J. Lipid Res.*)

m/z 627 and 662); 18:0–18:2 (10%, m/z 603 and 638); 18:0–18:1 (14%, m/z 605 and 640); and 18:0–20:3 (11%, m/z 629 and 664). Nine other molecular species were identified, which included 16:0–18:2 (2%, m/z 575 and 610); 16:0–18:1 (4%, m/z 577 and 612); 16:0–20:4 (4.5%, m/z 599 and 634); and 18:0–20:2 (2.6%, m/z 631 and 666). GLC analysis of fatty acid methyl esters obtained from the same sample agreed well with the calculated amounts of the fatty acid as determined by CIMS.

1.5.3.5 Sphingomyelin

The major high molecular weight ions in the positive-ion ammonia CIMS of bovine brain sphingomyelin (Fig. 1.12) were the ceramide ions M^+ − 182 and $[M^+ + 18] - 182$. The even-numbered ceramide ions are easily distinguished from the odd-numbered acylglycerol ions. The major sphingomyelin molecular species were C_{18}-sphingenine with 18:0 (48%, m/z 530 and 548); 16:0 (4%, m/z 502 and 520); 20:0 (5%, m/z 558 and 576); 22:0 (6%, m/z 586 and 604); 24:1 (7%, m/z 612 and 630); and 24:0 (7%, m/z 614 and 632). Small amounts of molecular species containing C_{18}-sphinganine and fatty acid 18:0 (10%, m/z 550 and 532), 20:0, 22:0, and 24:0 were also identified. The presence of C_{20}-sphingenine with 16:0 fatty acid cannot be resolved from C_{18}-sphingenine with 18:0 fatty acid. However, C_{18}-sphinganine and C_{20}-sphingenine-containing sphingomyelins are about 7 and 10%, respectively, in bovine brain sphingomyelin (Jungalwala et al., 1983). Fatty acid analyses by GLC and CIMS were in agreement.

1.5.4 HPLC–MS of Phospholipid Mixtures

HPLC–MS of standard phospholipid mixture was performed with a variety of solvents and columns. The MS monitoring was generally done with ammonia as a reagent gas in the positive-ion mode. When a silica gel column (Accupak 3 μm, 4.6 mm inside diameter × 10 cm) with a gradient solvent mixture of dichloromethane–methanol–water–acetic acid was used for HPLC, excellent separation of all the phospholipid standards was achieved initially. However, after repeated injections, the separation deteriorated and variable chromatographic resolution was obtained. The separation of PS and PI from each other and from PE was difficult under these conditions, possibly due to formation of various ionic forms of these phospholipids. This difficulty was resolved by performing HPLC with ammonia-containing solvent and by equilibration of the sample in ammonia-containing solvent prior to injection (Jungalwala et al., 1984).

A reconstructed plot of the total ion current after HPLC–MS analysis of standard phospholipids (5 μg each) is shown in Figure 1.13a. The sep-

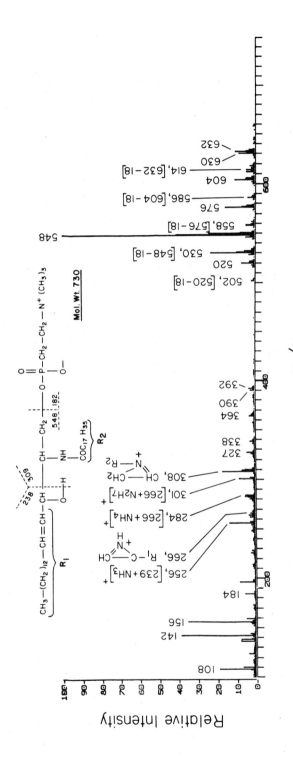

FIGURE 1.12 Ammonia CI mass spectrum of bovine brain sphingomyelin. The spectrum was obtained as described in the legend of Figure 1.8. Fragmentation of 18:0 fatty acid and C₁₈-sphingenine containing sphingomyelin is shown as an example. Ions m/z 364, 390, and 392 have the structure

, corresponding to 22:0, 24:1, and 24:0 fatty acids. (Reproduced by permission from

J. Lipid Res.)

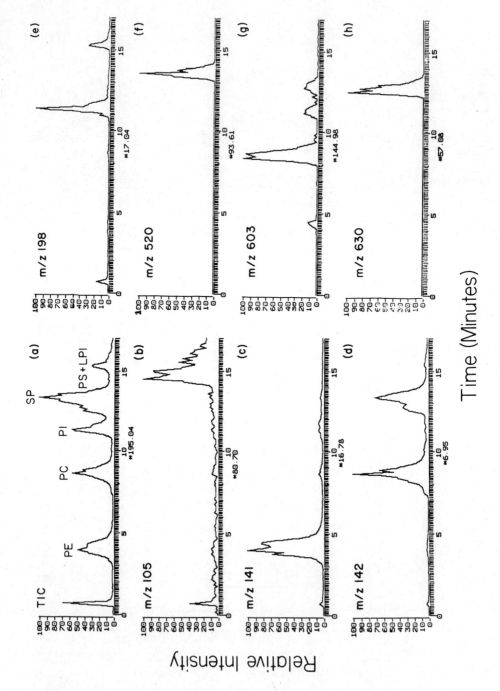

36

aration of phospholipids was achieved on a Brownlee silica gel (5 μm) cartridge column (2 × 60 mm). The column was developed with a linear gradient of solvent A, dichloromethane–methanol–water, 93:6.5:0.5 (by volume), and B, dichloromethane–methanol–water–15 M NH4OH, 65:31:4:0.2 (by volume), from 12% B to 45% B in 10 min and programming to 100% B in 2 min at a flowrate of 0.8 ml/min. Under these conditions, fairly good reproducibility was achieved. All the phospholipids were well resolved except PS, which tailed to some extent into the lysoPI peak. The specific ion plots for m/z 105, 141, 142, and 198 are given in Figure 13b–e. These ions are fairly specific for the individual phospholipid bases. Thus, m/z 105, specific for PS, is not found to be associated with other phospholipids. Similarly, m/z 141 is relatively specific for ethanolamine-containing phospholipids, whereas m/z 142 is specific for choline-containing phospholipids, and m/z 198 is found to be associated only with inositol-containing phospholipids. Individual phospholipids were chromatographically resolved to some extent based on molecular species. Thus, sphingomyelin was resolved into two peaks (Fig. 1.13d). Mass spectral analysis showed that the front peak contained mostly long-chain fatty acid–containing sphingomyelin such as 24:1, m/z 630 (Fig. 1.13h) whereas the later peak contained mostly short-chain fatty acid–containing sphingomyelin such as 16:0, m/z 520 (Fig. 1.13f). Similarly, the long-chain fatty acid–containing species of other phospholipids were eluted before the short-chain fatty acid–containing species. The diacylglycerol ion m/z 603 corresponding to 18:0–18:2 is predominantly in PC (Fig. 1.13g).

A reconstructed plot of the total ion current after HPLC–MS analysis of rat brain phospholipids (80 μg) is given in Fig. 1.14a. In general, the phospholipids were well resolved, as can be seen by the specific ion plots for m/z for phospholipid bases (Fig. 1.14b–d). The ethanolamine-containing phospholipids were resolved into two separate peaks (Fig. 1.14c). The mass spectral analysis of the earlier peak showed that it contained mostly alkenylacyl-GPE, m/z 561 (Fig. 1.14e) and 587 (Fig. 1.14g), m/z

---

FIGURE 1.13 Reconstructed plots of total ion current (a) and various specific ions (b–h) monitored after HPLC–CIMS of standard phospholipids. Bovine brain PE, PC, PS, PI, and SP (5 μg each) were injected on a Brownlee silica gel (5 μm) cartridge HPLC column and eluted as described in the text. The eluate was applied to the moving belt of a Finnigan HPLC–MS interface. The solvent was removed by heating the belt at 330°C under vacuum and the phospholipid was introduced into the ion source (150°C) of the mass spectrometer. Positive-ion mass spectra were continuously collected in the CI mode with ammonia as the reagent gas from m/z 100–900, every 7 s, under the control of Teknivent model 56K MS data system. The magnification factor (*) is given under each panel. LysoPI (LPI) is an impurity in PI sample. (Reproduced by permission from *J. Lipid Res.*)

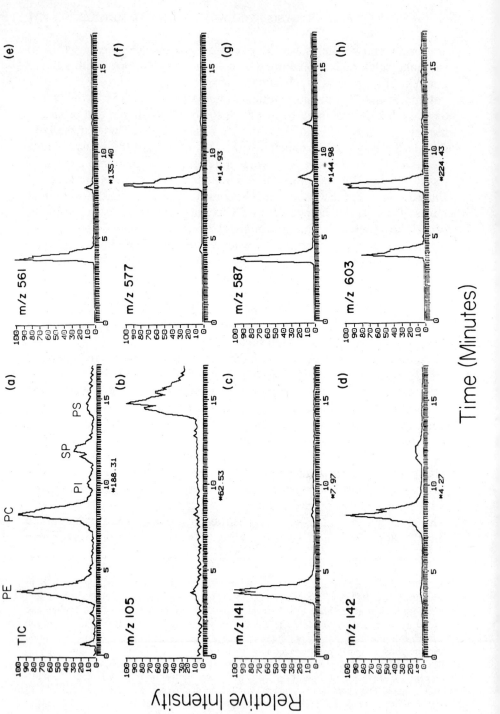

38

589 corresponding to plasmalogens with 16:1–18:1 (33%), 18:1–18:2 (36%), and 18:2–18:2 (31%), respectively. This peak also contained some diacyl-GPE, m/z 623, 627, and 651, corresponding to 16:0–22:6 (20%), 18:0–20:4 (28%), and 18:0–22:6 (19%), respectively. The later-eluting peak contained mostly diacyl-GPE with 18:0–18:1 (m/z 605, 15%) and 18:0–18:2 (m/z 603, 19%, Fig. 1.14h). The ratio of alkenylacyl-GPE to diacyl-GPE was 58:42. These results agree well with the previously published analysis (Jungalwala et al., 1975; Norton and Poduslo, 1973).

Rat brain PC peak also split into two major peaks; the earlier peak contained mostly long-chain fatty acid–containing species, whereas the latter contained short-chain fatty acid species. From the relative intensity of the diacylglycerol ions of PC, it was calculated that of the total rat brain PC, 5.4% was ether-containing PC, mostly 16:1–18:0 (m/z 563, 27%) and 18:0–20:4 (m/z 613, 25%) containing species. The major diacyl-containing PC species were 16:0–18:1 (m/z 577, 43%, Fig. 1.14f); 16:0–16:0 (m/z 551, 19%); 18:0–18:1 (m/z 605, 11%); 16:0–18:0 (m/z 579, 9%); 16:0–16:1 (m/z 549, 6%); and 14:0–16:0 (m/z 523, 6%). Eight other minor species were also recognized in the mass spectrum. It is surprising to note that rat brain PC contained several bis-saturated fatty acid–containing species in large amounts. Saturated species represented 35% of the total diacyl-PC. Freysz and Van den Bosch (1979) also reported high amounts of saturated fatty acid–containing PC in rat brain. The percentage composition of individual fatty acids in PC was calculated and found to be in good agreement with the previously reported amounts.

The amount of PI in rat brain phospholipids is very small (about 4%). The specific ion m/z 198, however, clearly identified the peak as PI. The relative intensity of the $[M + 35]^+ - 259$ ions indicated that the major species of rat brain PI were 18:0–20:4 (m/z 662 and 627, 90%), 18:0–20:3 (m/z 664, 5%), and 18:0–22:5 (m/z 688, 5%).

The rat brain sphingomyelin was resolved into two major peaks. The front peak was associated with sphingomyelin characterized by C_{18}-sphingenine and 22:0 (m/z 586 and 604, 4%), 24:1 (m/z 612 and 630, 12%), and 24:0 (m/z 614 and 632, 6%) fatty acids. The following peak contained C_{18}-sphingenine and 16:0 (m/z 502 and 520, 5%), 18:0 (m/z 530 and 548, 54%), 20:0 (m/z 558 and 576, 5%), and C_{18}-sphinganine with 16:0 (m/z 522, 1%)

FIGURE 1.14 Reconstructed plots of the total ion current (a) and various specific ions (b–h) monitored after HPLC–CIMS of rat brain phospholipids (80 µg). HPLC–CIMS data were collected as described in the legend of Figure 1.13. (Reproduced by permission from *J. Lipid Res.*)

and 18:0 (*m/z* 532 and 550, 10%) fatty acids. Small amounts (<3%) of other minor species of sphingomyelin were also identified.

The last peak in the chromatogram was due to PS (*m/z* 105). The major molecular species of rat brain PS was identified as the 18:0–18:1 species.

The percentage distribution of each phospholipid class molecular species as determined by MS agreed fairly well with that obtained by other methods. While these results indicate that MS has good potential for direct molecular species analysis, further work will be necessary using internal standards to confirm the accuracy of quantitative analysis. This should not be difficult since each phospholipid produces specific ions in the low-mass range. The limits of sensitivity have also not been explored; routinely we have injected about 5 µg of individual phospholipid for complete HPLC–MS analysis. However, sensitivity can be easily increased fivefold to obtain reliable molecular species analysis. The detection of subnanogram amounts of individual phospholipids in a mixture should be possible by means of specific ion monitoring in the low-mass range.

In summary, HPLC–CIMS overcomes the limitations of detection techniques encountered in HPLC. Moreover, the method provides within a few minutes extensive information on the molecular structure of each phospholipid and on the relative abundance of each molecular species of an individual class of phospholipids. In contrast, conventional and time-consuming molecular species analysis requires separation of large quantities of individual phospholipids by TLC or another chromatographic procedure, and enzymatic and chemical degradation of the isolated phospholipids followed by gas chromatography.

ACKNOWLEDGMENTS

This work was supported by USPHS grants MS-16447, CA-16853, NS-10437, and HD-05515. HPLC–MS results were obtained in collaboration with Dr. R. H. McCluer and Mr. J. E. Evans.

REFERENCES

Albro, P.W., and Ditmer, J.C., *J. Chromatogr.*, **38**, 230–239 (1968).

Alcock, N.J., Eckers, C., Games, D.E., Games, M.P.L., Lant, M.S., McDowall, M.A., Rossiter, M., Smith, R.W., Westwood, S.A., and Wong, H.Y., *J. Chromatogr.*, **251**, 165–174 (1982).

Allan, D., and Cockcroft, S. *J. Lipid Res.*, **23**, 1373–1374 (1982).

Althaus, H.H., and Neuhoff, V., *Hoppe-Seyler's Z. Physiol. Chem.*, **354**, 1073–1076 (1973).

Arvidson, G.A.E., *J. Lipid Res.*, **6**, 574–577 (1965).

Arvidson, G.A.E., *Eur. J. Biochem.*, **4**, 478–486 (1968).

Aveldano, M.I., and Bazan, N.G. *J. Lipid Res.*, **24**, 620–627 (1983).

Bartlett, G.R., *J. Biol. Chem.*, **234**, 466–468 (1959).

Batley, M., Packer, N.H., and Redmond, J.W., *J. Chromatogr.*, **198**, 520–525 (1980).

Bell, M.E., Peterson, R.G., and Eichberg, J., *J. Neurochem.* **39**,192–200 (1982).

Bernard, D.M., and Vercauteren, R.E., *J. Chromatogr.*, **120**, 211–212 (1976).

Blank, M.L., Cress, E.A., Piantadosi, C., and Snyder, F., *Biochim. Biophys. Acta*, **380**, 208–218 (1975).

Blass, K.G., Briand, R.L., Ng, D.S., and Harold, S., *J. Chromatogr.*, **182**, 311–316 (1980).

Blom, C.P., Deierkauf, F.A., and Riemersma, J.C., *J. Chromatogr.*, **171**, 331–338 (1979).

Briand, R.L., Harold, S., and Blass, K.G., *J. Chromatogr.*, **223**, 277–284 (1981).

Chen, S.S., Kou, A.Y., and Chen, H.Y., *J. Chromatogr.*, **208**, 339–346 (1981).

Chen, S.S., and Kou, A.Y., *J. Chromatogr.*, **227**, 25–31 (1982).

Clarke, N.G., and Dawson, R.M.C., *Biochem. J.*, *195*, 301–306 (1981).

Cook, A.M., and Daughton, C.G., *Methods in Enzymol.*, **72**, 292–295 (1981).

Crawford, C.G., and Plattner, R.D. *J. Lipid Res.* **24**, 456–460 (1983).

Dawson, R.M.C., *Biochim. Biophys. Acta*, **14**, 374–379 (1954).

Dawson, R.M.C., in G.V. Marinetti, Ed., *Lipid Chromatographic Analysis*, Vol. 1, 1st ed., Dekker, New York, 1967, pp. 163–189.

Dawson, R.M.C., in G.V. Marinetti, Ed., *Lipid Chromatographic Analysis*, 2nd ed., Dekker, New York, 1976, pp. 149–172.

Ditmer, J.C., and Wells, M.A., *Methods in Enzymol.*, **14**, 482–530 (1969).

Eichberg, J., Shein, H.M., Schwartz, M., and Hauser, G., *J. Biol. Chem.*, **248**, 3615–3622 (1973).

Evans, J.E., Jungalwala, F.B., and McCluer, R.H., Am. Soc. Mass. Spec. 31st Ann. Conference, Boston, 1983, pp. 160–161.

Felix, A.M., and Jimenez, M.H., *J. Chromatogr.*, **89**, 361–364 (1974).

Fine, J.B., and Sprecher, H., *J. Lipid Res.*, **23**, 660–663 (1982).

Folch-Pi, J., Lees, M., and Sloane-Stanley, G.H., *J. Biol. Chem.*, **226**, 497–509 (1957).

Foltz, R.L., *Lloydia*, **35**, 344–353 (1972).

Freysz, L., and Van den Bosch, H., Abst. 7th Meeting of Intl. Soc. Neurochem., Jerusalem, Israel, 1979, p. 334.

Getz, G.S., Jakovcic, S., Heywood, J., Frank, J., and Rabinowitz, M., *Biochim. Biophys. Acta*, **218**, 441–452 (1970).

Geurts van Kessel, W.S.M., Hax, W.M.A., Demel, R.A., and DeGier, J., *Biochim. Biophys. Acta*, **486**, 524–530 (1977).

Gilfillan, A.M., Chu, A.J., Smart, D.A., and Rooney, S.A., *J. Lipid Res.*, **24**, 1651–1656 (1983).

Gonzalez-Sastre, F., and Folch-Pi, J., *J. Lipid Res.*, **9**, 532–533 (1968).

Goswami, S.K., and Frey, C.F., *J. Lipid Res.*, **12**, 509–510 (1971).

Gross, R.W., and Sobel, B.E., *J. Chromatogr.*, **197**, 79–85 (1980).

Hanson, V.L., Park, J.Y., Osborn, T.W., and Kiral, R.M., *J. Chromatogr.*, **205**, 393–400 (1981).

Hara, A., and Radin, N.S., *Analyt. Biochem.*, **90**, 420–426 (1978).

Harrington, C.A., Fenimore, D.C., and Eichberg, J., *Analyt. Biochem.*, **106**, 307–313 (1980).

Hatch, F.W., *Amer. Soc. Mass Spectrom. Abstracts*, **30**, 157–158 (1982).

Hauser, G., and Eichberg, J., *Biochim. Biophys. Acta*, **326**, 201–209 (1973).

Hayes, M.J., Lankmayer, E.P., Vouros, P., Karger, B.L., and McGuire, J.M., *Anal. Chem.*, **55**, 1745–1752 (1983).

Hess, H.H., and Derr, J.E., *Analyt. Biochem.*, **63**, 607–613 (1975).

Heyneman, R.A., Bernard, D.M., and Vercauteren, R.E., *J. Chromatogr.*, **68**, 285 (1972).

Horrocks, L.A., *J. Lipid Res.*, **9**, 469–472 (1968).

Horvath, C., and Melander, W., *Chromatographia*, **11**, 262–273 (1978).

Hsieh, J.Y.K., Welch, D.K., and Turcotte, J.G., *J. Chromatogr.*, **208**, 398–403 (1981a).

Hsieh, J.Y.K., Welch, D.K., and Turcotte, J.G., *Lipids*, **16**, 761–763 (1981b).

Hubmann, F.H., *J. Chromatogr.*, **86**, 197–199 (1973).

James, J.L., Clawson, G.A., Chan, C.H., and Smuckler, E.A., *Lipids*, **16**, 541–545 (1981).

Jones, M., Keenan, R.W., and Horowitz, P., *J. Chromatogr.*, **237**, 522–524 (1982).

Jungalwala, F.B., Evans, J.E., Bremer, F., and McCluer, R.H., *J. Lipid Res.*, **24**, 1380–1388 (1983).

Jungalwala, F.B., Evans, J.E., Kadowaki, H., and McCluer, R.H., *J. Lipid Res.*, **25**, 209–216 (1984).

Jungalwala, F.B., Evans, J.E., and McCluer, R.H., *Biochem. J.*, **155**, 55–60 (1976).

Jungalwala, F.B., Evans, J.E., and McCluer, R.H., *J. Lipid Res.*, **25**, 738–749 (1984).

Jungalwala, F.B., Hayssen, V., Pasquini, J.M., and McCluer, R.H., *J. Lipid Res.*, **20**, 579–587 (1979).

Jungalwala, F.B., Sanyal, S., and LeBaron, F., in L. Horrocks, G.B. Ansell, and G. Porcellati, Eds., *Phospholipids in the Nervous System*, Vol. 1, *Metabolism*, Raven Press, New York, 1982, pp. 91–103.

Jungalwala, F.B., Turel, R.J., Evans, J.E., and McCluer, R.H., *Biochem. J.*, **145**, 517–526 (1975).

Kaduce, T.L., Norton, K.C., and Spector, A.A., *J. Lipid Res.*, **24**, 1398–1403 (1983).

Kaitaranta, J.K., and Bessman, S.P., *Anal. Chem.*, **53**, 1232–1235 (1981).

Kates, M., *Techniques in Lipidology*, Elsevier, Amsterdam, 1972, pp. 541–546.

Kishimoto, Y., and Hoshi, M., *Methods in Neurochem.*, **3**, 75–154 (1972).

Kiuchi, K., Ohta, T., and Ebine, H., *J. Chromatogr.*, **133**, 226–230 (1977).

Klien, R.A., *J. Lipid Res.*, **12**, 123–131 (1971).

Kuksis, A., in R.T. Holman, Ed., *Progress in Chemistry of Fats and Other Lipids*, Vol. 12, Pergamon Press, Oxford, England, 1972, pp. 1–164.

Kuksis, A., and Marai, L., *Lipids*, **2**, 217–224 (1967).

Kundu, S.K., Chakravarty, S., Bhaduri, N., and Saha, H.K. *J. Lipid Res.*, **18**, 128–130 (1977).

LeBaron, F.N., Sanyal, S., and Jungalwala, F.B., *Neurochem. Res.*, **6**, 1081–1089 (1981).

Lederer, M., *J. Chromatogr.*, **251**, 91–224 (1982).

Lehmann, W.D., and Kessler, M., *Chem. Phys. Lipids*, **32**, 123–135 (1983).

Lin, H.J., Jie, M.S.F., Lee, C.L.H., and Lee, D.H.S., *Lipids*, **12**, 620–625 (1977).

Luthra, M.G., and Sheltawy, A., *Biochem. J.*, **126**, 251–253 (1972).

Michell, R.H., in L. Horrocks, G.B.Ansell, and G. Porcellati, Eds., *Phospholipids in the Nervous System*, Vol. 1, *Metabolism*, Raven Press, New York, 1982, pp. 315–325.

Myher, J.J., and Kuksis, A., *Can. J. Biochem.*, **60**, 638–650 (1982).

Myher, J.J., Kuksis, A., Marai, L., and Yeung, S.K.F., *Anal. Chem.*, **50**, 557–561 (1978).

Nakagawa, Y., and Horrocks, L.A., *J. Lipid Res.*, **24**, 1268–1275 (1983).

Nelson, G.J., in E.G. Perkins, Ed., *Analysis of Lipids and Lipoproteins* American Oil Chem. Soc., Champaign, Il., 1975, pp. 1–22, 70–107.

Norton, W.T., and Poduslo, S.E., *J. Neurochem.*, **21**, 759–773 (1973).

Palmer, F.B., *J. Lipid Res.*, **22**, 1296–1300 (1981).

Patton, G.M., Fasulo, J.M., and Robins, S.J., *J. Chromatogr.*, **23**, 190–196 (1982).

Park, J.G., and Thompson, W., *J. Biol. Chem.*, **248**, 6655–6662 (1973).

Phillips, F., and Privett, O.S., *Lipids*, **14**, 590–595 (1979).

Pollet, S., Ermidou, S., Saux, F.L., Monge, M., and Baumann, N., *J. Lipid Res.*, **19**, 916–921 (1978).

Poorthuis, B.J.H.M., Yazaki, P.J., and Hostetler, K.Y., *J. Lipid Res.*, **17**, 433–437 (1976).

Portoukalian, J., Meisler, R., and Zwingelstein, G., *J. Chromatogr.*, **152**, 569–574 (1978).

Renkonen, O., *J. Amer. Oil Chem. Soc.*, **42**, 298–304 (1965).

Renkonen, O., *J. Lipid Res.*, **9**, 34–39 (1968).

Renkonen, O., in Eds. A. Niederwieser and G. Pataki, *Progress in Thin Layer Chromatography and Related Methods*, Ann Arbor Sc. Pub., Ann Arbor, Mich., 1971, pp. 143–181.

Renkonen, O., and Luukkonen, A., in G.V. Marinetti, Eds., *Lipid Chromatographic Analysis*, Dekker, New York, 1976, p. 1–58.

Ryu, E.K., and MacCoss, M., *J. Lipid Res.*, **20**, 561–563 (1979).

Schacht, J., *J. Lipid Res.*, **19**, 1063–1067 (1978).

Schiefer, H.G., and Neuhoff, V., *Hoppe-Seyler's Z. Physiol. Chem.*, **352**, 913–926 (1971).

Schmid, H.H.O., Bandi, P.C., and Su, K.L., *J. Chrom. Sc.*, **13**, 478–486 (1975).

Sheltawy, A., in N. Marks and R. Rodnight, Eds. *Research Methods in Neurochemistry*, Vol. 3, Plenum Press, New York, 1975, pp. 293–307.

Skipski, V.P., and Barclay, M., *Methods in Enzymol.*, **14**, 530–598 (1969).

Smith, M., and Jungalwala, F.B., *J. Lipid Res.*, **22**, 697–704 (1981).

Smith, M., Monchamp, P., and Jungalwala, F.B., *J. Lipid Res.*, **22**, 714–719 (1981).

Spanner, S., in G.B. Ansell, J.N. Hawthorne, and R.M.C. Dawson, Eds., *Form and Function of Phospholipids* Elsevier, Amsterdam, 1973, pp. 43–65.

Su, K.L., and Schmid, H.H.O., *Lipids*, **9**, 208–213 (1974).

Sugatani, J., Kino, M., Saito, K., Matsuo, T., Matsuda, H., and Katakuse, I., *Biomed. Mass Spectrom.*, **9**, 293 (1982).

Sugnaux, F.R., and Djerassi, C., *J. Chromatogr.*, **251**, 189–201 (1982).

Sundler, R., and Akesson, B., *J. Chromatogr.*, **80**, 233–240 (1973).

Vance, D.E., and Sweeley, C.C., *J. Lipid Res.*, **8**, 621–630 (1967).

Vaskovsky, V.E., and Kostetsky, E.Y., *J. Lipid Res.*, **9**, 396 (1968).

Vaskovsky, V.E., Kostetsky, E.Y., and Vasendin, I.M., *J. Chromatogr.*, **114**, 129–141 (1975).

Viswanathan, C.V., *J. Chromatogr.*, **98** 129–155 (1974).

Vitiello, F., and Zanetta, J.P., *J. Chromatogr.*, **166**, 637–640 (1978).

Wiegand, R.D., and Anderson, R.E., *Methods in Enzymol.*, **81** 297–304 (1982).

Wood, G.W., Lau, P.Y., Morrow, G., Rao G.N.S., Schmidt, D.E., and Tuebner, J., *Chem. Phys. Lipids*, **18**, 316–333 (1977).

Yandrasitz, J.R., Berry, G., and Segal, S., *J. Chromatogr.*, **225**, 319–328 (1981).

—— two ——

ENZYMIC PATHWAYS OF PHOSPHOLIPID METABOLISM IN THE NERVOUS SYSTEM

R. M. C. DAWSON

Department of Biochemistry
ARC Institute of Animal Physiology
Babraham, Cambridge, United Kingdom

CONTENTS

2.1   INTRODUCTION   46

2.2   BIOSYNTHESIS OF PHOSPHOLIPIDS IN THE NERVOUS
        SYSTEM   48

    2.2.1   Phosphatidylcholine and Phosphatidylethanolamine: *De
                  Novo* Synthesis, 48

    2.2.2   Phosphatidylcholine, Phosphatidylethanolamine,
                  Phosphatidylserine: Synthesis by Interconversion or
                  Exchange, 51

    2.2.3   Plasmalogen (Alkenyl-Acyl) and Glycerol Ether (Alkyl-
                  Acyl) Phospholipid Synthesis, 53

    2.2.4   Sphingomyelin Synthesis, 56

    2.2.5   Phosphatidic Acid Synthesis, 58

    2.2.6   CDP-Diacylglycerol Synthesis, 60

    2.2.7   Phosphatidylglycerol and Diphosphatidylglycerol
                  Synthesis, 60

    2.2.8   Phosphatidylinositol and Polyphosphoinositide
                  Synthesis, 62

2.3   CATABOLISM OF PHOSPHOLIPIDS IN THE NERVOUS
        SYSTEM   64

    2.3.1   Deacylating Phospholipases, 64

    2.3.2   Degradation of Plasmalogens and Glycerol Ether
                  Phospholipids, 67

    2.3.3   Sphingomyelin Degradation, 68

    2.3.4   Phosphoinositide Hydrolysis, 69

    2.3.5   Phospholipase D Enzymes, 72

    REFERENCES   73

2.1 INTRODUCTION

Before 1940 it was generally considered that phospholipids once laid down
in the nervous system of mammals during growth and development were
comparatively static entities. Even in extreme and prolonged states of

starvation the brain tenaciously retained its phospholipid content whereas that of liver was much more labile. The introduction of isotopes into research and especially [^{32}P]inorganic phosphate quickly dispelled this assumption. Although, in comparison with other tissues, the rate of entry of isotopic precursors of phospholipids into the brain from the blood is relatively slow due to the hindrance of the blood–brain barrier, it soon became clear that once available to the intracellular pool, such precursors became rapidly incorporated into the membrane phospholipids. Since such incorporation occurred even when the animal was adult, that is, virtually a nongrowth situation in the brain tissue, it was obvious that this biosynthesis of the phospholipids must be balanced by a continuous catabolism to maintain the turnover and the concentration equilibrium. All membranes of nervous tissue show this continual turnover of phospholipid components, although that of the myelin sheath tends to be somewhat slower possibly because its newly synthesized phospholipids arrive by lateral diffusion through the rolled-up membrane bilayer continuum ending in the plasmalemma of the oligodendrioglia or Schwann cells (Gould and Dawson, 1976). The turnover does not appear to be related in any way to cell division since the neurons appear to be at least as active in this respect as the glia.

By and large, the enzymic pathways for carrying out at least the last steps in the synthesis of the complete phospholipid molecules are located in the endoplasmic reticulum both rough and smooth. This means therefore that the newly synthesized phospholipid molecules incorporated into other membranes such as the mitochondrial, plasmalemma, Golgi, lysosomal, nuclear envelope, and so on, must be transported there in some fashion. We know now that a complex system of exchange proteins exists in the cytoplasm of the brain cells that can bring about the transfer of phospholipid molecules from synthetic to nonsynthetic sites, or vice versa (Miller and Dawson, 1972a; Helmkamp, 1980). It is also possible that some phospholipid molecules might be transported by lateral diffusion through a continuous bilayer system, although the electron microscope evidence for endoplasmic reticulum having direct connections with, for example, the outer membranes of mitochondria is still somewhat uncertain. The catabolic enzyme systems, or phospholipases in the first instance, that carry out the hydrolysis of the membrane phospholipids appear to have a much wider distribution through the structure of the cell, including the cytoplasm, possibly to degrade specific areas of the membrane which for some reason require repair and maintenance. The whole lipoprotein network of neurons and glial cells can therefore be considered as an integrated complex in dynamic equilibrium as far as phospholipids are concerned, with depletion at one point resulting in a net flow of phospholipid to this site. Such a dynamic system is clearly more resilient to damage and more capable of functional variation than one that is static.

As well as the *de novo* turnover of the whole phospholipid molecule, there is evidence that enzymic systems exist that are capable of removing and reinserting one of the molecular entities comprising the whole phospholipid structure as an independent operation. The deacylation and reacylation system whereby a fatty acid can be removed and replaced by a differing fatty acid (Corbin and Sun, 1978; Fisher and Rowe, 1980) is an example of such a process and this could have an important role in maintaining the membrane in a state of optimal fluidity. The exchange systems for removing and replacing base moieties or inositol are further examples, although their biological function is at present obscure. Theoretically such systems for replacing or substituting a part of the phospholipid molecule as the necessity arose would be much more economical in terms of energy expenditure than *de novo* turnover of the whole molecule.

Inositol-containing phospholipids appear to be catabolized more rapidly in the working state of the cell, and this is followed by a rapid incorporation of newly synthesized phosphoinositide into the area to maintain the status quo. The precise function, if any, of this enhanced turnover of phospholipid in response to stimulation is obscure, although it has been suggested that it could be associated with prostaglandin formation or divalent cation translocation (Michell, 1975; Irvine et al., 1982). There is no evidence that the enzymic pathways involved in the catabolism and subsequent resynthesis after cell stimulation differ from those involved in normal phospholipid turnover, although, of course, the question of the enzymic control mechanism becomes of paramount importance with a rapid turn on of activity and an equally rapid turn off as stimulation ceases.

2.2   BIOSYNTHESIS OF PHOSPHOLIPIDS IN THE NERVOUS SYSTEM

2.2.1   Phosphatidylcholine and Phosphatidylethanolamine: *De Novo* Synthesis

These nitrogen-containing glycerophospholipids constitute the bulk of the phospholipids in nervous tissue. Their biosynthetic pathways are depicted in Figure 2.1. When labeled choline is injected intracerebrally into the adult rat and the specific radioactivity-time sequences of phosphocholine, CDP-choline, and phosphatidylcholine are determined, it is apparent that the cytidine route is the principal pathway of *de novo* biosynthesis (Ansell and Spanner, 1968b). Equivalent experiments using [^{14}C]ethanolamine

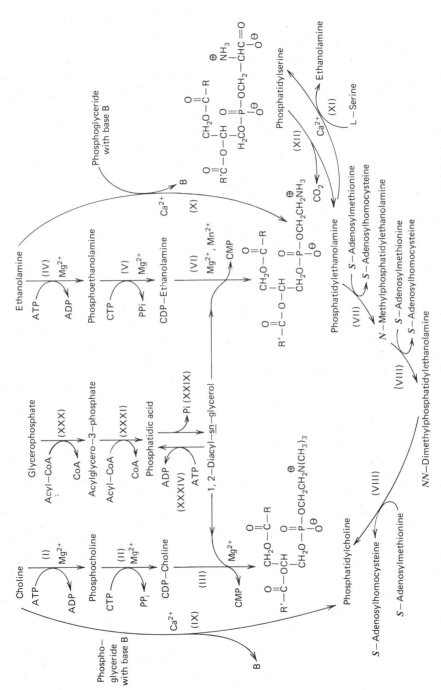

FIGURE 2.1 Pathways of phosphatidylcholine and phosphatidylethanolamine biosynthesis in nervous tissue.

indicate that that same pathway is also likely to be the principal route for phosphatidylethanolamine biosynthesis (Ansell and Spanner, 1967). Choline is though to be principally derived from the diet or by synthesis in the liver. On entering the brain, it is rapidly phosphorylated by the Mg^{2+}-requiring choline kinase system (I) which exists in all areas of the brain and peripheral nervous system (McCaman, 1962). Choline kinase is an enzyme of the cytosol. Recent evidence would suggest that it exists in a number of forms in the nervous system showing either a sensitivity or insensitivity to the inhibitor hemicholinium-3 (Ansell and Spanner, 1974; Burt, 1977).

The conversion of phosphocholine into CDP-choline by the Mg^{2+}-requiring enzyme CTP: cholinephosphate cytidylyltransferase (II) is essentially a soluble enzyme of the nervous system (Porcellati and Arienti, 1970). It exists in two forms, one with a molecular weight of 190,000 and another as a very high molecular weight component of $>5 \times 10^6$; the former is predominant in rat brain (Feldman et al., 1980). The activity of the enzyme is closely related to accompanying phospholipid and both phosphatidylglycerol and lysophosphatidylethanolamine appear to be very active in this respect. The final enzyme in the synthesis of phosphatidylcholine by the cytidine pathway, CDP-choline:1,2-diacylglycerol cholinephosphotransferase (III), has been demonstrated many times in brain and the peripheral nervous system (McCaman and Cook, 1966). It displays its highest activity *in vitro* in preparations from neonatal tissue and neuronal-rich gray matter has a much higher activity than that of the white matter. The enzyme is believed to be entirely confined to the endoplasmic reticulum, and previous reports of a wider distribution through the membranous structure of the cell are likely to be due to contamination of the isolated subcellular fractions with this membrane. A possible exception is the synaptic vesicles isolated from the nerve endings (Miller and Dawson, 1972b). The 1,2-diacylglycerol used in phosphatidylcholine biosynthesis is believed to be largely derived by the dephosphorylation of phosphatidic acid. The enzyme involved, phosphatidic acid phosphatase (XXIX), is much more active in gray than white matter from rabbit brain (McCaman et al., 1965). It increases during early development of the rabbit brain and also during demyelination.

The enzymic steps in the biosynthesis of phosphatidylethanolamine by the cytidine pathway have all been demonstrated in nervous tissue. As in liver, the phosphorylation of ethanolamine (IV) in nerve ending cytosol appears to be distinct from that of choline with differing requirements for Mg^{2+} and ATP and a lack of inhibition by hemicholinium-3 (Spanner and Ansell, 1979). This suggests that two separate enzymes may be involved in the phosphorylation of choline or ethanolamine, but whether choline kinase can phosphorylate both bases as occurs in liver (Weinhold and Rethy, 1974) must await the physical separation of the two activities. The formation of CDP-ethanolamine seems to be the rate-limiting enzyme in the formation of phosphatidylethanolamine; the CTP:ethanolamine phosphate cytidylyltransferase (V) appears not to be stimulated by lipid cofactors as is the analogous CTP:phosphocholine cytidylyltransferase (Porcellati et al., 1970a). CDP-ethanolamine:1,2-diacylglycerol ethanolaminephosphotransferase (VI), the final enzyme in the synthetic chain, appears to be located in the microsomal fraction of rat brain (Ansell and Metcalfe, 1971), of chicken brain (Porcellati et al., 1970b), and rat spinal cord (Toews et al., 1976) and the incorporation of CDP-ethanolamine-^{14}C into phosphatidylethanolamine is greatly stimulated by adding saturating concentrations of diacylglycerol. Chicken brain mitochondria (Porcellati et al., 1970a,b) and also rat brain mitochondria (Miller and Dawson, 1972b) seem to be totally unable to synthesize phosphatidylethanolamine.

Recent evidence would suggest that highly purified myelin from rat brain contains some CDP-ethanolamine: 1,2-diacylglycerol ethanolaminephosphotransferase at approximately 12–16% of the specific activity found in microsomes from the same tissue (Wu and Ledeen, 1980). The enzyme has a requirement for Mg^{2+} or Mn^{2+} ions (Ansell and Metcalfe, 1971).

The cytidine pathway in brain shows absolute specificity for cytidine and deoxycytidine nucleotides although the phosphate esters of dimethylaminoethanol and monomethylaminoethanol can be incorporated from their cytidine diphosphate esters into the phospholipids of brain homogenates (Ansell and Chojnacki, 1966). However, the cytidylyltransferases of brain are less effective in forming the cytidine diphosphate esters of these two phosphorylated bases than those of ethanolamine and choline, and presumably this is, at least, partly responsible for maintaining the specific base composition of brain phospholipids.

2.2.2 Phosphatidylcholine, Phosphatidylethanolamine, and Phosphatidylserine: Synthesis by Interconversion or Exchange

The synthesis of phosphatidylcholine by the stepwise methylation of phosphatidylethanolamine using S-adenosyl methionine as donor does not appear to be a major pathway for the synthesis of this phospholipid in nervous tissue. Early studies in which [^{14}C]ethanolamine was injected intracerebrally (Ansell and Spanner, 1967) or when S-adenosyl methionine was incubated with rat brain cortex preparations (Chojnacki et al., 1964) indicated negligible methylation of phosphatidylethanolamine. More recent studies have suggested that brain synaptosome preparations and also the microsomal fraction do possess methyltransferases (Blusztajn and Wurtman, 1981; Crews et al., 1980). In synaptosomes at least two methyltransferases occur. One, tightly bound to membranes, methylates phosphatidylethanolamine to its N-monomethyl derivative (VII); it has a pH optimum at 7.4 and a partial requirement for Mg^{2+}. The second enzyme catalyzes successive methylations of this N-monomethyl derivative giving phosphatidyl-N,N-dimethylethanolamine and eventually phosphatidylcholine (VIII) This enzyme is easily solubilized, it has a high pH optimum, and no requirement for Mg^{2+}. An active formation of phosphatidylcholine by the methylation pathway has also been reported in frog retina generally considered to be part of the central nervous system (CNS) (Anderson et al., 1980).

The quantitative significance of these reactions has yet to be assessed, but it is apparent that from the *in vitro* rates so far presented they amount to only a few percent of the choline synthesis observed in liver by the same pathway, and they probably account for only a small proportion of the total phosphatidylcholine synthesized by brain. However, several groups have produced evidence for a net efflux of unesterified choline from the brain (e.g., Choi et al., 1975) and it is possible that the methylation pathway may contribute to this release.

It is now known that in nervous tissue base-exchange enzymes exist that are responsible for the energy-independent incorporation of choline (IX), ethanolamine (X), and serine (XI) into the membrane phospholipid fraction with the formation of phosphatidylcholine, phosphatidylethanolamine, and phosphatidylserine, respectively (Porcellati et al., 1971; Kanfer, 1972). The enzymes appear to be tightly membrane bound especially to the microsomal fraction. However, they have been solubilized with detergents and fractionated into independent entities by chromatography on Sepharose 4B Affi-Gel 102 and DEAE cellulose (Miura and Kanfer, 1976). The enzymes have a strict requirement for calcium and consequently their significance in an intracellular environment with very low levels of Ca^{2+} has been questioned. However, it is apparent that their effect may be modulated by calmodulin especially that of the choline-exchange protein (Buchanan and Kanfer, 1980a). It is suggested that in the brain microsomal membranes, the enzymes are asymmetrically distributed with the choline-exchange activity (trypsin sensitive) being on the cytoplasmic side and the serine and ethanolamine exchange activities (trypsin insensitive) being located on the luminal side (Buchanan and Kanfer, 1980b). In rabbit brain the ethanolamine and serine exchange enzymes seem to be specifically associated with neuronal fractions (Goracci et al., 1973).

As to the precise function of these base-exchange proteins little is known. The serine base-exchange enzyme seems to be the sole route for phosphatidylserine production in brain as well as other tissues and phosphatidylethanolamine seems to be the preferred substrate for exchange (Yavin and Zeigler, 1977; Taki and Kanfer, 1978). Surprisingly the phosphatidylserine can be readily converted to phosphatidylethanolamine by a decarboxylase (XII) (Anderson et al., 1980) so the whole forms a cyclical system that can presumably alter the phosphatidylethanolamine and phosphatidylserine complement of an individual membrane according to requirements. Recent evidence from brain cells in culture would suggest that a not inconsiderable part of the total ethanolamine phosphoglyceride biosynthesis occurs via the decarboxylation reaction (Yavin and Zeigler, 1977; Bradbury, 1982).

The mechanism by which the fatty acids in phosphatidylcholine and ethanolamine can be changed by deacylating enzymes followed by reacylation of the lysophospholipids will be discussed in the section on deacylating phospholipases.

2.2.3 Plasmalogen (Alkenyl-Acyl) and Glycerol Ether (Alkyl-Acyl) Phospholipid Synthesis

Ethanolamine plasmalogen is a major component of the phospholipids in the nervous system. Its metabolism is shown in Figure 2.2. When chicken or rat brain microsomes or homogenates are incubated with CDP-ethanolamine-^{14}C, there is a notable increase in the labeling of 1-alkenyl-2-acyl-glycerophosphoethanolamine (ethanolamine plasmalogen) when the system is supplemented with 1-alkenyl-2-acyl-glycerol or of 1-alkyl-2-acyl-glycerophosphoethanolamine (glycerol ether phospholipid) when 1-alkyl-2-acyl-glycerol is added (Porcellati, 1970b; Ansell and Metcalfe, 1971; Radominska-Pyrek and Horrocks, 1972; Radominska-Pyrek et al., 1977). Analogous reactions occur with CDP-choline as acceptor nucleotide (Radominska-Pyrek et al., 1977) even though little choline plasmalogen is present in brain tissue.

Although the synthesis of ethanolamine plasmalogen can occur in this way in brain preparations *in vitro* presumably catalyzed by ethanolaminephosphotransferase (VI) or an analogous enzyme, it is by no means certain that an equivalent route participates in plasmalogen formation *in vivo*. Instead there is very good isotopic evidence that the vinyl ether bond is introduced by a direct *cis*-hydrogen elimination of the alkyl group of the 1-alkyl-2-acyl-glycerophosphoethanolamine present (Stoffel and LeKim, 1971; Radominska-Pyrek and Horrocks, 1972; Paltauf, 1972). The desaturation appears to be carried out by a mixed-function oxidase system

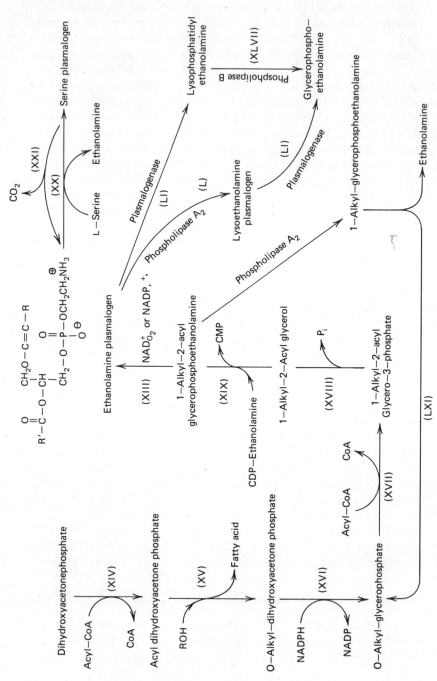

FIGURE 2.2 Metabolism of 1-alkenyl-2-acyl-glycerophosphoethanolamine (plasmalogen) and 1-alkyl-2-acyl-glycerophosphoethanolamine (glycerol ether phospholipid) in nervous tissue.

54

similar to that involved in fatty acid desaturation (XIII). This requires molecular oxygen, NAD, or NADP but not ATP or divalent metal cations (Wykle and Schremmer-Lockmiller, 1975).

The synthesis of the 1-alkyl-2-acyl-glycerol precursor required to form the immediate precursor (1-alkyl-2-acyl-glycerophosphoethanolamine) of ethanolamine plasmalogen is believed to occur through the acylation of dihydroxyacetone phosphate, an intermediate in glycolysis, by acyl transfer from acyl-CoA (XIV). The fatty acid residue is then replaced by a long-chain alcohol residue by a unique alkyl-acyl displacement reaction resulting in O-alkyl dihydroxyacetone phosphate and free fatty acid (XV). This reaction, which occurs in brain microsomes, seems to be stimulated by ATP and Mg^{2+} but coenzyme A is not necessary (Hajra, 1970). The ketone group is then reduced by a NADPH-linked oxidoreductase to form 1-alkylglycerol-3-phosphate (XVI). In rat brain this reaction seems to occur in both mitochondria and microsomes; the requirement for NADPH is highly specific and NADH will not substitute (LaBelle and Hajra, 1972). After acylation at position 2 with acyl-CoA as donor (XVII), the subsequent analog of phosphatidic acid formed can be dephosphorylated to form the 1-alkyl-2-acylglycerol derivative (XVIII) for subsequent reaction with CDP-ethanolamine to form 1-alkyl-2-acylglycerophosphoethanolamine (XIX) and subsequent reduction to ethanolamine plasmalogen (XIII). During early postnatal development the specific activity of NADPH alkyldihydroxyacetone phosphate oxidoreductase in rat brain microsomes is maximal at 4–5 days after birth, when the specific activity of the enzyme that synthesizes alkyldihydroxyacetone phosphate also peaks (El-Bassiouni et al., 1975). The enzyme in brain microsomes which dephosphorylates 1-alkyl-2-acylglycerol-3-phosphate appears to be different from equivalent enzymes that dephosphorylate alkyldihydroxyacetone phosphate and 1-alkylglycerol-3-phosphate. These latter enzymes can prevent the formation of alkyl phospholipids, and consequently they may be important regulators of plasmalogen biosynthesis in brain. Whether the Mg^{2+}-requiring enzyme involved in 1-alkyl-2-acylglycerol-3-phosphate dephosphorylation is the same as that in membranes responsible for phosphatidic acid dephosphorylation (XXIX) is not clear.

The brain usually has a small percentage of its phospholipid complement as serine plasmalogen. This is almost certainly formed by the serine-exchange enzyme (XX) discussed above since ethanolamine plasmalogen has proved to be a very effective lipid acceptor for serine catalyzed by the exchange enzyme prepared from brain tissue (Taki and Kanfer, 1978). Present evidence is strong that the serine plasmalogen formed can also be decarboxylated to reform ethanolamine plasmalogen (XXI) (Yavin and Zeigler, 1977; Bradbury, 1982).

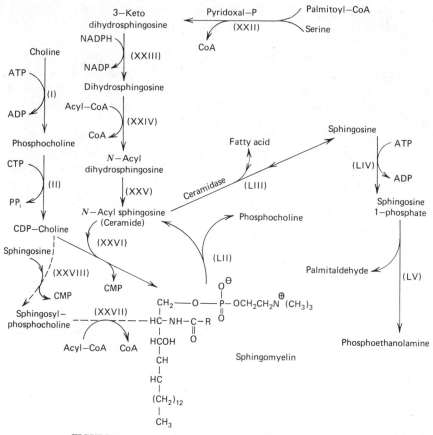

FIGURE 2.3   Metabolism of sphingomyelin in nervous tissue.

2.2.4   Sphingomyelin Synthesis

The pathways of sphingomyelin biosynthesis in nervous tissue (Fig. 2.3) have largely been elucidated, although there are still a number of unsolved problems and in particular the relative importance *in vivo* of the possible pathways of sphingomyelin assembly. Dihydrosphingosine appears to be formed by the same pathway as exists in other tissues, namely the reaction of palmitoyl-CoA and a pyridoxal-P-bound serine which results in the formation of 3-ketodihydrosphingosine (XXII) (Braun et al., 1970; Kanfer and Bates, 1970). The 3-ketodihydrosphingosine is reduced in the presence of NADPH to yield dihydrosphingosine (XXIII). However, the most common sphingosine base occurring in brain sphingomyelin is not dihydrosphingosine but sphingosine. It would seem that the free base is not reduced but instead the dihydrosphingosine is acylated to form N-acyl-dihydrosphingosine or dihydroceramide (XXIV). This compound is desaturated by an enzyme present in brain which introduces a 4-*trans* double bond into the base moiety forming N-acylsphingosine or ceramide (XXV) (Ong and Brady, 1973; Stoffel and Bister, 1974). The ceramides formed contain C18–C26 nonhydroxy and C22–C26 hydroxy fatty acids, the precise composition depending on the species and age of the animal. The specificity of the acyl-CoA long-chain base acyltransferase probably accounts for the distribution of fatty acids in brain ceramides, although it is possible that a separate pool of ceramide containing C18 and C20 acids is largely used for sphingomyelin biosynthesis (Svennerholm, 1970; Morell and Radin, 1970).

Ceramide can be converted to sphingomyelin by the donation of a phosphocholine unit from CDP-choline by an enzyme CDP-choline:N-acylsphingosine choline phosphotransferase which has been demonstrated in liver, brain, and kidney (XXVI) (Sribney and Kennedy, 1958). Originally it was believed that this enzyme, which is highly specific for CDP choline, must have a sphingosine base in the ceramide with a *trans* configuration of the double bond and a hydroxy group on carbon 3 with a *threo* relationship to the amino group on carbon 2. Subsequently, it was shown that *erythro*-ceramide could also act as a substrate *in vitro* provided it was dispersed adequately (Fujino et al., 1968a; Sribney, 1968). However, only *erythro*-sphingosine is introduced into the sphingomyelin molecule *in vivo*. Evidence for the ceramide cholinephosphotransferase pathway occuring in the intact brain has been obtained by Kopaczyk and Radin (1965) who injected emulsions of labeled N-acyl-linoceroyl- and stearoyl-N-acyl-sphingosine directly into rat brain. Although ceramide was rapidly hydrolyzed, there did nevertheless appear to be a rapid incorporation into sphingomyelin.

A possible alternative route for sphingomyelin synthesis has been demonstrated in homogenates of young rat brain and monkey brain (Brady et al., 1965; Portman et al., 1973). In this pathway sphingosylphosphocholine is directly acylated by an acyl transfer from acyl-CoA (XXVII). Both *erythro*- and *threo*-sphingosylphosphocholine can act as lipid acceptors. The sphingosylphosphocholine itself can be formed by a direct reaction involving the transfer of a phosphocholine unit from CDP-choline to sphingosine catalyzed by an enzyme present in many tissues (XXVIII) (Fujino et al., 1968b). However, experiments with doubly labeled sphingenyl-1-phosphocholine (sphingosyl) and sphinganyl-1-phosphocholine (dihydrosphingosyl) cause doubt as to whether this pathway is of significance *in vivo* at least in the liver (Stoffel and Assmann, 1972). It has even been suggested that the results obtained by earlier workers could result from some of the substrates acting as detergents rather than participating in the reaction (Ullman and Radin, 1974). A reaction whereby a phosphocholine unit can be directly transferred from phosphatidylcholine to ceramide without the intermediary of CDP-choline is present in many tissues but apparently not in brain (Ullman and Radin, 1974).

2.2.5 Phosphatidic Acid Synthesis

Although present in low concentration, phosphatidic acid plays a central role as an intermediate in the synthesis of most phospholipids in the nervous system (Fig. 2.1 and 2.4). Not only does its dephosphorylation (XXIX) (McCaman et al., 1965) provide the diacylglycerol substrate needed for phosphatidylcholine and phosphatidylethanolamine biosynthesis from the CDP-base derivatives (III, VI) but also, after reaction with CTP, the CDP-diacylglycerol formed is utilized for the synthesis of the phosphoinositides and the polyglycerophospholipids (phosphatidylglycerol and diphosphatidylglycerol). There are a number of routes by which phosphatidic acid can be formed in the nervous system, and at present there is a lack of evidence as to the quantitative importance of these in the functioning of the brain *in vivo*.

Rat brain contains an enzymic system whereby *sn*-glycerol-3-phosphate, a substrate formed from dihydroxyacetone phosphate through the reversible action of glycerophosphate dehydrogenase, is successively acylated to form lysophosphatidic acid (XXX) and then phosphatidic acid (XXXI) (Sánchez de Jiménez and Cleland, 1969; Pieringer and Hokin, 1962b; Binaglia et al., 1978). By analogy with liver the acylation is probably mainly via 1-acyl-*sn*-glycerol-3-phosphate (Tamai and Lands, 1974). The enzyme is located exclusively in the microsomes (Possmayer et al., 1973) and acyl-CoA is the acyl donor. The specificity of the acyl-CoA:*sn*-glycerol-3-phosphate acyltransferase in isolated brain microsomes has been determined and acyl-CoAs containing saturated fatty acid with 15–18 carbons were good substrates while the unsaturated fatty acid derivatives were less so. However, the kinetics of such reactions are complicated since Michaelis kinetics only apply below the critical micelle concentration of the fatty acid CoA derivatives and free monomeric molecules prevail while micelles can inhibit through their detergent properties (Zahler and Cleland, 1969).

In 1968 Hajra and Agranoff described a new pathway for phosphatidic acid formation whereby dihydroxyacetone phosphate is directly acylated (XIV) and the acyldihydroxyacetone phosphate so formed is subsequently reduced to 1-acyl-*sn*-glycerol-3-phosphate with NADPH specifically supplying the hydrogen (XXXIII). This can then be further acylated to form phosphatidic acid (XXXI). Although originally demonstrated in liver, microsomal fractions of rat brain show the same enzymes (LaBelle and Hajra, 1972; Hajra and Burke, 1978). According to Hajra and Burke (1978), the enzymes bringing about the acylation of glycerophosphate and dihydroxyacetone phosphate in rat brain are different, whereas in some tissues the enzymes show rather similar properties (Schlossman and Bell, 1976). The quantitative significance of the two pathways for forming phosphatidic acids by acylation of either glycerophosphate or dihydroxyacetone phosphate remains unknown and may depend on the availability of these substrates according to the metabolic conditions pertaining *in vivo*. Brain homogenates show an apparently greater capacity to synthesize phosphatidic acid via glycerophosphate than via acyldihydroxyacetone phosphate but did not express the potential (Pollock, Hajra, and Agranoff, 1975).

Another pathway for the synthesis of phosphatidic acid in brain is via the direct phosphorylation of diacylglycerol by ATP catalyzed by diacylglycerol kinase (XXXIV). Originally this enzyme was demonstrated in brain microsomes which had been solubilized by the careful addition of deoxycholate (Hokin and Hokin, 1959). Too much deoxycholate completely inhibited the phosphorylation. Diacylglycerol kinase appeared to require Mg^{2+} for full activity; Ca^{2+} also activated but was inhibitory in the presence of optimum Mg^{2+} (Lapetina and Hawthorne, 1971). In rat brain the enzyme seems to be concentrated in both the supernatant and microsomal fractions. Its specificity regarding fatty acid composition *in vitro* has recently been examined and there is no evidence that it produces the phosphatidic acid required for phosphatidylinositol synthesis (1-arachidonyl-2-stearoyl) (Bishop and Strickland, 1980). It perhaps should be emphasized that this pathway of phosphatidic acid formation is, as far is known, only used for recycling diacylglycerol which has itself been formed from phosphatidic acid either after dephosphorylation (XXIX) or alternatively after the conversion of the phosphatidic acid into the phosphoinositides followed by direct phosphodiesterase action on such substrates. Phosphatidic acid can also be formed directly from CDP-diacylglycerol by a hydrolase that splits off CMP (Rittenhouse et al., 1981). The enzyme involved (LXII) is of lysosomal origin and has a pH optimum of 4.8: it has been purified considerably from guinea pig cerebral cortex.

Preparations of brain microsomes can also catalyze the direct phosphorylation of monoacylglycerols using ATP (XXXV) (Bishop and Strickland, 1980). Both 1- and 2-monoacylglycerols can be utilized as substrates but phosphorylation only takes place at a terminal hydroxy of the glycerol molecule (Pieringer and Hokin, 1962a). The lysophosphatidic acid formed can then be rapidly acylated to form phosphatidic acid (Pieringer and Hokin, 1962b). To what extent monoacylglycerols are normally present in the brain *in vivo* to act as substrates for this pathway is unknown.

Finally, it should be mentioned here that phosphatidic acid can be formed in brain by the action of phospholipase D (XXXVI), which will be discussed in a later section. Again this, in reality, is a means of recycling phosphatidic acid and diacylglycerol, since presumably phosphatidic acid has already been synthesized to supply the diacylglycerol for the formation of the substrates of phospholipase D, for example, phosphatidylcholine and phosphatidylethanolamine.

2.2.6 CDP-Diacylglycerol Synthesis

Phosphatidic acid can be converted to CDP-diacylglycerol, which acts as an active intermediary for the donation of a "phosphatidyl" unit to various acceptors resulting in the formation of other membrane phospholipids (Fig. 2.4). The enzyme involved, CTP:1,2-diacylglycerophosphatecytidylyl transferase, was originally shown to be in guinea pig liver (XXXVII) (Carter and Kennedy, 1966). It has a high specificity for cytidine triphosphate although deoxycytidine triphosphate can substitute to a limited extent (Ter-Schegget et al., 1971). Petzold and Agranoff (1967) found the same enzyme in a particulate fraction from embryonic chicken brain and showed that palmitoyl-CoA inhibited the reaction. More recently Hauser and Eichberg (1975) showed a rapid formation of CDP-diacylglycerol in rat pineal gland, and the liponucleotide has also been isolated in small quantities from bovine brain (Thompson and McDonald, 1976). In the latter brain 1-stearoyl-2-arachidonyl was the major species of CDP-diacylglycerol present, and its fatty acid composition was quite unlike that of the phosphatidic acid in the same tissue and much more akin to that of phosphatidylinositol. This raises the possibility that CDP-diacylglycerol is synthesized from a selected pool of phosphatidic acid, or alternatively its composition is determined by the back reaction of CDP-diacylglycerol:inositol phosphatidyl transferase (see Section 2.2.8.).

2.2.7 Phosphatidylglycerol and Diphosphatidylglycerol Synthesis

The studies of Possmayer et al. (1968) have shown that the pathways existing in liver particles for the synthesis of phosphatidylglycerol (Kiyasu et al., 1963) also occur in rat brain (Fig. 2.4). In these CDP-diacylglycerol donates a phosphatidyl unit to glycerophosphate forming 3-*sn*-phosphatidyl-1'-glycero-3-phosphate and CMP (XXXVIII). Subsequently a dephosphorylation occurs with the formation of phosphatidylglycerol

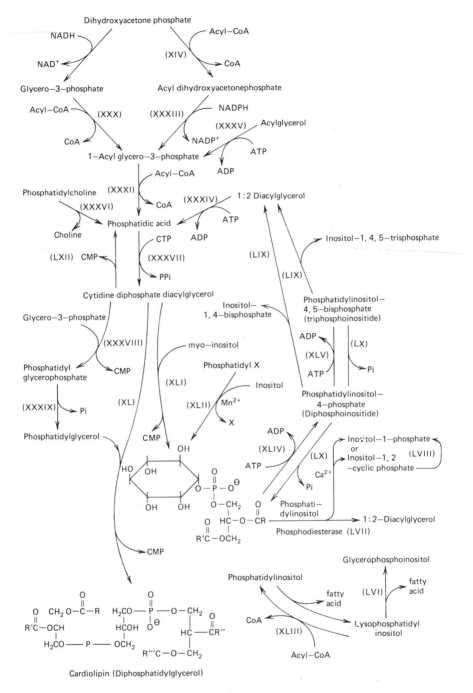

FIGURE 2.4 Metabolism of phosphoinositides in nervous tissue.

(XXXIX). The Mg^{2+}-dependent enzyme involved in the dephosphorylation is highly sensitive to reagents that react with thiol groups (Chang and Kennedy, 1967) and consequently phosphatidylglycerophosphate accumulates if $HgCl_2$ is added to the system. These reactions occur in mitochondria, consistent with phosphatidylglycerol being an intermediary in the synthesis of diphosphatidylglycerol since in brain, as in other tissues, this phospholipid is almost exclusively mitochondrial (Eichberg et al., 1964). Diphosphatidylglycerol is synthesized in the inner membrane of liver mitochondria by a mechanism by which CDP-diacylglycerol donates a phosphatidyl unit to the vacant terminal hydroxy group of phosphatidylglycerol (XL) (Hostetler et al., 1972; Stanacev et al., 1972; McMurray and Jarvis, 1980); presumably a similar reaction occurs in brain mitochondria.

2.2.8   Phosphatidylinositol and Polyphosphoinositide Synthesis

These pathways are outlined in Figure 2.4. Probably the most important acceptor for a phosphatidyl unit from CDP-diacylglycerol is the cyclitol, *myo*-inositol, which exists in brain at concentrations well above that in blood. The newly synthesized phosphatidylinositol is not only required to support normal turnover but also probably to replenish any of the phospholipid broken down in response to stimulation (Michell, 1975). The enzyme involved, CDP-diacylglycerol:*myo*-inositol phosphatidyl transferase (XLI), exists predominantly in brain microsomes (Benjamins and Agranoff, 1969), and any found in other particulate fractions can probably be ascribed to microsomal contamination (Miller and Dawson, 1972b). Presumably any replacement phosphatidylinositol required in the cell is transferred from the endoplasmic reticulum using the specific cytoplasmic exchange proteins that exist in brain (Helmkamp, 1980). The enzyme shows high selectivity for *myo*-inositol but is partially inhibited by galactinol, a *myo*-inositol galactoside (Benjamins and Agranoff, 1969). Its activity cannot be correlated with any particular phase of brain development (Salway et al., 1968). The enzyme seems to be tightly bound to brain membranes and it has proved difficult to solubilize it with detergents without appreciable inactivation (Rao and Strickland, 1974). Nevertheless, some purification has been achieved although the product appeared to be a membrane fragment with a molecular weight above 300,000.

Phosphatidylinositol can also be synthesized by an exchange reaction whose significance is not yet understood, involving an energy-independent incorporation of inositol into the microsomal fraction, which is catalyzed by manganese and stimulated by cytidine nucleotides (XLII)

(Holub, 1975). Although this reaction undoubtedly occurs in brain, it is not known whether phosphatidylinositol is the preferred substrate for the exchange and whether as in liver the products of the Mn^{2+}-stimulated exchange reaction are largely the tetraenoic species of phosphatidylinositol (Holub, 1974).

Washed brain microsomes can bring about the rapid reacylation of lysophosphatidylinositol when CoA and ATP are provided, presumably to synthesize acyl-CoA as acyl donor (XLIII) (Keenan and Hokin, 1962). Lysophosphatidylinositol can be formed in brain by the action of phospholipases A_1 and A_2 (Section 2.3.1). It is known that, as in liver, the acyl-CoA: 1-acylglycerophosphoinositol acyltransferase shows some specificity for arachidonoyl-CoA (Baker and Thompson, 1973; Holub, 1976). This substantiates earlier findings of double-label experiments which indicated that in brain *in vivo* the entry of arachidonate into phosphatidylinositol can occur without the synthesis of the corresponding phosphatidic acid (Baker and Thompson, 1972).

Phosphatidylinositol in brain can undergo successive phosphorylations with ATP as donor at the 4 and then 5 vacant hydroxy groups of the inositol ring producing phosphatidylinositol-4-phosphate (diphosphoinositide) and phosphatidylinositol-4,5-bisphosphate (triphosphoinositide) (XLIV and XLV). This was indicated in the early experiments of Saunders and Ballou (1966) using rabbit brain slices incubated with [^{32}P] and [^{3}H]inositol. Colodzin and Kennedy (1965) found phosphatidylinositol kinase (XLIV) widely distributed in rat tissues including brain; the enzyme required Mg^{2+} or Mn^{2+} and was substantially inhibited by Ca^{2+} and reagents that react with thiol groups. Prottey et al. (1968) showed that the phosphatidylinositol kinase present in a rat brain homogenate synthesized the expected phosphatidylinositol-4-phosphate and the phosphatidylinositol-4-phosphate kinase in a rat brain supernatant synthesized phosphatidylinositol-4,5-bisphosphate. The enzyme seems to be enriched in the plasma membrane fraction of rat brain homogenates (Kai et al., 1966a; Harwood and Hawthorne, 1969) and its activity rapidly rises prior to myelination (Salway et al., 1968).

In contrast, phosphatidylinositol-4-phosphate kinase (XLV) appears to be a supernatant enzyme in rat brain tissue (Kai et al., 1968), phosphatidylinositol-4,5-bisphosphate being formed in the presence of ATP and Mg^{2+}. Other cations (Mn^{2+}, Ca^{2+}) can substitute for Mg^{2+}, but on the other hand Ca^{2+} inhibits in the presence of optimum levels of Mg^{2+}. Unlike phosphatidylinositol kinase, the activity of the enzyme is not increased with detergents (Kai et al., 1966b).

2.3 CATABOLISM OF PHOSPHOLIPIDS IN THE NERVOUS SYSTEM

It was pointed out in the introduction that normal turnover of phospholipid in the fully developed nervous system requires a catabolism of equal magnitude to that of the synthesis to maintain concentration equilibrium. There is a good deal of information available concerning the types of phospholipases present in the nervous system, but it is not always easy to decide on whether individual reports are concerned with the same enzyme. Thus, the pH optimum and substrate specificity of a phospholipase can depend substantially on the way the enzyme is assayed (Dawson, 1973). Furthermore, it is often not clear whether the stimulatory effect certain divalent cations such as Ca^{2+} have on an individual activity is due to an obligatory role of this metal in the enzyme substrate interaction or if its action can be ascribed to an effect on the electrokinetic parameters of the substrate's surface.

At the present time there is little information available on what controls the phospholipases in an *in vivo* situation since many of them have a potential activity for degradation which if uninhibited would rapidly bring about dissolution of the membrane structure. Nor do we have much information concerning the quantitative importance of various possible routes in bringing about hydrolysis of an individual phospholipid in the intact nervous system.

2.3.1 Deacylating Phospholipases

Enzymes that hydrolyze fatty acids from the phospholipid structure (Fig. 2.5) produce initially lysophospholipids that have been detected in low concentrations in the brain. Lysophospholipids such as lysophosphatidylcholine, lysophosphatidylethanolamine, and lysophosphatidylinositol can be reacylated by acyl-CoA transferases in brain (XLIII, XLVI) (Keenan and Hokin, 1962; Webster, 1965; James et al., 1979; Fisher and Rowe, 1980; Corbin and Sun, 1978), thus providing a mechanism for rapidly changing the fatty acid composition of individual phospholipids according to membrane requirements. Both in the central nervous system (Fisher and Rowe, 1980) and the peripheral nervous system (Doherty and Rowe, 1979) the reacylation of lysophosphatidylcholine from acyl-CoA appears to be largely a function of the endoplasmic reticulum. Alternatively, lysosphospholipids can undergo further deacylation (XLVII) resulting in the nonhydrophobic backbone of the original phospholipid. In the intact nervous system glycerophosphoryl derivatives of choline, ethanolamine, and inositol can be detected and presumably these are bro-

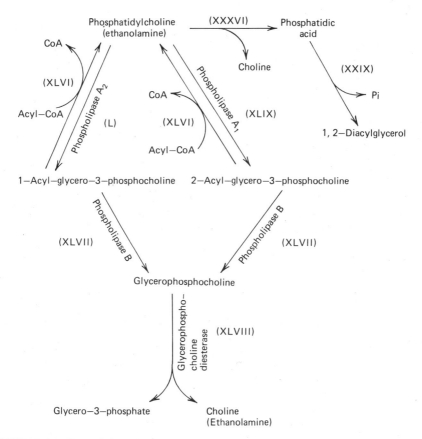

FIGURE 2.5 Degradation of phosphatidylcholine and phosphatidylethanolamine in brain.

ken down into glycerophosphate and the free bases or inositol by phosphodiesterases present (XLVIII). Thus, the individual molecular components would be available for recycling back into the membrane phospholipids during the normal processes of biosynthesis.

Gallai-Hatchard et al. (1962) were perhaps the first to show phospholipase A activity in brain tissue and Eyrich et al. (1976) in squid axon and sciatic nerve. Using extracts of acetone-dried human brain and substrates of phosphatidylcholine, phosphatidylethanolamine, and phosphatidylserine, Gallai-Hatchard et al. (1962) demonstrated the release of the corresponding lysophospholipids on incubation at neutral pH values. Subsequent workers have shown that both phospholipases of the A_1 (XLIX) and A_2 (L) types exist in brain tissue (Webster, 1970). Cooper and Webster (1970, 1972) showed that human and rat brains contained phospholipases

A_1 with pH optima of 4.6 and 4.2, respectively, which were active against phosphatidylcholine, phosphatidylethanolamine, and phosphatidylserine, as well as heat-stable phospholipases A_2 with pH optima of 5.0 and 5.5, respectively. Neither the A_1 nor the A_2 activity required Ca^{2+}, and both were widely distributed in white and gray matter; only the phospholipase A_1 could be detected in peripheral nerve.

The phospholipase A_1 described by these authors is probably the same as Ca^{2+}-independent phospholipase A_1 previously isolated and purified 50-fold from rat and calf brain which had a pH optimum of 4 (Gatt et al., 1966; Gatt, 1968) and an analogous enzyme obtained from human brain which had a pH optimum of 4.2 and a molecular weight of 75,000 as determined by gel filtration (Woelk et al., 1972). The low pH optima registered for all these enzymes suggests they could be of lysosomal origin. The rat brain phospholipase A_1 had limited action on neutral lipids and is therefore unlikely to be a lipase displaying some phospholipase A_1 activity (Gatt, 1968). Subcellular distribution studies by Woelk and Porcellati (1973) suggested, however, that phospholipase A_1 in rat brain was almost exclusively located in the microsomal fraction, while phospholipase A_2 predominated in the mitochondria, confirming previous preliminary results of Bazan (1971). However, the pH optima recorded for these enzymes was 6.8 for A_1 and 8.4 for A_2 (Woelk and Porcellati, 1973). Choline plasmalogen and ethanolamine plasmalogen acted as competitive inhibitors of the breakdown of phosphatidylcholine and phosphatidylethanolamine, respectively, by the phospholipase A_1.

A similar microsomal location for phospholipase A_1 was observed in neuronal cell–enriched fractions of the rabbit cerebral cortex although considerable activity could still be observed in the plasma membrane fraction (Woelk et al., 1979). Previously Woelk et al. (1973) had shown that both phospholipases A_1 and A_2 were highly concentrated in neuronal cell fractions compared with the glial cells isolated from rabbit brain. The phospholipase A_1 in the plasma membrane fraction of both glia and neuronal components seemed to possess higher pH optima ranging between 8.0 and 9.0 (Woelk et al., 1981).

Recently Gray and Strickland (1982a,b) have isolated and purified to homogeneity a phospholipase A_2 with a pH optimum of 7.5 from bovine brain microsomes which has some action on phosphatidylcholine, phosphatidylethanolamine, and phosphatidylserine although phosphatidylinositol was the preferred substrate. The enzyme was stimulated by calcium ions and the molecular weight was in the neighborhood of 18,400 (Gray and Strickland, 1982b). In addition, Hirasawa et al. (1981) have found a phospholipase A_1 in rat brain supernatant and microsomal fractions that attacked phosphatidylinositol at a pH optimum of 8.0 yet did not attack triolein or phosphatidycholine under the same incubation conditions. Clearly, therefore, the precise location of the various membrane-bound phospholipase A enzymes existing in nervous tissue still requires further study.

In 1976, Rooke and Webster extracted and purified a phospholipase A_1 enzyme from acetone-dried human brain that was most active at pH 9.25, had a high molecular weight of approximately 5×10^5, and was stimulated by Ca^{2+}. Phosphatidylethanolamine was the preferred substrate and phosphatidylcholine was hydrolyzed at a much slower rate. Doherty and Rowe (1980) showed that this enzyme was located in the cytoplasm of rat brain and confirmed the stimulation brought about by Ca^{2+}. Recently it has been shown that the function of the Ca^{2+} is not as a metallic coenzyme but rather to reduce the negative surface zeta potential existing on the phosphatidylethanolamine substrate at the high optimum pH used for assay (Dawson et al., 1982). Thus, Mg^{2+}, NaCl at higher concentrations, and even Na EDTA could produce an equivalent stimulation and, with the same enzyme isolated from liver, long-chain quaternary nitrogen cations could also (Dawson, 1982).

There have been many reports of the presence of lysophospholipases in brain tissue, although most of these do not establish unequivocally that this activity is due to a true phospholipase B (XLVII) unable to act on the equivalent diacylated substrates (e.g., Marples and Thompson, 1960; D'Amato et al., 1975). Leibovitz-BenGershon and Gatt (1968) purified an enzyme from rat brain that hydrolyzed both 1-acylglycerophosphocholine and 1-acylglycerophosphoethanolamine, yet was without action on the fully acylated phospholipids. There was no evidence for any cofactor requirements including Ca^{2+} or Mg^{2+} and the molecular weight was low (15–20,000). Most of the activity was contained in the "microsomal" pellet and was difficult to solubilize; only minimal activity was present in the 100,000g supernatant (Leibovitz-BenGershon et al., 1972). Apparently the enzyme utilized molecular solutions of lysophosphatidylcholine and was inhibited by its micellar aggregates (Leibovitz-Ben Gershon and Gatt, 1974).

2.3.2 Degradation of Plasmalogens and Glycerol Ether Phospholipids

The main plasmalogen in brain is ethanolamine containing. It was shown by Ansell and Spanner (1965, 1968) that an enzyme was present in mitochondrial and microsomal particles obtained from rat brain that when incubated with this plasmalogen released a fatty aldehyde and 2-acyl-*sn*-glycerol-3-phosphoethanolamine (LI) (Fig. 2.2). Normally this enzyme, which probably accounts for the main turnover of ethanolamine plasmalogen in brain (Horrocks and Fu, 1978), is assessed by substrate disappearance but it can be determined by coupling the aldehyde released to alcohol dehydrogenase (Freeman and Carey, 1980). The enzyme was inhibited by EDTA and stimulation was observed with Mg^{2+}, but it is by no means certain that this divalent cation is obligatory. Lysoethanolamine plasmalogen was cleaved although at a slower rate. The plasmalogenase was almost exclusively located in white matter so it could be mainly present in glial cells. In mouse brain plasmalogenase activity correlates well with the degree of myelination (Dorman et al., 1978) and is much higher in oligodendroglia than in neuronal perikarya or in astroglia (D'Amato et al., 1975).

The plasmalogenase was extracted in a soluble form from acetone-dried beef brain (D'Amato et al., 1975). This preparation hydrolyzed ethanolamine plasmalogen, while phosphatidylcholine, phosphatidylethanolamine, and choline plasmalogen competitively inhibited substrate breakdown. Conversely, using choline plasmalogen as substrate, competitive inhibition was observed with phosphatidycholine and ethanolamine plasmalogen. This suggests that the same enzyme may be responsible for the hydrolysis of both plasmalogens. Once the lysophospholipid is released from the plasmalogen, it can be rapidly deacylated by any phospholipase B present.

In addition, Woelk et al. (1974) showed that the phospholipase A_2 (L) mentioned in the previous section and present in rat brain mitochondria or extracted from acetone-dried cerebral cortex was capable of deacylating choline plasmalogen and alkyl-acyl-glycerophosphocholine, albeit at a slower rate than phosphatidycholine. Presumably any lysoplasmalogen formed could be further hydrolyzed either by the enzyme degrading the vinyl ether linkage as discussed in the previous two paragraphs or possibly by phospholipase D action (Section 2.3.5). The pteridine-dependent enzyme that brings about the oxidation of the glycerol ether bond of simple lipids seems to be relatively absent from brain tissue (Pfleger et al., 1967). Finally Yavin and Gatt (1972a,b) reported that brain tissue contained a soluble factor that could bring about the cleavage of the vinyl ether linkage of plasmalogens coupled with the reduction of molecular oxygen. The factor is nonenzymic and is probably an iron–ascorbate complex. Its significance, if any, in brain plasmalogen degradation *in vivo* is unknown.

2.3.3 Sphingomyelin Degradation

Two distinct forms of sphingomyelinase that split sphingomyelin into ceramide and phosphocholine (LII) (Fig. 2.3) have been identified in the nervous system. The lysosomal form possesses properties (acid pH optimum, no metal requirement) that distinguishes it from the microsomal form (neutral pH optimum, metal requirement). The lysosomal form has a pH optimum of 5 and prefers sphingomyelins with a D-*erythro*-sphingosine rather than a D-*threo* or L-*erythro* configuration (Barenholtz et al., 1966). It can be prepared by isolating lysosomal-rich fractions from rat brain and solubilizing the enzyme by detergent treatment or freezing and thawing (Gatt and Gottesdiner, 1976). It has been extensively purified from human brain (e.g., Yamaguchi and Suzuki, 1977; Barenholtz et al., 1966) and appears to exist in a number of aggregated forms with the minimum molecular weight so far reported being 67,000. It has been shown that the lysosomal sphingomyelinase is nearly absent from the brain of patients with the infantile form of Niemann-Pick disease (Fredrickson and Sloan, 1972; Gatt et al., 1978), a condition in which sphingomyelin accumulates in the gray matter. On the other hand, in other types of Niemann-Pick diseases (Type C) there appears to be no difference in the properties of sphingomyelinase from pathological and normal tissue (Müller and Harzer, 1980).

The neutral sphingomyelinase of brain shows a pH optimum of 7.4 and has a requirement for Mg^{2+} (Rao and Spence, 1976; Gatt, 1976). It is very enriched (9- to 13-fold) in human gray matter compared with white and is present in the brains of patients with infantile Niemann-Pick disease at a time when the lysosomal activity is virtually absent (Gatt et al., 1978).

The ceramide released by sphingomyelinase can be hydrolyzed by ceramidase (LIII), an enzyme that has been purified 200-fold from young rat brain (Yavin and Gatt, 1969). It would appear that this enzyme can also catalyze the synthesis of ceramide from its individual molecular components. Further degradation of the sphingosine liberated takes place via a preliminary phosphorylation by an ATP-dependent kinase (LIV). The resulting sphingosine-1-phosphate is then split by a pyridoxal phosphate–dependent lyase with the formation of phosphoethanolamine and palmitaldehyde (LV). While the phosphoethanolamine can be used for phosphatidylethanolamine synthesis, the palmitaldehyde is both reduced to alcohol and incorporated into the alk-1-enyl ether chains of plasmalogens or oxidized to fatty acid (Stoffel et al., 1970; Stoffel, 1971).

2.3.4 Phosphoinositide Hydrolysis

The degradation of the phosphoinositides (Fig. 2.4) appears to be somewhat different from the rest of the glycerophospholipids in that the main pathway or potential for catabolism is by phosphodiesterase action. However, as previously mentioned (Section 2.3.1), both phospholipases A_1

and A_2 occur in brain and are capable of breaking down phosphatidylinositol, with some degree of specificity in the case of the A_2 enzyme. It is known that the lysophosphatidylinositol formed can be further deacylated to form glycerophosphoinositol (LVI) (Shum et al., 1979; Hirasawa et al., 1981) and since brain tissue contains the latter phosphodiester, it is reasonable to assume that the deacylation pathway plays some part in the total turnover of the phosphoinositide molecule *in vivo*. It also seems likely that reacylation of the lysophosphatidylinositol produced (XLIII) can complete the deacylation–reacylation cycle for the generation of specific molecular species of phosphatidylinositol (Shum et al., 1979; Gray and Strickland, 1982b).

The cytoplasm of brain tissue contains a very active calcium-requiring phosphatidylinositol phosphodiesterase which cleaves the substrate into 1,2-diacylglycerol and either inositol-1-phosphate (hydrolysis) or inositol-1,2-cyclic phosphate (cyclization) (LVII). Both these water-soluble phosphate esters can be detected in brain tissue quickly frozen to minimize postmortem artefacts so it can be assumed the cyclization reaction is not a test tube artefact. Animal tissues also contain a specific phosphodiesterase that hydrolyzes inositol-1,2-cyclic phosphate liberating inositol-1-phosphate (LVIII), and this enzyme is widely distributed in different areas of the brain and spinal cord. In the rat, brain has the highest activity after kidney (Dawson and Clarke, 1972).

There is some evidence that the phosphatidylinositol phosphodiesterase in nervous tissue cells is responsive to stimulation by agents such as receptor agonists (Michell, 1975) (see Chapter 7). It was originally believed the enzyme had a bimodal distribution in brain with a component being located in the membrane fractions (Friedel et al., 1969; Lapetina and Michell, 1973), but more recent evidence has suggested that it is probably entirely cytoplasmic (Irvine and Dawson, 1978). The pH optimum of the ammonium sulfate–fractionated enzyme in rat brain has been reported as 5.8 (Thompson, 1967; Keough and Thompson, 1970, 1972), but distinct activity with a pH optimum in the alkaline range is also apparent, and this is lost on ammonium sulfate purification (Hirasawa et al, 1981). Recent studies (Hirasawa et al., 1982; Irvine and Dawson 1983) employing chromatofocusing to separate proteins on the basis of their isoelectric points have demonstrated several distinct activity peaks of the enzyme activity assayed at pH 5.5 (Hofmann and Majerus (1982) have also obtained immunological evidence for heterogeneity of the acid pH optimum enzyme) but only a single distinct peak (pI 4.6) assayed at neutral pH values in the presence of 1 mM Ca^{2+}. This latter activity is highly sensitive to other phospholipids mixed with the phosphatidylinositol substrate; in general phospholipids containing a phosphocholine head group, for example, phosphatidylcholine or sphingomyelin are strongly inhibitory and acidic phospholipids, especially phosphatidic acid, produce marked activation (Irvine et al., 1979).

As well as this cytoplasmic Ca^{2+}-requiring phosphatidylinositol phosphodiesterase, brain tissue also possesses a similar enzyme present in the lysosomal fraction that has no requirement for Ca^{2+} (Irvine et al., 1977, 1978). The metabolic products are inositol-1-phosphate and diacylglycerol; no inositol-1,2-cyclic phosphate is formed. The lysosomal enzyme from liver tissue that has been more fully characterized preferentially hydrolyzes phosphatidylinositol, although phosphatidylcholine and phosphatidylethanolamine can be attacked at a much slower rate. The pH optimum is 4.8 and the enzyme can be released from a purified lysosomal fraction by osmotic shocking (Irvine et al., 1977). Such results were confirmed subsequently by Matsuzawa and Hostetler (1980).

Enzymes are present in the brain that can bring about the hydrolysis of phosphatidylinositol-4-phosphate and phosphatidylinositol-4,5-bisphosphate, and disappearance of the latter from brain tissue postmortem can be rapid (Eichberg and Hauser, 1967). These are of two types, a phosphodiesterase that can split off diacylglycerol and the corresponding polyphosphorylated inositol (inositol trisphosphate, inositol bisphosphate) (LIX) and a phosphomonoesterase that can successively dephosphorylate phosphatidylinositol bisphosphate, producing phosphatidylinositol phosphate and eventually phosphatidylinositol (LX) (Thompson and Dawson, 1964a,b; Dawson and Thompson, 1964). It has been shown that the first dephosphorylation is specific for the phosphate in the 5-position of the inositol ring, thus producing a phosphatidylinositol phosphate of the same structure as that on the synthetic pathway (Chang and Ballou, 1967; Prottey et al., 1968). The phosphatidylinositol bisphosphate phosphomonoesterase of rat brain has been purified to homogeneity; it has a low molecular weight, an isoelectric point of 6.8, and no absolute requirement for Ca^{2+} or Mg^{2+}, although these divalent cations stimulated its activity (Nijjar and Hawthorne, 1977). It was predominantly located in the cytoplasm and also hydrolyzed phosphatidylinositol phosphate although at a slower rate. In guinea pig brain Sheltawy et al. (1972) reported that the enzyme was enriched in the plasma membrane fractions and also that KCl stimulated the activity. Such a stimulation by a variety of cations is perhaps due to modification of the high negative zeta potential near the substrate's surface, and in this respect long-chain cations can stimulate the enzymic activity (Dawson and Thompson, 1964).

Brain phosphatidylinositol bisphosphate phosphodiesterase also had no absolute requirement for metallic cations, although these as well as long-chain cations and basic proteins could activate under certain conditions, suggesting a similar effect on the zeta potential (Thompson and Dawson, 1964b). Subcellular fractionation suggested that the enzyme might be located in the plasma membrane, although some was present in the supernatant fraction (Keough and Thompson, 1970). The membrane-bound enzyme in ox brain can be solubilized with 2 M KCl, and when partially purified, it appears to have properties similar to that of the cytoplasmic enzyme; the pH optimum was 6.0 for phosphatidylinositol phosphate as substrate and 7.2–7.8 with phosphatidylinositol bisphosphate (Keough and Thompson, 1972). Both the phosphomonoesterase and phosphodiesterase seem to increase during myelination (Salway et al., 1968; Keough and Thompson, 1970) and on subfractionation of guinea pig brain nerve-ending particles (synaptosomes) the enzymes are found in the cytoplasm (Harwood and Hawthorne, 1969).

2.3.5 Phospholipase D Enzymes

Phospholipase D types of enzyme are known to be widely distributed in the tissues of higher plants, but until recently there was no firm evidence that they occurred in mammalian tissues, although such enzymes had been postulated and sought for. Wykle and Schremmer in 1974 and Gunawan et al. in 1979 described a lysophospholipase D tightly bound to rat brain microsomes which removed the base from the 1-alkyl derivatives of glycerophosphocholine and glycerophosphoethanolamine and also from 1-alkenylglycerophosphoethanolamine (LXI) (Fig. 2.2). The reaction was stimulated by Mg^{2+} but not by Ca^{2+} which, in fact, inhibited the Mg^{2+}-stimulated reaction. The removal of the base appears to be specific for simple alkyl or alkenyl derivatives—the plasmalogens, or the monoacyl and diacyl esters of glycerophospho "bases," are not hydrolyzed (Wykle et al., 1980). Presumably, therefore, this enzyme only operates after the acyl group has been removed from the parent phospholipids by phospholipase A_2.

A more conventional phospholipase D has been demonstrated in a solubilized preparation from a rat brain particulate preparation (Saito and Kanfer, 1975). Phosphatidylcholine was converted into phosphatidic acid and choline (XXXVI) (Fig. 2.5). The pH optimum was around 6 and calcium produced a small stimulation of the activity. Taki and Kanfer (1979) were able to extract the enzyme from rat brain particles under conditions that left most of the base-exchange enzymes behind and subsequently to purify it 240 times. The enzyme seems to be distinct from that of the Ca^{2+}-catalyzed base-exchange activity, which could theoretically have phosphatidic acid as an intermediary. The purified enzyme had a molecular weight of around 200,000, hydrolyzed both phosphatidylcholine and phosphatidylethanolamine, and was stimulated somewhat by Ca^{2+} and Fe^{2+}, but not by Mg^{2+} or Mn^{2+}. It differs from the similar enzyme in higher plants in not having an absolute requirement for Ca^{2+} and in its profound inhibition by agents such as diethyl ether and deoxycholates, which cause activation of the plant enzyme. Like the plant enzyme, it can carry out phosphatidyl transferase reactions to acceptors such as glycerol (Kanfer, 1982). Its precise significance in overall brain phospholipid turnover is entirely unknown.

REFERENCES

Anderson, R.E., Kelleher, P.A., and Maude, M.B., *Biochim. Biophys. Acta*, *620*, 227–235 (1980).

Ansell, G.B., and Chojnacki, T., *Biochem. J.*, *98*, 303–310 (1966).

Ansell, G.B., and Metcalfe, R.F., *J. Neurochem.*, *18*, 647–665 (1971).

Ansell, G.B., and Spanner, S., *Biochem. J.*, *94*, 252–258 (1965).

Ansell, G.B., and Spanner, S., *J. Neurochem.*, *14*, 873–885 (1967).

Ansell, G.B., and Spanner, S., *Biochem. J.*, *108*, 207–209 (1968a).

Ansell, G.B., and Spanner, S., *Biochem. J.*, *110*, 201–206 (1968b).

Ansell, G.B., and Spanner, S.G., *J. Neurochem.*, *22*, 1153–1155 (1974).

Baker, R.R., and Thompson, W., *Biochim. Biophys. Acta*, *270*, 489–503 (1972).

Baker, R.R., and Thompson, W., *J. Biol. Chem.*, *248*, 7060–7065 (1973).

Barenholz, Y., Roitman, A., and Gatt, S., *J. Biol. Chem.*, *241*, 3731–3737 (1966).

Bazán, N.G., *Acta Physiol. Latinoam.*, *21*, 101–106 (1971).

Benjamins, J.A., and Agranoff, B.W., *J. Neurochem.*, *16*, 513–527 (1969).

Binaglia, L., Roberti, R., and Porcellati, G., in S. Gatt, I.. Freysz, and P. Mandel, Eds., *Enzymes of Lipid Metabolism*, Plenum Press, New York, 1978, pp. 353–366.

Bishop, H.H. and Strickland, K.P., *Lipids*, *15*, 285–291 (1980).

Blusztajn, J.K. and Wurtman, R.J., *Nature, Lond.*, *290*, 417–418 (1981).

Bradbury, K., in L.A. Horrocks, G.B. Ansell, and G. Porcellati, Eds., *Phospholipids in the Nervous System*, Vol 1, *Metabolism*, Raven Press, New York, 1982, p. 328.

Brady, R.O., Bradley, R.M., Young, O.M., and Kaller, H., *J. Biol. Chem.*, *240*, PC3693–3694 (1965).

Braun, P.E., Morell, P., and Radin, N.S., *J. Biol. Chem.*, *245*, 335–341 (1970).

Buchanan, A.G., and Kanfer, J.N., *J. Neurochem.*, *35*, 814–822 (1980a).

Buchanan, A.G., and Kanfer, J.N., *J. Neurochem.*, *34*, 720–725 (1980b).

Burt, A.M. *J. Neurochem.*, *28*, 961–966 (1977).

Carter, J.R., and Kennedy, E.P., *J. Lipid Res.*, *7*, 678–683 (1966).

Chang, M., and Ballou, C.E., *Biochem. Biophys. Res. Commun.*, *26*, 199–205 (1967).

Chang, Y.Y., and Kennedy, E.P., *J. Lipid Res.*, *8*, 456–462 (1967).

Choi, R.L., Freeman, J.J., and Jenden, D.J., *J. Neurochem.*, *24*, 735–741 (1975).

Chojnacki, T., Korzybski, T., and Ansell, G.B., *Biochem. J.*, *90*, 18–19P (1964).

Colodzin, M., and Kennedy, E.P., *J. Biol. Chem.*, *240*, 3771–3780 (1965).

Cooper, M.F., and Webster, G.R., *J. Neurochem.*, *17*, 1543–1554 (1970).

Cooper, M.F., and Webster, G.R., *J. Neurochem.*, *19*, 333–340 (1972).

Corbin, D.R., and Sun, G.Y., *J. Neurochem.*, *30*, 77–82 (1978).

Crews, F.T., Hirata, F., and Axelrod, J., *J. Neurochem.*, *34*, 1491–1498 (1980).

D'Amato, R.A., Horrocks, L.A., and Richardson, K.E., *J. Neurochem.*, *24*, 1251–1255 (1975).

Dawson, R.M.C., G.B. Ansell, R.M.C. Dawson, and J.N. Hawthorne, Eds., in *Form and Function of Phospholipids*, Elsevier, Amsterdam, 1973, pp. 97–116.

Dawson, R.M.C., *J. Amer. Oil Chem. Soc.*, *59*, 401–406 (1982).

Dawson, R.M.C., and Clarke, N., *Biochem. J.*, *127*, 113–118 (1972).

Dawson, R.M.C., Irvine, R.F., Hemington, N., and Hirasawa, K., *Neurochem. Res. 7*, 1149–1161 (1982).

Dawson, R.M.C., and Thompson, W., *Biochem. J.*, *91*, 244–250 (1964).

Doherty, F.J., and Rowe, C.E., *J. Neurochem.*, *33*, 819–822 (1979).

Doherty, F.J., and Rowe, C.E., *Brain Res.*, *197*, 113–122 (1980).

Dorman, R.V., Freysz, L., Mandel, P., and Horrocks, L.A., *J. Neurochem.*, *30*, 157–159 (1978).

Eichberg, J., and Hauser, G., *Biochim. Biophys. Acta*, *144*, 415–422 (1967).

Eichberg, J., Whittaker, V.P., and Dawson, R.M.C., *Biochem. J.*, *92*, 91–100 (1964).

El-Bassiouni, E.A., Piantadosi, C., and Snyder, F., *Biochim. Biophys. Acta*, *388*, 5–11 (1975).

Eyrich, T.L., Barrett, D., and Rock, P.A., *J. Neurochem.*, *26*, 1079–1085 (1976).

Feldman, D.A., Dietrich, J.W., and Weinhold, P.A., *Biochim. Biophys. Acta*, *620*, 603–611 (1980).

Fisher, S.K., and Rowe, C.E., *Biochim. Biophys. Acta*, *618*, 231–241 (1980).

Fredrickson, D.S., and Sloan, H.R., in J.B. Stanbury, D.S. Wyngaarden, and D.S. Fredrickson, Eds., *The Metabolic Basis of Inherited Disease*, 3rd ed. McGraw Hill, New York, 1972, pp. 783–807.

Freeman, N.M., and Carey, E.M., *Biochem. Soc. Trans.*, *8*, 612–613 (1980).

Friedel, R.O., Brown, J.D., and Durell, J., *J. Neurochem.*, *16*, 371–378 (1969).

Fujino, Y., Nakano, Mo., Negishi, T., and Ito, S., *J. Biol. Chem.*, *243*, 4650–4651 (1968a).

Fujino, Y., Negishi, T., and Ito, S., *Biochem. J.*, *109*, 310–311 (1968b).

Gallai-Hatchard, J., Magee, W.L., Thompson, R.H.S., and Webster, G.R., *J. Neurochem.*, *9*, 545–554 (1962).

Gatt, S., *Biochim. Biophys. Acta*, *159*, 304–316 (1968).

Gatt, S., *Biochem. Biophys. Res. Commun.*, *68*, 235–241 (1976).

Gatt, S., Barenholz, Y., and Roitman, A., *Biochem. Biophys. Res. Commun.*, *24*, 169–172 (1966).

Gatt, S., Dinur, T., and Kopolovic, J., *J. Neurochem.*, *31*, 547–550 (1978).

Gatt, S., and Gottesdiner, T., *J. Neurochem.*, *26*, 421–422 (1976).

Goracci, G., Blomstrand, C., Arienti, G., Hamberger, A., and Porcellati, G., *J. Neurochem.*, *20*, 1167–1180 (1973).

Gould, R.M., and Dawson, R.M.C., *J. Cell Biol.*, *68*, 480–496 (1976).

Gray, N.C.C., and Strickland, K.P., *Lipids*, *17*, 91–96 (1982a).

Gray, N.C.C., and Strickland, K.P., *Can. J. Biochem.*, *60*, 108–117 (1982b).

Gunawan, J., Vierbucken, M., and Debuch, H., *Hoppe-Seyler's Z. Physiol. Chem.*, *360*, 971–978 (1979).

Hajra, A.K., *Biochem. Biophys. Res. Commun.*, *39*, 1037–1044 (1970).

Hajra, A.K., and Agranoff, B.W., *J. Biol. Chem.*, *243*, 1617–1622 (1968).

Hajra, A.K., and Burke, C., *J. Neurochem.*, *31*, 125–134 (1978).

Harwood, J.L., and Hawthorne, J.N., *Biochim. Biophys. Acta*, *171*, 75–88 (1969).

Hauser, G., and Eichberg, J., *J. Biol. Chem.*, *250*, 105–112 (1975).

Helmkamp, G.M., *Biochim. Biophys. Acta*, *595*, 222–234 (1980).

Hirasawa, K., Irvine, R.F., and Dawson, R.M.C., *Eur. J. Biochem.*, *120*, 53–58 (1981).

Hirasawa, K., Irvine, R.F., and Dawson, R.M.C., *Biochem. J.*, *205*, 437–442 (1982).

Hofmann, S.L., and Majerus, P.W., *J. Biol. Chem.*, *257*, 6461–6469 (1982).

Hokin, M.R., and Hokin, L.E., *J. Biol. Chem.*, *234*, 1381–1386 (1959).

Holub, B.J., *Biochim. Biophys. Acta*, *369*, 111–122 (1974).

Holub, B.J., *Lipids*, *10*, 483–490 (1975).

Holub, B.J., *Lipids*, *11*, 1–5 (1976).

Horrocks, L.A., and Fu, S.C., *Adv. Exp. Med. Biol.*, *101*, 397–406 (1978).

Hostetler, K.Y., van den Bosch, H., and van Deenen, L.L.M., *Biochim. Biophys. Acta*, *260*, 507–513 (1972).

Irvine, R.F., and Dawson, R.M.C., *J. Neurochem.*, *31*, 1427–1434 (1978).

Irvine, R.F., and Dawson, R.M.C., *Biochem. J.*, *215*, 431–432 (1983).

Irvine, R.F., Dawson, R.M.C., and Freinkel, N., *Contemporary Metabolism*, *2*, 301–342 (1982).

Irvine, R.F., Hemington, N., and Dawson, R.M.C., *Biochem. J.*, *164*, 277–280 (1977).

Irvine, R.F., Hemington, N., and Dawson, R.M.C., *Biochem. J.*, *176*, 475–484 (1978).

Irvine, R.F., Hemington, N., and Dawson, R.M.C., *Eur. J. Biochem.*, *99*, 525–530 (1979).

James, O.A., MacDonald, G., and Thompson, W., *J. Neurochem.*, *33*, 1061–1066 (1979).

Kai, M., Salway, J.G., and Hawthorne, J.N., *Biochem. J.*, *106*, 791–801 (1968).

Kai, M., White, G.L., and Hawthorne, J.N., *Biochem. J.*, *101*, 328–337 (1966a).

Kai, M., Salway, J.G., Michell, R.J., and Hawthorne, J.N., *Biochem. Biophys. Res. Commun.*, *22*, 370–375 (1966b).

Kanfer, J.N., *J. Lipid Res.*, *13*, 468–476 (1972)

Kanfer, J.N., in L.A. Horrocks, G.B. Ansell, and G. Porcellati, Eds., *Phospholipids in the Nervous System*, Vol. 1, Raven Press, 1982, pp. 13–20.

Kanfer, J.N., and Bates, S., *Lipids*, *5*, 718–720 (1970).

Keenan, R.W., and Hokin, L.E., *Biochim. Biophys. Acta*, *60*, 428–430 (1962).

Keough, K.M.W., and Thompson, W., *J. Neurochem.*, *17*, 1–11 (1970).

Keough, K.M.W., and Thompson, W., *Biochim. Biophys. Acta*, *270*, 324–336 (1972).

Kiyasu, J.Y., Pieringer, R.A., Paulus, H., and Kennedy, E.P., *J. Biol. Chem.*, *238*, 2293–2298 (1963).

Kopaczyk, K.C., and Radin, N.S., *J. Lipid Res.*, *6*, 140–145 (1965).

LaBelle, E.F., and Hajra, A.K., *J. Biol. Chem.*, *247*, 5825–5834 (1972).

Lapetina, E.G., and Hawthorne, J.N., *Biochem. J.*, *122*, 171–179 (1971).

Lapetina, E.G., and Michell, R.H., *Biochem. J.*, *131*, 433–442 (1973).

Leibovitz-BenGershon, Z., and Gatt, S., *Biochim. Biophys. Acta*, *164*, 439–441 (1968).

Leibovitz-BenGershon, Z., and Gatt, S., *J. Biol. Chem.*, *249*, 1525–1529 (1974).

Leibovitz-BenGershon, Z., Kobiler, I., and Gatt, S., *J. Biol. Chem.*, *247*, 6840–6847 (1972).

McCaman, R.E., *J. Biol. Chem.*, *237*, 672–676 (1962).

McCaman, R.E., and Cook, K., *J. Biol. Chem.*, *241*, 3390–3394 (1966).

McCaman, R.E., Smith, M., and Cook, K., *J. Biol. Chem.*, *240*, 3513–3517 (1965).

McMurray, W.C., and Jarvis, E.C., *Can. J. Biochem.*, *58*, 771–776 (1980).

Marples, E.A., and Thompson, R.H.S., *Biochem. J.*, *74*, 123–127 (1960).

Matsuzawa, Y., and Hostetler, K.Y., *J. Biol. Chem.*, *255*, 646–652 (1980).

Michell, R.H., *Biochim. Biophys. Acta*, *415*, 81–147 (1975).

Miller, E.K., and Dawson, R.M.C., *Biochem. J.*, *126*, 823–835 (1972a).

Miller, E.K., and Dawson, R.M.C., *Biochem. J.*, *126*, 805–821 (1972b).

Miura, T., and Kanfer, J., *Arch. Biochem. Biophys.*, *175*, 654–660 (1976).

Morell, P., and Radin, N.S., *J. Biol. Chem.*, *245*, 342–350 (1970).

Müller, H., and Harzer, K., *J. Neurochem.*, *34*, 446–448 (1980).

Nijjar, M.S., and Hawthorne, J.N., *Biochim. Biophys. Acta*, *480*, 390–402 (1977).

Ong, D.E., and Brady, R.N., *J. Biol. Chem.*, *248*, 3884–3888 (1973).

Paltauf, F., *FEBS Lett.*, *20*, 79–82 (1972).

Petzold, G.L., and Agranoff, B.W., *J. Biol. Chem.*, *242*, 1187–1191 (1967).

Pfleger, R.C., Piantadosi, C., and Snyder, F., *Biochim. Biophys. Acta*, *144*, 633–648 (1967).

Pieringer, R.A., and Hokin, L.E., *J. Biol. Chem.*, *237*, 653–660 (1962a).

Pieringer, R.A., and Hokin, L.E., *J. Biol. Chem.*, *237*, 659–663 (1962b).

Pollock, R.J., Hajra, A.K., and Agranoff, B.W., *Biochim. Biophys. Acta*, *380*, 421–435 (1975).

Porcellati, G., and Arienti, G., *Brain Res.*, *19*, 451–464 (1970).

Porcellati, G., Arienti, G., Pirotta, M., and Giorgini, D., *J. Neurochem.*, *18*, 1395–1417 (1971).

Porcellati, G., Biasion, M.G., and Arienti, G., *Lipids*, *5*, 725–733 (1970a).

Porcellati, G., Biasion, M.G., and Pirotta, M., *Lipids*, *5*, 734–742 (1970b).

Portman, O.W., Illingworth, D.R., and Alexander, M., *J. Neurochem.*, *20*, 1659–1667 (1973).

Possmayer, F., Balakrishnan, G., and Strickland, K.P., *Biochim. Biophys. Acta*, *164*, 79–87 (1968).

Possmayer, F., Meiners, B., and Mudd, J.B., *Biochem. J.*, *132*, 381–394 (1973).

Prottey, C., Salway, J.G., and Hawthorne, J.N., *Biochim. Biophys. Acta*, *164*, 238–251 (1968).

Radominska-Pyrek, A., and Horrocks, L.A., *J. Lipid Res.*, *13*, 580–587 (1972).

Radominska-Pyrek, A., Strosznajder, J., Dabrowiecki, Z., Goracci, G., Chojnacki, T., and Horrocks, L.A., *J. Lipid Res.*, *18*, 53–58 (1977).

Rao, B.G., and Spence, M.W., *J. Lipid Res.*, *17*, 506–515 (1976).

Rao. R.H., and Strickland, K.P., *Biochim. Biophys. Acta*, *348*, 306–314 (1974).

Rittenhouse, H.G., Seguin, E.B., Fisher, S.K., and Agranoff, B.W., *J. Neurochem.* *36*, 991–999 (1981).

Rooke, J.A., and Webster, G.R., *J. Neurochem.*, *27*, 613–620 (1976).

Saito, M., and Kanfer, J., *Arch. Biochem. Biophys.*, *169*, 318–323 (1975).

Salway, J.G., Harwood, J.L., Kai, M., White, G.L., and Hawthorne, J.N., *J. Neurochem.*, *15*, 221–226 (1968).

Sánchez de Jiménez, E., and Cleland, W.W., *Biochem. Biophys. Acta*, *176*, 685–691 (1969).

Saunders, R.M., and Ballou, C.E., *Biochemistry*, *5*, 352–358 (1966).

Schlossman, D.M., and Bell, R.M., *J. Biol. Chem.*, *251*, 5738–5744 (1976).

Sheltawy, A., Brammer, M., and Borrill, D., *Biochem. J.*, *128*, 579–586 (1972).

Shum, T.Y.P., Gray, N.C.C., and Strickland, K.P., *Can. J. Biochem.*, *57*, 1359–1367 (1979).

Spanner, S., and Ansell, G.B., *Biochem. J.*, *178*, 753–760 (1979).

Sribney, M., *Arch. Biochem. Biophys.*, *126*, 954–955 (1968).

Sribney, M., and Kennedy, E.P., *J. Biol. Chem.*, *233*, 1315–1322 (1958).

Stanacev. N.Z., Davidson, J.B., Stuhne-Sekalec, L., and Domazet, Z., *Biochim. Biophys. Res. Commun.*, *47*, 1021–1027 (1972).

Stoffel, W., *Am. Rev. Biochem.*, *40*, 57–82 (1971).

Stoffel, W., and Assman, G., *Hoppe-Seyler's Z. Physiol. Chem.*, *353*, 65–74 (1972).

Stoffel, W., and Bister, K., *Hoppe-Seyler's Z. Physiol. Chem.*, *355*, 911–923 (1974).

Stoffel, W., and LeKim, D., Hoppe-Seyler's Z. Physiol. Chem., *352*, 501–511. (1971).

Stoffel, W., LeKim, D., and Heyn, G., *Hoppe-Seyler's Z. Physiol. Chem.*, *351*, 875–883 (1970).

Svennerholm, L., *Compr. Biochem.*, *18*, 201–227 (1970).

Taki, T., and Kanfer, J.N., *Biochim. Biophys. Acta*, *528*, 309–317 (1978).

Taki, T., and Kanfer, J.N., *J. Biol. Chem.*, *254*, 9761–9765 (1979).

Tamai, Y., and Lands, W.E.M., *J. Biochem.*, *76*, 847–860 (1974).

Ter-Schegget, J., van den Bosch, H., van Baak, M.A., Hostetler, K.Y., and Borst, P., *Biochim. Biophys. Acta.*, *239*, 234–242 (1971).

Thompson, W., *Can. J. Biochem.*, *45*, 853–861 (1967).

Thompson, W., and Dawson, R.M.C., *Biochem. J.*, *91*, 233–236 (1964a).

Thompson, W., and Dawson, R.M.C., *Biochem. J.*, *91*, 237–243 (1964b).

Thompson, W., and MacDonald, G., *Eur. J. Biochem.*, *65*, 107–111 (1976).

Toews, A.D., Horrocks, L.A., and King, J.S., *J. Neurochem.*, *27*, 25–31 (1976).

Ullman, M.D., and Radin, N.S., *J. Biol. Chem.*, *249*, 1506–1512 (1974).

Webster, G.R., *Biochim. Biophys. Acta*, *98*, 512–519 (1965).

Webster, G.R., *Biochem. J.*, *117*, 10–11P (1970).

Weinhold, P.A., and Rethy, V.B., *Biochemistry*, *13*, 5135–5141 (1974).

Woelk, H., Fürniss, H., and Debuch, H., *Hoppe-Seyler's Z. Physiol. Chem.*, *353*, 1111–1119 (1972).

Woelk, H., Goracci, G., Gaiti, A., and Porcellati, G., *Hoppe-Seyler's Z. Physiol. Chem.*, *354*, 729–736 (1973).

Woelk, H., Goracci, G., and Porcellati, G., *Hoppe-Seyler's Z. Physiol. Chem.*, *355*, 75–81 (1974).

Woelk, H., and Porcellati, G., *Hoppe-Seyler's Z. Physiol. Chem.*, *354*, 90–100 (1973).

Woelk, H., Porcellati, G., and Gaiti, A., *Neurochem. Res.*, *4*, 535–543 (1979).

Woelk, H., Rubly, N., Arienti, G., Gaiti, A., and Porcellati, G., *J. Neurochem.*, *36*, 875–880 (1981).

Wu, P., and Ledeen, R.W., *J. Neurochem.*, *35*, 659–666 (1980).

Wykle, R.L., Kraemer, W.F., and Schremmer, J.M., *Biochim. Biophys. Acta*, *619*, 58–67 (1980).

Wykle, R.L., and Schremmer, J.M., *J. Biol. Chem.*, *249*, 1742–1746 (1974).

Wykle, R.L., and Schremmer-Lockmiller, J.M., *Biochim. Biophys. Acta*, *380*, 291–298 (1975).

Yamaguchi, S., and Suzuki, K., *J. Biol. Chem.*, *252*, 3805–3813 (1977).

Yamanaka, T., Hanada, E., and Suzuki, K., *J. Biol. Chem.*, *256*, 3884–3889 (1981).

Yavin, E., and Gatt, S., *Biochemistry*, *8*, 1692–1698 (1969).

Yavin, E., and Gatt, S., *Eur. J. Biochem.*, *25*, 431–436 (1972a).

Yavin, E., and Gatt, S., *Biochemistry*, *25*, 437–446 (1972b).

Yavin, E., and Zeigler, B.P., *J. Biol. Chem.*, *252*, 260–267 (1977).

Zahler, W.L., and Cleland, W.W., *Biochim. Biophys. Acta*, *176*, 699–703 (1969).

=three

PHOSPHOLIPID COMPOSITION AND METABOLISM IN THE DEVELOPING AND AGING NERVOUS SYSTEM

GRACE Y. SUN
LAURIE L. FOUDIN

Sinclair Comparative Medicine Research Farm and Biochemistry Department
University of Missouri
Columbia, Missouri

CONTENTS

3.1   INTRODUCTION   81

3.2   PHOSPHOLIPID COMPOSITION OF BRAIN   82

      3.2.1   Whole Brain, 82
      3.2.2   Brain Regions, 85
      3.2.3   Isolated Cells and Brain Subcellular Fractions, 89

3.3   ACYL GROUP COMPOSITION OF PHOSPHOLIPIDS IN
      BRAIN   93

      3.3.1   Acyl Groups of Total Phospholipids, 93
      3.3.2   Acyl Group Profiles of Individual Phospholipids, 94

3.4   COMPOSITION OF PHOSPHOLIPIDS AND THEIR ACYL
      GROUP PROFILES IN SPINAL CORD   104

3.5   COMPOSITION OF PHOSPHOLIPIDS AND THEIR ACYL
      GROUPS IN PERIPHERAL NERVE   106

3.6   DIETARY EFFECTS ON BRAIN PHOSPHOLIPIDS   107

      3.6.1   Essential Fatty Acid (EFA) Deficiency, 107
      3.6.2   Effects of Perinatal Undernutrition and Protein
               Malnutrition, 112
      3.6.3   Effects of Other Dietary Abnormalities, 114

3.7   PHOSPHOLIPID METABOLISM IN BRAIN   115

      3.7.1   Enzymes for Phospholipid Biosynthesis, 115
      3.7.2   Turnover of Brain Membrane Phospholipids during
               Development, 117
      3.7.3   Incorporation of Fatty Acids into Brain
               Phosphoglycerides, 118
      3.7.4   Incorporation of *Trans*-unsaturated Fatty Acids into
               Brain Phosphoglycerides, 123
      3.7.5   Release of Free Fatty Acids from Membrane
               Phospholipids, 124

3.8   CONCLUSIONS   125

3.9   SUMMARY   128

      REFERENCES   129

3.1 INTRODUCTION

There is little doubt that since phospholipids form an integral part of the lipid bilayer of membranes, they also play an important role in regulating cell membrane functions. Numerous studies have indicated that some of the membrane phospholipids undergo active metabolic turnover, and the lipid intermediates which are generated from metabolism of the phospholipids may, in fact, exert great influence on membrane properties and functions (Sun et al., 1983). In mammalian brain phospholipids comprise nearly half of the total dry weight. Although there is no large difference in the types of phospholipids present in different brain regions, obvious distinctions in the phospholipids and acyl group profiles are found among different subcellular membranes (Sun and Horrocks, 1970).

Frequently the phospholipids and their acyl group profiles give good indications of the functional activity of the membranes. These cellular membranes undergo compositional and metabolic changes during development and aging. Davison and Dobbing (1968) showed that the time schedule for development of brain membrane components varies widely among individual animal species. Frequently these changes reflect the structural organization of the nervous system during growth and development. Synaptogenesis and myelination, two separate processes that occur almost concurrently, are reflected by concomitant changes in lipid composition and acyl group profiles. In the past various aspects of the biochemical development of the nervous system have been studied with animal species such as rat, mouse, and rabbit. Investigations on humans have been limited in scope, mainly due to the difficulty of obtaining suitable tissues for study. Whereas there are voluminous amounts of information on lipid changes in brain during development, studies on brain lipid changes during aging are less numerous. Frequently a direct comparison of data from different laboratories is difficult because of major variations in isolation procedures and lack of proper controls for monitoring purity of subcellular preparations, as well as differences in analytical methods and animal species used for study. In this chapter we review the compositional and metabolic changes in phospholipid and acyl groups of membranes from nervous tissue of mammals, including man, with respect to development and aging. It is important to record these changes so that abnormal events occurring during brain maturation or aging may be readily revealed. Several reviews on the subject have been published (Rouser and Yamamoto, 1969; Rouser et al., 1971, 1972; Ramsey and Nicholas, 1972; Horrocks et al., 1975, 1982).

3.2 PHOSPHOLIPID COMPOSITION OF BRAIN

3.2.1 Whole Brain

The study of whole-brain composition during development and aging reveals the overall changes occurring in the brain; however, chemical analyses of whole brain normally do not take into consideration the complexity of the system or differences in the timing of maturation in different regions (Matthieu et al., 1973). It is known that in all vertebrate species examined, the concentration of each lipid class in brain and their fatty acid profiles change continuously from fetal life to old age (Rouser et al., 1972).

3.2.1.1 Human

In human fetus phospholipids vary from 13 to 17% of the dry weight of the brain but increase to about 50% from the third fetal month to term (Svennerholm, 1964). Among the individual phospholipids, phosphatidylcholine (PC) comprises about half of the total phospholipids of the fetal brain. Sphingomyelin, which is largely present in the myelin, is found in very small amounts (less than 3%) during the fetal stage and at birth (Brante, 1949; Balakrishnan et al., 1961; Svennerholm, 1964). Plasmalogens, another phospholipid class highly enriched in myelin, are present only in trace amounts during fetal life (Clausen et al., 1965). Rouser and Yamamoto (1968, 1969) studied the phospholipids of male human brain ranging in age from birth to 98 years. The phospholipid composition changes continuously throughout aging, and the change follows a curvilinear regression line. Most of the phospholipids increase up to age 30 and then start to decline. However, phosphatidylserine (PS) remains stable from 10 to 33 years while phosphatidylinositol (PI) starts to decline from 20 to 40 years and then increases again. Changes in phosphatidic acid (PA) are very small with no decline, and diphosphatidylglycerol (DPG) reaches a high level at 2 years. In general, the greatest increase in phospholipids occurs during the first year of life, 5–14 times greater than any other year. Using the equations of Rouser and Yamamoto (1968, 1969), Horrocks et al. (1982) calculated the lipid content of human whole brain. When expressed as mmol/kg fresh weight, the concentration of total lipid phosphorus at age 40 is about 70, while PC is 21; ethanolamine plasmalogen (PEpl), 15; phosphatidylethanolamine (PE), 9.2; PS, 11.9; and sphingomyelin, 10.

3.2.1.2 Rodents

Total phospholipid in rat brain increases markedly from birth up to 50 days, with a twofold increase by about 10 days. After this period the level

TABLE 3.1 Phospholipid Composition of Developing Rat Brain

Phospholipid	Concentration (μmol/g wet wt.)				
	3[a]	12[a]	24[a]	42[a]	180[a]
PC	14.7	20.4	24.8	25.0	25.0
diacyl-PE	5.3	8.0	9.4	10.9	10.7
PEpl	2.2	4.7	11.3	13.5	13.0
PI	1.2	1.6	2.0	2.2	2.2
PS	2.9	4.5	7.0	8.3	8.5
PA	0.1	0.3	0.7	1.0	1.3
Sphingomyelin	0.2	1.0	3.2	3.6	3.7

Source: Wells and Dittmer (1967).

[a] Age (days).

starts to plateau (Erickson and Lands, 1959; Spence and Wolf, 1967; Cuzner and Davison, 1968). The appearance and rate of deposition of rat brain lipids were correlated to morphological changes by Wells and Dittmer (1967), who examined the concentration of 24 lipid classes, including 17 types of phospholipids, in rats ranging from 3 to 330 days of age (Table 3.1). The study revealed that phospholipids associated primarily with myelination, such as sphingomyelin, phosphatidylinositol-4,5-bisphosphate (PIP$_2$), and PA, are present at concentrations of less than 10% of that of adult brain up to the onset of myelination (birth to 10 days) but then increase rapidly (two- to fourfold) throughout the period of active myelination (10th to 20th day). On the other hand, PEpl, choline plasmalogen (PCpl), DPG, and PS comprise a group of lipids which vary from 17 to 34% of the adult level shortly after birth and show marked elevations in concentration prior to and during myelination. Therefore, the latter group of lipids may be associated with changes in nonmyelin membrane structures during early development as well as during the period of myelination. PC, PE, and PI are present in concentrations of 49–60% of adult brain prior to myelination and rise only moderately throughout the period of development. These lipids are thought to be only minimally involved in the developmental process.

Recently the polyphosphoinositides in developing rat brain were studied by Uma and Ramakrishnan (1983). The concentration of PIP$_2$ rises from 100 nmol/g wet wt. at birth to 500 nmol/g at 63 days with a peak increase between 21 and 34 days. In the case of PIP the newborn level is 84 nmol/g, which increases to a peak of 234 nmol/g at 34 days. A period of rapid increase occurs between 14 and 21 days. A similar developmental pattern for polyphosphoinositides was previously reported by Eichberg and Hauser (1967). They suggested that the polyphosphoinositides present in unmyelinated newborn rat brain come from membranes that later give rise to myelin, as well as from other neuronal cells.

When the phospholipids are considered as a percentage of the total lipid, there is a fall from 74 to 56% during brain maturation (Norton and Poduslo, 1973) after a small increase from birth to 10 days (Sperry, 1955). Relative to the total lipid, PE and PS remain practically constant during development at about 25 and 6%, respectively, whereas PC decreases from 30 to 18% (Norton and Poduslo, 1973; Galli and Cecconi, 1967). Sphingomyelin increases from less than 1% at 8 days to a high of 3–4% at 37 days, consistent with the results of Wells and Dittmer (1967) and others (Ansell and Spanner, 1961; Marshall et al., 1966). Plasmalogens (primarily PE) represent about 8–10% of total phospholipid at birth and increase to 17–25% (the adult level) at 50 days (Erikson and Lands, 1959; Korey and Orchen, 1959).

Little is known regarding the phospholipid changes in mouse brain during development. Total phospholipids are higher in mouse than in rat brain at comparable ages (Folch-Pi, 1955). The rate of phospholipid deposition in mouse brain is highest between the 8th and 14th days but drops rapidly after 20 days (Matthieu et al., 1973). Nevertheless, the phospholipid concentration rises steadily (about 10%) from 3 to 8 months of age and then undergoes no further change upon reaching old age (Sun and Samorajski, 1972).

3.2.1.3 Rabbit

In rabbit whole brain the percentage of phospholipids relative to total lipids remains nearly constant throughout development to maturity, but individual phospholipids show different rates of deposition (Odutuga et al., 1973). Therefore, the percentage distribution of different lipid classes may vary according to different stages of development. In general, the maximum rate of lipid accumulation occurs between 3 and 11 days. Expressed as percentage of total lipid, PC decreases from 25 to 8.7%, PE remains constant at about 17.5%, and sphingomyelin increases twofold (Davison and Wajda, 1959; Dalal and Einstein, 1969; Odutuga et al., 1973). These results are comparable to the changes reported for rat whole brain; however, unlike rats, the PS in rabbit brain decreases with age (Dalal and Einstein, 1969).

3.2.2   Brain Regions

3.2.2.1   Human

Different regions of the human brain have been analyzed for their phospholipid content during development and aging. These regions include the cerebrum, cerebellum, and brain stem. The concentration of total lipid phosphorus was found to be highest in brain stem and lowest in cerebellum (Vanier et al., 1971; Yusuf and Dickerson, 1977; Martinez, 1982). These features occur throughout fetal development and at least up to 2 years of age.

The concentration of total phospholipids in cerebral white matter is generally higher than in cortex from early fetal stages to advanced age (Brante, 1949; Cumings et al., 1958; Fillerup and Mead, 1967; Svennerholm, 1968; Vanier et al., 1971; Svennerholm and Vanier, 1972). However, two reports have indicated that the concentrations of lipid P are the same at birth in the two tissues (Svennerholm, 1968; Vanier et al., 1971). In both cerebral cortex and white matter maximum levels of phospholipids are attained at about 2 years of age (Brante, 1949; Vanier et al., 1971; Svennerholm and Vanier, 1972), although the maximum rates of deposition for individual phospholipids are different and occur at different ages during the developmental period. A small decrease in the phospholipids of white matter may occur in individuals over 70 years of age (Brante, 1949).

Yusuf and Dickerson (1977) analyzed brains from 25 fetuses and 9 infants at 13 weeks gestation to 26 months. They found that with the exception of a few quantitative differences, the pattern of change of individual phospholipids in cerebrum, cerebellum, and brain stem during fetal development is remarkably similar. In general, the proportion of PC (about 60% of total phospholipid) declines, while the proportions of PE and sphingomyelin increase (from 20 to 30% and from 3 to 10%, respectively), and PS + PI remains constant at 15%. Most of the changes in the forebrain occur between the 13th and 25th fetal week, while in cerebellum the changes occur between the 30th week and term, and in brain stem the changes occur over the entire period of fetal development. These changes are similar to earlier reports on whole brain (Svennerholm, 1964; Clausen et al., 1965). During postnatal development the phospholipid patterns are similar in cerebrum and cerebellum but different in brain stem (Yusuf and Dickerson, 1977). In cerebrum and cerebellum the PC continues to decrease until the 9th month, while PE increases concomitantly, so that the two phospholipid classes are present in nearly equal proportions. On the other hand, PC in brain stem continues to decrease up to about 26 months, while PE increases to the 10th month to become the predominant phospholipid, at least through 2 years of age. Sphingomyelin also continues to increase up to the 9th month in forebrain and cerebellum, but in brain stem this increase is observed through the 26th month. PS + PI remain constant in all three regions.

Martinez and Ballabriga (1978) reported that changes in plasmalogens of cerebrum and cerebellum are similar during fetal development, although the amounts in cerebellum are slightly higher than that in cerebrum. The concentrations double between 20 and 44 weeks of gestation. After birth the plasmalogen level in cerebrum continues to increase until 2 years of age, but in cerebellum it starts to level off between the 4th and 6th postnatal months. The concentrations of plasmalogen range from 3 µmol/g fresh wt. to about 11 µmol/g for the developmental period studied. In a later study Martinez (1982) included data for brain stem, as well as cerebrum and cerebellum. The developmental changes in plasmalogens of cerebrum and cerebellum paralleled those of the earlier study. A similar pattern of increase during fetal and postnatal development occurs in brain stem, but the amount levels off after 14 months. The concentration in brain stem ranges from 4 to 23 µmol/g.

Comparisons of gray and white matter of the cerebrum (Cumings et al., 1958; Balakrishnan et al., 1961; O'Brien and Sampson, 1965a; Svennerholm, 1968; Svennerholm and Vanier, 1972) indicate a pattern of change similar to those reported by Yusuf and Dickerson (1977) for whole cerebrum. The phospholipid composition of fetal cerebrum is PC, 50%; PE, nearly 30%; PS, 13%; PI, 5%; and sphingomyelin, 3% (Svennerholm, 1968; Svennerholm and Vanier, 1972). Table 3.2 compares the distribution of phospholipids in cerebral cortex and white matter. During maturation of cortex, PC declines slightly to about 45% at term and to 38% at 2 years, PE and PS increase only slightly, and sphingomyelin increases significantly during the entire maturation period. Analysis of cerebral white matter indicates relatively larger changes in PC, PS, and sphingomyelin. Plasmalogens, 90% of which are the ethanolamine type, increase almost fourfold from birth up to 1 year in white matter (Balakrishnan et al., 1961). Except for a slight decrease in sphingomyelin of white matter in aged brain (Svennerholm, 1968), there is little change in lipid composition among different adult age groups (Fillerup and Mead, 1967).

3.2.2.2 Primate

A study on phospholipid composition of nonhuman primate brain has been reported (Portman et al., 1972). Lipids and other biochemical parameters were determined from cerebral cortex and pons of rhesus monkeys rang-

TABLE 3.2 Phospholipid Composition of Human Cerebrum During Development and Aging

Phospholipid	Tissue[a]	New-born	1 mo	7 mo	4 yr	16 yr	52 yr	82 yr
				Molar Percentage				
PC	CC	46.7	41.0	39.2	37.9	37.1	36.9	35.5
	WM	45.0	38.3	34.5	25.6	24.6	25.1	25.3
PE	CC	28.0	34.9	34.4	35.4	36.1	35.6	36.8
	WM	31.0	34.5	33.7	35.9	35.2	33.9	36.4
PI	CC	3.4	3.0	2.8	2.2	2.6	3.2	4.1
	WM	4.3	3.2	2.6	1.9	2.3	2.4	2.7
PS	CC	14.4	14.4	14.2	13.6	13.3	13.9	12.7
	WM	14.2	16.0	16.0	20.5	21.1	20.3	19.3
Sphingomyelin	CC	7.4	6.8	9.4	10.9	10.9	10.4	10.9
	WM	5.5	8.1	13.2	16.1	16.9	18.3	16.3

Source: Svennerholm (1968).

[a] CC = cerebral cortex; WM = white matter.

ing from 58 days gestational age to over 10 years. The concentration of total phospholipids in cerebral cortex is about twofold higher than those in pons. In both brain regions phospholipids accumulate most rapidly shortly before and after birth, and the increase continues after 1 year in pons but not in cerebral cortex. In addition to total phospholipid, five phospholipid subclasses were analyzed from pons. The concentrations of sphingomyelin and PEpl, two major components of myelin, are extremely low in midgestation (60–90 days) but increase rapidly shortly before birth and up to 3 months postnatal age and even continue to increase after 1 year. PC, PE, and PS are present in significant concentrations early in gestation and increase at a more moderate rate than PEpl or sphingomyelin. The levels of PC and PE seem to remain constant after about 3 months.

3.2.2.3 *Rodents*

Reports on the changes in phospholipid composition of specific brain regions of rodents are relatively few. The concentration of total phospholipids of rat cerebrum increases throughout development up to about 35 days of age with the most rapid increases occurring during the second and third weeks of life (Vanier et al., 1971; Alling and Karlsson, 1973; De Sousa and Horrocks, 1979). Marked changes in phospholipid composition occur in rat cerebrum during maturation (De Sousa and Horrocks, 1979). The proportion of PEpl rises from 9% at 2 days to 19% at 127 days, whereas PE increases only slightly. PC declines from 58 to 33%, whereas PS and PI remain relatively constant at 12 and 4%, respectively. Sphingomyelin also increases from the 11th day to about the 25th day, reaching a maximum of about 6%. Manukyan et al. (1962) reported large increases in sphingomyelin, PIP, and PS in cerebral cortex, cerebellum, and medulla oblongata of rat brain. The changes are similar in all brain regions up to 6 days, but the amount of sphingomyelin in the medulla increases sharply between 6 and 30 days of age. The concentrations of PC, comprising 40–50% of the total phospholipids at birth, and of PI are practically unchanged (on a dry-weight basis) throughout the postnatal period in all brain regions, although the relative proportions decline.

In guinea pigs ranging from fetus to 2 months old, total phospholipids increase significantly (from 16 to 23%) in cerebral white matter, whereas the increase in gray matter is not significant (Wender, 1965). The sphingomyelins of both tissues also increase, but the change is most obvious in white matter between birth and the 9th day of life, the period corresponding to rapid myelination in guinea pig brain.

Sheltawy and Dawson (1969) reported on the accumulation and metabolism of polyphosphoinositides in cerebrum of developing rat and guinea pig. These lipids are found mainly in the nervous system and are localized primarily in white matter. The newborn rat forebrain contains 18 and 30% of the adult levels of PIP and PIP_2, respectively. The patterns of change are slightly different, with the adult level for PIP_2 (45 µg P/g wet wt.) attained at 40 days and the level of PIP (15 µg P/g) at 30 days. In contrast, guinea pigs are born with a much higher content of PIP_2, which increases sharply shortly after birth to a level of 30 µg P/g and gradually continues to rise during adult life (to 40 µg P/g). On the other hand, the full complement of PIP (7 µg P/g) is present at birth and remains stable. In a later study Hauser and Eichberg (1973), using a modified technique for the recovery of the polyphosphoinositides, found that the level of PIP in rat brain was twice as high as reported previously (Sheltawy and Dawson, 1969), although the PIP_2 levels were similar. These patterns reflect the degree of neonatal neurogenesis in the two species, the rat brain which is not myelinated at birth and the guinea pig which is partially myelinated.

3.2.2.4 Rabbit

In the prenatal cerebral pallium (consisting of gray and white matter) of rabbit, phospholipids comprise about 19% of the dry weight and remain unchanged throughout gestation and postnatal development (Dekaban et al., 1971). On a dry weight basis the proportions of individual phospholipids of the cerebral pallium change little during fetal development. However, accelerated deposition of all the phospholipid classes occurs between 28 and 30 days gestation, just prior to birth. After birth PC decreases slightly, PE increases slightly, and PS + PI do not change. Sphingomyelin, however, declines slightly just before birth and then rises dramatically from birth to adult. This general lack of change in the percentage weight during prenatal development suggests that deposition of lipids is keeping pace with the general increase in brain size.

3.2.3 Isolated Cells and Brain Subcellular Fractions

Rouser et al. (1972) reviewed the changes in lipid composition with age occurring in brain subcellular membranes and whole cells. They pointed out the difficulties involved in comparing the various data in the literature. Although the lipid compositions of purified preparations of neurons, astrocytes, oligodendroglia, and capillaries in adult brain have been reported (see Rouser et al., 1972, for review), only a handful of papers are concerned with the changes occurring during development.

3.2.3.1 *Neurons and Astroglia*

Norton and Poduslo (1971) analyzed neuronal and astroglial cell preparations from rat brains during the period of rapid myelination (10–20 days). They found that the lipid composition of these two cell types is quite similar. Both cell types have a high phospholipid content (71% of total lipid), and neither cell types exhibit obvious changes with age. The glial cells have less PI and more PS than neuronal cells, and both cell types have less PS and total plasmalogens than whole brain at any age. Sphingomyelin levels are similar in the two cell types and do not seem to vary with age, although an increase of 45% in whole brain is observed. The only lipids that increase during development in both cell types are the plasmalogens. Similar findings have been obtained for rabbit neuronal cells (Baker, 1979). The results indicate that in contrast to tissues, these cells remain relatively unchanged in quantity and composition during development.

3.2.3.2 *Capillary Endothelial Cells*

The brain capillary endothelial cell fraction is of interest because of its presumed role in the formation of the blood brain barrier. The accumulation of these cells during development is independent of the processes

TABLE 3.3 Phospholipid Composition of Human Cerebral Myelin During Development

	Percent of Total Phospholipid						
Phospholipid	New-born	3 mo	5 mo	11 mo	3 yr	7 yr	17 yr
PC	38.3	33.3	34.5	31.5	29.3	27.2	23.0
PE	9.2	9.8	9.4	7.3	8.2	7.6	7.4
PEpl	27.0	23.5	26.9	30.6	29.3	28.8	30.7
PS	17.3	17.6	20.7	19.3	19.3	17.8	21.0
Sphingomyelin	8.3	10.2	8.5	11.3	13.9	16.1	18.0

Source: Fishman et al. (1975).

of myelination and synaptogenesis. The changes in phospholipids and their acyl group composition in these cells from developing rat brain have been described by Matheson et al. (1980, 1981a). During development the proportion of phospholipids remains relatively constant but the individual lipid species seem to change with age. As in most other brain fractions, PC is the major phospholipid (45%) in the young rat and diminishes with age to 30%. On the other hand, PE rises from 16 to 26%, and the proportion of PEpl increases about fourfold. Although the proportions of some phospholipids increase while others decrease, nearly all of the lipid classes are increasing in actual amount per brain throughout development. Therefore, the change in proportion actually reflects different rates of accumulation of the lipids.

3.2.3.3 Myelin

Among the subcellular fractions, the myelin fraction has been most extensively studied because of its distinctive role in brain function, its involvement in neurological disorders, and its unique process of *de novo* formation during the early part of development. Other subcellular fractions are generally included with studies on myelin for comparison. In human cerebral myelin the phospholipids comprise 40–45% of the total lipids and show a slight tendency to diminish with age (Eng et al., 1968; Fishman et al., 1975). Distinct developmental profiles for the individual phospholipids are found (Table 3.3). There is a twofold increase in sphingomyelin from neonate to old age (70+ years) and a decrease in PC from 35 to 25% (Eng et al., 1968; Fishman et al., 1975; Svennerholm and Vanier, 1977; Svennerholm et al., 1978). In contrast, Gerstl et al. (1967) reported an increase in PE but not in the other phospholipids. Although the relative concentration of total ethanolamine phosphoglyceride (PE + PEpl) remains constant at about 40%, the plasmalogen component increases slightly with age and ranges from 75 to 84% of the total PE (Fishman et al., 1975; Svennerholm et al., 1978). The adult pattern of lipid distribution is reached around 5 years of age.

The amount of human myelin apparently decreases during aging (Berlet and Volk, 1980), starting from about 60 years and older. This decrease is also reflected by a loss of myelin lipids in whole brain (Rouser et al., 1971). Sun and Samorajski (1973) analyzed the phospholipids of myelin from corpus callosum of rhesus monkey during aging. PC, PE, and PEpl are the major phosphoglycerides and together constitute more than 70% of the total phosphoglycerides. The least common constituents, PCpl and PA, each comprise 2% or less. There are only minor differences in the distribution of phospholipids in relation to age after maturity. The most notable change is a decrease in PE with a concomitant increase in PEpl, which occurs in the oldest age group.

Unlike humans, rodent myelin in the brain continues to increase beyond maturity, although the rate of accumulation decreases with age (Eng and Noble, 1968; Rawlins and Smith, 1971; Sun and Samorajski, 1972; Horrocks, 1973; Norton and Poduslo, 1973; Smith, 1973). Evidence from rats and mice indicates that in addition to mature myelin, an immature or "myelinlike" fraction is also found in developing rat brain (Davison et al., 1966; Banik and Davison, 1969). This early myelin was found to have a lower concentration of cerebroside and a higher level of phospholipids, especially PC, as compared to the adult myelin. Thus, the early myelin resembles the lipid composition of cellular membranes. Davison and co-workers (Davison et al., 1966; Banik and Davison, 1969) have suggested that the myelin isolated from very young rats is a heterogeneous mixture consisting of adult myelin and immature myelin derived from the oligodendroglial plasma membrane. Thus, a larger variance for myelin composition would be obtained from young rats due to differences in time of maturation of different brain regions.

In purified myelin from rats 15 days old to more than 1 year of age, phospholipids constitute over 50% of the total lipids and the proportion decreases with increasing age up to 2 months (Eng and Noble, 1968; Norton, 1971; Norton and Poduslo, 1973). Most of the decrease is attributed to a 30–40% decrease in PC during development. The ethanolamine phosphoglycerides are the major component at 15–20%. However, the proportion of plasmalogen relative to total PE increases continuously up to 5 months of age before leveling off (Norton and Poduslo, 1973). The observed changes are not obvious in myelin fractions of rats younger than

15 days, which include the immature myelin (Eng and Noble, 1968). Besides the major phospholipids, some minor components have also been measured. Eichberg and Hauser (1973) examined the subcellular distribution of polyphosphoinositides in rats 7 and 34 days old. At 34 days more than 50% of the total PIP and more than 75% of the total PIP_2 were recovered in the myelin fraction. However, it appears that in unmyelinated brain from very young rats, the PIP and PIP_2 are concentrated in the neuronal and glial plasma membranes instead.

Smith (1973) compared myelin composition during development in four brain regions of rats aged 20 days to 20 months. Purified myelin from the forebrain areas (cerebral cortex, thalamus) indicated a composition characteristic of immaturity of greater duration than did myelin from the hindbrain areas (cerebellum, brain stem). This pattern of chemical maturity also reflects the morphological observations on the course of myelination in the brain (Jacobson, 1963). At 20 days of age total phospholipid, which is at least 50% of the total lipids in all regions, is higher in the forebrain areas than the hindbrain areas. Most of this can be attributed to a higher amount of PC, which is the major constituent. In all brain regions the proportion of PC decreases during maturation, but this drop is more obvious in cortex and thalamus. By 6 months of age the myelin from all brain regions becomes quite similar.

In mouse brain the phospholipids of myelin increase continuously from 14 days into old age (Horrocks, 1968; Sun and Samorajski, 1972), although the proportion of phospholipid relative to total lipid remains stable after about 24 days. In contrast to rat brain myelin, the lipid composition of mouse brain myelin shows the adult pattern at 24 days and does not change thereafter (Horrocks, 1968). PC and PE are the predominant species, and the proportions and changes are similar to that of rat myelin. PC decreases 30% with age while PE increases 17%. The proportion of PEpl relative to total ethanolamine phosphoglycerides increases from 55 to 75–80%. Sphingomyelin and other acidic phospholipids do not vary extensively with age.

Rabbit brain myelin shows more dramatic changes during maturation (Dalal and Einstein, 1969). Phosphoglycerides comprise about 57% of the total lipid in the neonate and decrease 30% during maturation. Among them, PC and PE decline 30–50%, whereas sphingomyelin + PI increase about twofold during maturation.

3.2.3.4 Other Subcellular Fractions

Cuzner and Davison (1968) analyzed the lipids of subcellular fractions (nuclei, myelin, synaptosomes, mitochondria, microsomes, and cytosol) of rat brain during development. However, with respect to phospholipids, only total phosphoglycerides were measured. There is an early rise in phospholipids in all fractions, which reflects the general increase in whole brain, but the increase is sustained only in the myelin fraction. There are some differences in the absolute amount of phospholipid per brain in each fraction, but this may partially reflect the relative contribution of each fraction to the whole-brain weight. The phospholipids of myelin and synaptosomes together constitute about 50% of the phospholipids in whole homogenate, while microsomes constitute 11.5%.

Microsomal phospholipids in rat brain increase from birth through 47 days but begin to decline by 70 days (Cuzner and Davison, 1968; Horrocks, 1968). Horrocks (1968) found that microsomes have higher levels of PC and lower levels of PE than myelin, and PEpl is substantially lower. Changes in composition with age are not as obvious in microsomes.

3.3 ACYL GROUP COMPOSITION OF PHOSPHOLIPIDS IN BRAIN

Not only do different regions of the brain have unique phospholipid profiles that change during development but the fatty acid compositions of these lipids are also distinct and exhibit changes with age. Some investigators have reported on acyl group compositional changes in the total phospholipid fraction, while others have analyzed the fatty acids of individual phospholipids. Both kinds of information may provide new insight into the influence of lipids on brain function.

3.3.1 Acyl Groups of Total Phospholipids

Crawford et al. (1977) derived a computer projection curve based on analysis of postmortem material from 27 human fetuses and infants up to 2 years of age. Their result indicates that 60–70% of the adult complement of long-chain polyenoic acids are accumulated at birth; thereafter the rate of accumulation drops off during development. On the other hand, the rate of accumulation of the long-chain saturated and monoenoic acids (24:0 and 24:1) involved in myelination rises during the first 6 months of postnatal life.

The fatty acid and fatty aldehyde (mainly from PEpl) compositions of total phospholipids in human prenatal and postnatal whole brain were analyzed by Altrock and Debuch (1968). The fatty aldehydes are comprised mainly of 16:0, 18:0, and 18:1. Both the C16 fatty acids and aldehydes decrease, while the C18 derivatives increase with increasing postnatal age. However, 16:0 fatty acid increases slightly until the seventh fetal month, whereas both 18:1 derivatives decrease from the third fetal month until term. The amounts of long-chain polyenoic fatty acids remain relatively constant during the fetal period but increase at term or shortly after birth.

In cerebrum of developing human fetal brain (Srinivasa Rao and Subba Rao, 1973) 16:1 increases from the fourth fetal month to the sixth month and 18:1 decreases steadily to term. At birth there is a dramatic increase in the proportions of the long-chain polyenes, apparently at the expense of shorter-chain fatty acids. The fatty acid patterns of cerebellum are somewhat different from those of cerebrum, but the acyl group change is similar in cerebellum and medulla oblongata (Srinivasa Rao and Subba Rao, 1973).

Martinez et al. (1974) reported lower percentage values for the unsaturated and monounsaturated fatty acids and higher values for the polyenoic acids in human brain. Their results emphasize changes in families of fatty acids and indicate an increase of the $n - 3$ series, mainly $22:6(n - 3)$, with increasing gestational age. The total $n - 6$ fatty acids did not vary during the prenatal period.

Biran and Bartley (1961) and Kishimoto et al. (1965) studied the fatty acid composition of total phosphoglycerides in developing rat brain. They suggested that comparison of fatty acid ratios can be used as an estimation of maturity. For example, the 16:0/18:0 ratio drops with increasing age while the ratio of 18:1/18:0 increases. Sinclair and Crawford (1972) were able to correlate the myelination process with development by comparing the accumulation of 20:4 and 22:6, fatty acids characteristic of gray matter, with 24:1 and 20:1, which are characteristic of myelin.

Banik and Davison (1969) compared the phosphoglyceride fatty acid patterns of myelin and microsomes from developing and adult rats. In myelin 16:0 comprises 44% of the total fatty acids in younger rats, but declines to 13% in the adult, whereas 18:1 doubles to 41%. The "immature" myelin fraction has a higher proportion of short-chain fatty acids (16 carbon and below) as compared to adult rat myelin and thus resembles the fatty acid pattern of other cellular membranes (Biran and Bartley, 1961). In microsomes the major fatty acid is 16:0, which decreases during the period of rapid myelination from 40 to 30%. There is an increase at 3 weeks in 18:0 to the adult level of 26% and in 18:1 from 18 to 23%.

3.3.2 Acyl Group Profiles of Individual Phospholipids

The first report of the fatty aldehyde and acid compositions of the individual major lipid classes in human brain was that of O'Brien and Sampson

(1965b), who analyzed gray and white matter and myelin from four brains with widely different ages. The fatty aldehyde patterns of ethanolamine and serine plasmalogens are similar: mainly 16:0 and 18:0 with lesser amounts of 18:1. Like the fatty acids, the proportions of 18:0 and 16:0 aldehydes decrease with age, while the proportion of 18:1 increases. The proportion of 18:0 aldehyde is twofold higher in gray matter than in white matter, whereas the opposite is found for the 18:1 aldehyde.

The authors reported that PE and PS contain high proportions of polyunsaturated fatty acids, especially 20:4, 22:5, and 22:6, whereas PC contains only 20:4 in any significant amounts. On the other hand, PC contains 31–55% of 16:0, while PE and PS have 5–14% and 1–3%, respectively. The proportion of polyenes is highest in gray matter and lowest in myelin, but the reverse is true for the monoenes.

Svennerholm and co-workers (1963, 1964, 1968, 1973a,b, 1977, 1978) published more extensive studies on changes in acyl group profiles of the major phospholipids during maturation of human brain. Several other reports have focused on the acyl group profile of just one or a few of the phospholipids in brain from human, rat, mouse, and rabbit. For this reason, acyl group changes in individual phosphoglycerides are discussed separately in the next five sections. For a comparison, the acyl group profiles of the major phospholipids in human cerebral cortex are shown in Table 3.4.

3.3.2.1   Choline Phosphoglycerides

The fatty acid composition of PC in human fetal cerebrum and cerebellum has been described (Martinez et al., 1974; Ballabriga and Martinez, 1978). The major fatty acids are 16:0 and 18:1, comprising 51–54% and 23%, respectively, and they show little change during fetal development in cerebrum. In cerebellum 18:1 increases from 21 to 28%, while 18:0 increases from about 7% to nearly 11% in both brain regions. Arachidonate, the only significant polyunsaturated fatty acid found in this phosphoglyceride, increases in cerebrum to 6% but remains stable at 4% in cerebellum.

Differences in the acyl group profiles of PC are found in cerebral cortex and white matter during development (Svennerholm, 1968; Svennerholm and Vanier, 1973a). In cerebral cortex the proportion of 16:0 is constant during the fetal period and decreases only slightly during maturation to the adult level of 46%. Stearic acid (18:0) starts to increase during the fetal period to a peak (13%) at 4 years of age and then gradually declines in old age to 10%. Oleic acid (18:1) increases from 24 to 30% during maturation. Fatty acids of the linoleate series, mainly 20:4(n − 6), are low during the fetal period but increase shortly after birth. In white matter

TABLE 3.4 Acyl Group Concentration of Phosphoglycerides in Developing Human Cerebral Cortex

Acyl Group[a]	New-born	1 mo	7 mo	4 yr	16 yr	52 yr	82 yr
PC (%, wt.)							
16:0	52.4	46.6	47.1	43.5	48.9	45.9	45.7
16:1	6.5	5.4	3.8	2.7	2.6	2.4	2.5
18:0	9.1	9.6	12.1	13.5	11.7	11.2	9.9
18:1	21.5	25.9	25.7	29.0	29.0	30.3	29.0
20:3 (n − 6)	0.4	0.7	0.8	1.1	0.5	0.6	0.8
20:4 (n − 6)	4.2	6.1	5.0	5.2	3.8	3.6	4.7
22:6 (n − 3)	0.9	1.7	1.5	1.5	0.8	2.5	3.6
PE (including plasmalogen) (%, wt.)							
16:0	7.6	6.4	6.5	5.0	6.0	5.7	6.8
18:0	32.8	34.6	27.8	30.1	29.8	28.4	27.2
18:1	8.5	8.7	10.3	8.8	10.2	10.3	9.8
20:3 (n − 6)	1.0	1.2	1.5	1.6	1.1	1.0	1.0
20:4 (n − 6)	14.9	16.5	16.4	16.7	13.0	11.2	10.3
22:4 (n − 6)	10.6	11.1	11.7	9.9	8.4	7.7	6.3
22:5 (n − 6)	4.4	2.7	5.0	2.4	1.7	1.2	0.9
22:6 (n − 3)	17.1	16.1	16.9	22.3	27.0	30.5	33.9
PI (%, wt.)							
16:0	18.1	14.0	11.4	10.4	15.9	9.0	11.0
16:1	2.3	1.6	1.0	1.3	1.0	0.2	6.5
18:0	33.7	40.2	41.5	39.7	37.8	39.1	37.5
18:1	9.9	8.2	8.6	8.0	12.7	13.0	8.9
20:3 (n − 6)	1.0	0.6	1.2	1.3	0.9	1.3	1.6
20:4 (n − 6)	29.5	29.0	27.2	31.6	22.5	28.5	33.2
22:4 (n − 6)	1.3	1.4	1.7	1.2	1.4	1.6	1.4
22:6 (n − 3)	1.5	2.5	3.6	3.0	5.3	4.8	5.3
PS (%, wt.)							
16:0	4.2	3.0	4.6	5.4	3.6	4.2	3.7
18:0	47.4	49.9	48.6	47.4	50.1	45.3	40.6
18:1	6.8	9.6	9.5	12.0	17.5	17.5	14.2
20:3 (n − 6)	1.1	1.3	1.4	1.4	0.7	0.9	0.8
20:4 (n − 6)	4.3	3.8	3.1	2.4	1.8	1.8	1.9
22:4 (n − 6)	10.7	7.7	6.3	4.6	3.5	3.0	3.2
22:5 (n − 6)	5.8	3.5	6.3	3.0	1.7	0.7	1.0
22:6 (n − 3)	18.2	18.7	18.1	21.5	18.1	23.2	27.5

Source: Svennerholm (1968).

[a] Fatty acids not shown constitute less than 1% each at any age.

the proportion of 16:0 is similar to cortex at birth but decreases rapidly shortly after birth to remain stable at 30% by 4 years of age. This decrease is marked by a concomitant increase in 18:1. Stearic acid in white matter also decreases during aging. Unlike cortex, fatty acids of the linoleate series in white matter decline during the first year of life.

Like human, the major fatty acids of PC in rat brain are 16:0 and 18:1 (Marshall et al., 1966; Skrbic and Cumings, 1970; Alling and Karlsson, 1973; Crawford and Wells, 1979; Ogino et al., 1979). The 16:0 level falls from a high of 58% at 5 days of age to 42% in the adult, whereas 18:1 increases from 23 to 32% between 17 days and 4.5 weeks and 18:0 increases from 8 to 15%. The polyunsaturated fatty acids (mainly 20:4) together constitute about 10–13% during the developmental period. Since the fatty acid pattern observed is similar to that for total brain lipids (Biran and Bartley, 1961), it has been suggested that the fatty acid pattern in immature whole brain is reflective of the high proportion of PC present (Marshall et al., 1966).

The fatty acid pattern of PC from rabbit brain is quite different from that of human and rat (Odutuga et al., 1973). In the newborn rabbit 16:0 and 18:1 are present in nearly equal proportions (about 36%), and 16:0 does not change with age. Oleic acid increases to 46%. The proportion of 18:0 declines slightly after maturity to 10%.

The distribution of molecular species of PC in rat cerebrum (Ogino et al., 1979) and whole brain (Crawford and Wells, 1979) has been examined. The relative amounts of different classes of PC were 35% saturated, 40% monoenoic, 6% dienoic, 11% tetraenoic, 2% pentaenoic, and 5% hexaenoic (Crawford and Wells, 1979). These proportions remain relatively constant, although the acyl group composition of individual molecular species show distinct changes with development. During the prenatal period, the main molecular species are 32:0 (16:0/16:0), 34:1 (16:0/18:1), 34:0 (16:0/18:0), and 32:1 (16:0/16:1). From birth to the 10th day, there are increases in 32:0 and 30:0 (14:0/16:0) and decreases in 34:1, 32:1, and 34:0. During the period of rapid myelination there are increases in 34:1, 34:0, and 36:1. During the latter part of development (3 weeks to adult) 34:1 and 34:0 continue to increase (to 30 and 14%) (Ogino et al., 1979).

In a study on human myelin during development (Svennerholm and Vanier, 1977; Svennerholm et al., 1978), the proportion of polyunsaturated fatty acids in PC did not change, but the saturated fatty acids decreased with a concomitant increase in monoenes. In aging human myelin (Horrocks, 1973; Horrocks et al., 1982) there is a slight increase in both 18:1 and 20:1. The proportions of fatty acids in mature myelin from rhesus monkey are similar to human, and there is relatively little compositional change with increasing age (Sun and Samorajski, 1973).

The fatty acid profile of PC in rat myelin is rich in 18:1 (44%), 16:0 (32–35%), and 18:0 (16–18%) (Skrbic and Cumings, 1970). These proportions tend to remain relatively constant throughout the developmental period. The PC fatty acid profiles of mitochondria, microsomes, and cytosol follow the trend of whole homogenate in amount and in pattern of developmental change (Skrbic and Cumings, 1970).

Mouse myelin PC is also composed mainly of 16:0, 18:1, and 18:0 with polyunsaturated fatty acids constituting less than 4% each (Sun and Yau, 1976a). There is a slight decrease in 16:0 and slight increases in 18:0 and 18:1 from 2 to 8 weeks. PC of microsomes is composed mainly of 16:0, which increases to 57% at 7 days and then declines to 50% by 3 weeks, and 18:1, which does not exhibit any age-related changes. Both $20:4(n - 6)$ and $22:6(n - 3)$ increase during development, to 7% at 2 weeks and 5% at 4 months, respectively.

The acyl group composition of PC from the rat capillary endothelial cell fraction was reported by Matheson et al. (1980, 1981a). The proportion of saturated fatty acids as a group remains constant, although 16:0 decreases from 50 to 33% and 18:0 increases from 6 to 20%. The monoenes also do not change, although 16:1 decreases and 20:1 increases. In contrast, the proportions of polyenes, mainly 18:2 and 20:4, increase at least twofold between 8 and 20 days.

In neuronal cell bodies from rabbit cerebral cortex (Baker, 1979) the major fatty acid of PC is 16:0, which diminishes from 46 to 39% with increasing age. Palmitoleic acid (16:1) also falls (from 6 to 2%), while 18:0 rises slightly to 28%.

3.3.2.2   Ethanolamine Phosphoglycerides

Reports on the acyl group composition of ethanolamine phosphoglycerides seem rather confusing since diacyl compounds and the plasmalogens are analyzed as a single component in some cases and the two phosphoglycerides are treated separately in others. Unless the diacyl and plasmalogen compounds are described separately, the reader should assume that the analysis was performed on the combined lipids.

In human cerebrum and cerebellum of prenatal brain the ethanolamine phosphoglycerides are comprised mainly of 18:0 (27–34%) and polyunsaturated fatty acids (Martinez et al., 1974; Ballabriga and Martinez, 1978). With time of maturation, 18:0 decreases in cerebellum from 29 to 22% but remains constant in cerebrum. Oleic acid (18:1) decreases with maturation from 12 to 7%, whereas in cerebellum it decreases from 29 to

22%. The proportion of 20:4 also decreases. During postnatal development of cerebrum (White et al., 1971a) 16:0 falls from 11 to 6% and 18:0 from 26 to 17% with a corresponding rise in 18:1 (11–28%) and 20:1 (0.6–4%). In the linoleic acid series the proportions of 20:4 and 22:5 decrease (15–10% and 5–1%, respectively), while 22:4 increases to 15%. Changes from adolescence into old age are relatively small; most notable is a small increase in 18:1 and 20:1.

The fatty acid profiles of PE in human pre- and postnatal cerebral cortex and white matter were examined (Svennerholm, 1968; Svennerholm and Vanier, 1973a). In cerebral cortex 18:0 is the major fatty acid at all ages and contributes about 30% with a peak of 35% at 1 month of age. Palmitic acid (16:0) decreases during prenatal development but remains constant after birth and during aging. The monoenes (primarily 18:1) decrease during the prenatal period to 10% at term and then remain constant. In younger brains polyunsaturated fatty acids of the linoleate series predominate, with $20:4(n-6)$ and $22:4(n-6)$ constituting about 25%. With increasing age these fatty acids decline with a corresponding increase in the linolenic acid $(n-3)$ series (22:5, 22:6) from 18 to 35%. In white matter 18:0 is also the major fatty acid of PE at birth (29%) but declines thereafter. Oleic acid (18:1) becomes the major fatty acid shortly after birth and reaches a peak of 43% at maturity. Unlike cortex, the proportion of $22:4(n-6)$ is greater than $20:4(n-6)$, and $22:5(n-3)$ and $22:6(n-3)$ decrease shortly after birth.

In the developing rat the acyl group composition of PE in cerebrum during development was analyzed by Alling and Karlsson (1973). The saturated fatty acids increase slightly to 44% during the first week of life, mainly due to an increase of 18:0, the major fatty acid. From the 8th day 16:0 declines rapidly, while 18:0 increases slightly, resulting in a net decrease of the saturated fatty acids. The monoenes, primarily 18:1, diminish from 12 to 10% during the first 8 days and then increase to 17% during the period studied. The sum of the linoleic and linolenic acid series is constant at 48–52%. However, the concentration of the two series varies inversely. Changes in the linoleate series are mainly due to $20:4(n-6)$, which increases to a peak at 10 days and then declines continuously after 16 days. At this time $22:6(n-3)$, the major linolenate series constituent, increases continuously to exceed the $n-6$ series concentration.

Crawford and Wells (1979) reported the acyl group composition of PE in developing rat brain. In the newborn rat the major fatty acids are 18:0 (27%), 20:4 (18%), 22:6 (17%), 16:0 (15%), and 18:1 (11%). The polyenes together constitute 45% of the total fatty acids, but they decrease to 39% during development. Both 18:0 and 18:1 increase moderately while 16:0 and $20:4(n-6)$ decrease about the same and $22:6(n-3)$ declines slightly between the 3rd and 6th days. The acyl group profile of PE indicates 1% saturated, 8% monoenoic, 3% dienoic, 40% tetraenoic, 9% pentaenoic, and 37% hexaenoic species. The $20:4(n - 6)$ and $22:6(n - 3)$ are predominantly paired with $18:0$. Joffe (1969) compared the molecular species of PE and PEpl in rat brain. He found that the fatty aldehydes and alkyl ethers in the 1-position of PEpl are distinct from the acyl groups. The predominant fatty acid in the 1-position is $18:0$ (65%) with moderate amounts of $16:0$ and $18:1$, whereas in the plasmalogen $16:0$ and $18:0$ contribute almost equally (40%). As expected, 95% of the fatty acids in the 2-position are unsaturated, and the profile is similar in diacyl-PE and plasmalogen, except that $20:4(n - 6)$ is 40% higher in the diacyl-PE. In contrast to other reports, Joffe (1969) found few developmental changes with this phosphoglyceride; however, his samples were obtained from animals ranging only from 17 to 22 days of age.

As with PC, the acyl group profile of PE from rabbit brain is quite different from human or rat (Odutuga et al., 1973). At birth the major fatty acids of PE are $18:0$ (32%), $18:1$ (15%), $20:4$ (15%), and $16:0$ (13%). During development, both $16:0$ and $18:0$ decrease to one-half the level at birth, whereas the proportion of $18:1$ doubles. Among the polyenes, $20:4(n - 6)$ decreases, while $18:2$ and $22:5(n - 6)$ increase. The monoene $20:1$ increases most dramatically from less than 1 to 6%.

In a study on human myelin by Svennerholm's group (Svennerholm and Vanier, 1977; Svennerholm et al., 1978), ethanolamine phosphoglycerides showed the largest changes in acyl group composition with increasing age among the phosphoglycerides analyzed. The proportion of saturated fatty acids decreases rapidly with a corresponding increase in monoenes. The linoleic acid series constitute 40% of the total fatty acids at 1 year and then decline to 25%. The polyunsaturated fatty acid $22:4(n - 6)$, which is the major polyene of this phospholipid, rises from 15% at birth to 25% at 1 year and then declines to 17–19%. Of the monoenes, $18:1$ increases from 25 to 48% and $20:1$ from 4 to 10%. Palmitic acid $(16:0)$ and $18:0$ are present in relatively small proportions and decrease with increasing age. Similar results were obtained by Sun and Horrocks (1971; see also Horrocks et al., 1982). In aging monkey brain myelin (Sun and Samorajski, 1973) $18:1$ and $20:1$ increase from the adult levels of 36 and 9% to 38 and 12%, respectively. Arachidonate $(20:4)$, which comprises 11% of the total, changes very little, while $22:4$ decreases from 19 to 16%, $22:5$ from 1.4 to 0.8%, and $24:4$ from 4 to 2%.

The fatty acid compositions of ethanolamine phosphoglycerides of mouse myelin during development and aging have been reported (Sun and Samorajski, 1972; Sun and Yau, 1976a). The major fatty acid is $18:1$, which increases from 24% at 2 weeks of age to 34% at maturity and then remains constant. Other major fatty acids are 18:0, which decreases from 15 to 12% at maturity; 20:4($n - 6$), which decreases up to 8 weeks and then increases to 14% at maturity; 22:4($n - 6$), which decreases continuously during development and aging after a short spurt (to 11%) between the 2nd and 3rd weeks; and 22:6($n - 3$), which decreases to 11% at 8 weeks and then increases with age.

Samorajski and Rolsten (1973) compared the acyl group compositions of PE from brain myelin of mouse, rhesus monkey, and human at three age levels corresponding to late development, maturity, and early senescence. In this study there is no apparent change in levels of the saturated fatty acids during aging. Monoenes constitute the largest proportion of fatty acids of PE in all three species and appear to increase with age in monkey and human but not in mouse. There is a concomitant decrease in the polyenes in monkey and human.

Major differences in profiles are observed when PE and PEpl are analyzed separately. Sun and Horrocks (1971; see also Horrocks et al., 1982) found that the PE of adult human myelin is enriched in 18:0 (20%), 18:1 (40%), 20:4($n - 6$) (9%), and 22:4($n - 6$) (10%), and there are no obvious age-related changes during aging. The 2-acyl groups of PEpl are almost exclusively unsaturated and are especially rich in 18:1 (43%) and 22:4 (22%) with moderate amounts of 20:1 (8%) and 20:4 (10%). Age-related changes observed include an increase in 18:1 and 20:1 and a corresponding decrease in 20:4($n - 6$) and 22:4($n - 6$). The alkenyl group composition from the 1-position of PEpl is comprised mainly of 16:0, 18:0, and 18:1, a profile similar to that reported for human whole brain (Altrock and Debuch, 1968).

In monkey myelin (Sun and Samorajski, 1973) the PE profile is similar to human, except that the proportions are slightly different. There is a small decrease in 18:0 and a small increase in 18:1 during aging. The acyl group profile and age-related changes in PEpl are also similar to human, except that 20:4($n - 6$) does not change with age.

In mouse myelin (Sun and Yau, 1976a) most of the age-related changes observed in the total PE fraction are related to changes in the acyl groups of PEpl. This fraction is especially enriched in 18:1 (40% at maturity) and 20:1 (25%) with equal proportions of 20:4($n - 6$), 22:4($n - 6$), and 22:6($n - 3$) (9–10%). Generally, 18:1 and 20:1 increase with age during development while the polyenes decrease. The diacyl-PE fraction has nearly equal proportions of 18:0 and 18:1 at maturity (28–31%) and moderate proportions of 20:4 and 22:6 (10 and 14%, respectively).

Sun and Yau (1976a) also analyzed the total ethanolamine phosphoglycerides and separate lipid species from mouse microsomes. There is a large increase in 22:6($n - 3$) of total PE during maturation (from 30 to

42%), which is related to an increase in the diacyl-PE fraction. Arachidonic acid [20:4(n − 6)] increases during the first week to 20% and then declines to 12% at maturity. A similar developmental pattern is observed in both diacyl-PE and PEpl.

The acyl group composition of the diacyl-PE from rat capillary endothelial cells undergoes relatively small changes during development (Matheson et al., 1980, 1981a). The most notable change is an increase in 18:0 from 10 to 16%. On the other hand, the PEpl changes significantly. There is a marked decline in saturated fatty acids, from 41 to 5%, which is due mainly to a fall in the 16:0 and 18:0 levels. There is also a twofold increase in 20:4(n − 6) (to 48%) and 22:4(n − 6) (to 8%) and a threefold increase in 18:1 (to 25%).

In rabbit neuronal cells (Baker, 1979) 18:0, the major fatty acid of PE, remains relatively constant at 22–23%, whereas 20:4(n − 6) decreases slightly to 21% and 22:6(n − 3) increases from 11 to 17%.

3.3.2.3   Serine Phosphoglycerides

Human cerebral PS (Svennerholm, 1968; Svennerholm and Vanier, 1973a) has a much lower concentration of fatty acids of the linoleic acid series and a much higher concentration of 18:0 as compared to PE. During fetal development the saturated fatty acids remain unchanged in both cerebral cortex and white matter. However, shortly after birth 18:0 increases to the adult levels of 45–50% and then decreases during old age. In cerebral cortex 18:1 declines during the fetal period and then remains at about 10% through the first year. By 4 years of age there is an increase to the adult level of 12–17%. Arachidonic acid [20:4(n − 6)] and 22:4(n − 6) increase during fetal development to term and then decrease with age into maturity. On the other hand, 22:6(n − 3) increases from 18% at puberty to 30% during aging. In white matter 18:1 increases from less than 8 to 41% in the adult. The proportions of 22:4(n − 6) and 22:6(n − 3) are higher than in cortex at birth and decrease by 50% shortly after birth. Along with 20:4(n − 6), they continue to decrease more gradually to puberty.

The fatty acid pattern of PS from human myelin is very similar to that of white matter and undergoes changes similar to, but less pronounced than, the ethanolamine phosphoglycerides (Svennerholm and Vanier, 1977; Svennerholm et al., 1978). Saturated fatty acids (primarily 18:0) decrease slightly with age, while the monoenes double, reflecting the increase in 18:1 seen in white matter. The polyunsaturated fatty acids decrease almost twofold with age. Adult human myelin has nearly equal proportions of 18:0 and 18:1 (90% of total fatty acids) with very small proportions of 16:0 and polyunsaturated fatty acids (Horrocks, 1973). During aging, there is a small increase in 18:0 and 20:1 and a small decrease in 18:1. An aging study on myelin from rhesus monkey (Sun and Samorajski, 1973) revealed that there is very little compositional change in a PI + PS mixture. Stearic (18:0) and 18:1 acids together comprise more than 80% of the total fatty acids.

3.3.2.4 Sphingomyelin

Human cerebral sphingomyelin (Svennerholm, 1963; Ställberg-Stenhagen and Svennerholm, 1965) contains about 20 different fatty acids. This phospholipid class is especially enriched in myelin, and alterations of its fatty acid composition have been correlated to demyelinating diseases. The major fatty acid of sphingomyelin is 18:0, which increases from 70% in the fetus to 85% at term and then decreases to 40–48% at 4 years of age and older. Palmitic acid (16:0) decreases steadily from 12% in the fetus to 3% at 14 months. The long-chain fatty acids (mainly 22–26 carbon chain length) increase from 13 to 46–56% from 4 years of age and older. Among these, 24:1 rises from 6 to 23–30% in the adult.

Distinct differences in the acyl composition of sphingomyelins in cerebral gray and white matter were observed (O'Brien and Sampson, 1965b; Ställberg-Stenhagen and Svennerholm, 1965; Svennerholm and Vanier, 1973b; Heipertz et al., 1977; Svennerholm et al., 1978). In gray matter 18:0 comprises about 75% of the total fatty acids, 24:1, 15%, 16:0 up to 8%, and the remaining ones less than 2%. The long-chain fatty acids (C22–C26) as a group increase from 7 to 36% during maturation. In white matter 18:0 decreases during maturation to about 30% at 2 years of age and then starts to rise slightly in old age. The proportion of 24:1 increases dramatically from 4 to 30% in young children and then declines with aging. The proportion of C22–C26 is about threefold higher in white matter than gray matter, and the amounts decrease during aging. Thus, there appears to be a reversal of composition in old age to resemble the immature pattern (Heipertz et al., 1977).

In purified myelin (Svennerholm and Vanier, 1977; Svennerholm et al., 1978), the proportion of saturated long-chain (C16–C22) fatty acids declines from birth to about 40% in old age (70 years), whereas saturated very long chain (C23–C26) fatty acids remain constant. The monoenes increase from 17% in the newborn to 50% in old age and are higher in myelin at all ages as compared to white matter.

Sphingomyelin from rat whole brain (Marshall et al., 1966) also contains mainly 18:0, which increases rapidly until the fifth week of development to 50% of the total fatty acids and then appears to decrease in proportion.

Palmitic acid (16:0) decreases slightly from 17% in the fetus to about 10% at 5 weeks. The long-chain fatty acids (C22–C26) in general are present in small proportions and show little variation with age. The proportions of 22:0 and 26:1 also decrease, the latter from 15% in the fetus to 3% in the adult, while 24:1 increases modestly.

The fatty acid profile of rabbit brain sphingomyelin (Odutuga et al., 1973) differs from both human and rat. Stearic acid (18:0) comprises 63% of the total fatty acid in newborns and decreases slightly during maturation, whereas 16:0 contributes only 5% at birth, and this proportion decreases during maturation. Among the long-chain fatty acids, 24:1 is the only acyl group that increases in the adult.

3.3.2.5 *Inositol Phosphoglycerides and Phosphatidic Acid*

The fatty acid composition of PI from human brain during fetal development and postnatal maturation into aging has been reported (Svennerholm, 1968; Svennerholm and Vanier, 1973a). PI is characterized by high concentrations of 18:0 (36%, average) and 20:4($n - 6$) (29%) and moderate concentrations of 16:0 and 18:1 (9–25%). Fatty acids of the linolenic acid series, mainly 22:6($n - 3$), constitute only 6% or less of the total. Arachidonic acid [20:4($n - 6$)] in cerebral cortex increases up to 4 years of age, whereas it decreases in white matter. The proportion of 18:1 also increases into maturity in both brain regions but declines into old age in cortex.

The acyl group composition of PI from mouse brain (Su and Sun, 1978) is similar to human with high 18:0 (36%) and 20:4($n - 6$) (43%). The acyl group proportions seem to remain relatively constant throughout development. There is, however, a twofold decrease in 16:0 and a 67% increase in 18:1 between 5 and 10 days.

Very little information about PA in brain is available. Su and Sun (1978) analyzed the acyl group composition of PA in mouse brain. The level of 18:0 is highest at 1 day (41%) but decreases to 28% at 40 days, and 18:1 increases from 20 to 36% between 5 and 40 days. Palmitic acid increases to a maximum of 27% at 10 days and then decreases to newborn levels (about 14%) at maturity.

3.4 COMPOSITION OF PHOSPHOLIPIDS AND THEIR ACYL GROUP PROFILES IN SPINAL CORD

Although studies on various biochemical parameters of spinal cord during maturation have been reviewed (Levi, 1969; Rouser et al., 1972), infor-

TABLE 3.5 Phospholipid Composition of Rat Spinal Cord during
Development

Phospholipid	Percent of Total Phospholipid							
	2[a]	7[a]	11[a]	15[a]	20[a]	30[a]	90[a]	127[a]
PC	53.6	47.2	44.3	37.1	34.2	30.1	24.8	25.3
PE	13.1	16.0	16.5	16.8	16.1	18.5	20.4	19.3
PEpl	18.1	23.3	24.5	28.7	26.3	28.6	30.4	29.1
PS	10.6	8.0	9.4	10.3	13.5	12.7	12.9	12.5
PI	3.5	4.1	3.6	2.9	3.3	3.8	3.9	3.9
Sphingomyelin	0.6	1.4	2.3	4.1	4.9	6.0	5.8	6.4

Source: De Sousa and Horrocks (1979).

[a] Age (days).

mation on changes in phospholipid composition during maturation is limited. In rat the concentrations of cholesterol, galactolipids, and phospholipids are higher in spinal cord than in brain at all ages (De Sousa and Horrocks, 1979) and the spinal cord reaches maturity sooner (Smith, 1973; De Sousa and Horrocks, 1979). The phospholipids increase up to 90 days, with the greatest increase occurring during the second and third weeks of life (Brante, 1949; De Sousa and Horrocks, 1979). In rhesus monkey (Portman et al., 1972) the greatest rate of increase in phospholipids occurs in the first 2 months, but a more gradual increase occurs at least to 2 years of age.

De Sousa and Horrocks (1979) found marked changes in the proportions of individual phospholipids occurring during maturation (1–127 days) of rat spinal cord (Table 3.5). PEpl increases from 18 to 30% at 40 days, whereas diacyl-PE increases only slightly to about 20%. Sphingomyelin increases moderately throughout development. PC decreases from 54 to 25%, while PS and PI undergo little change.

The phospholipid composition of spinal cord myelin from rat (Smith, 1973; Sun et al., 1983) and rabbit (Dalal and Einstein, 1969) and of microsomes from rat (Sun et al., 1983) during development have been reported. As in brain myelin, PC is the major phospholipid constituent of both rabbit and rat, comprising 48 and 53% of total phospholipids, respectively, and it decreases during maturation. PEpl in rat spinal cord myelin increases from 17 to 30%, while diacyl-PE remains relatively constant throughout development. However, in rabbit the total ethanolamine phosphoglycerides show a decline between 30 and 170 days of age. Sphingomyelin increases about threefold in both species.

The phospholipids in the microsomal fraction from rat spinal cord differ from those in myelin (Sun et al., 1983). During development PC from the microsomes decreases almost twofold, while both ethanolamine phosphoglycerides increase by the same amount. The proportion of PEpl is lower at all ages in microsomes as compared to myelin. PS also increases in the microsomes, but only trace amounts of PI are present in either subcellular fraction.

Sun et al. (1983) also reported on changes in the course of development in the acyl group profiles of individual phospholipid classes from rat spinal cord myelin and microsomal subcellular fractions. The acyl groups of PC from microsomes are enriched in 16:0, 18:0, and 18:1. Palmitic acid decreases from 57 to 34%, while 18:0 increases from 8 to 14% and 18:1 from 26 to 39%. PC from myelin has a lower proportion of 16:0 and a higher proportion of 18:1 with no change during development. The proportions of polyenes in both fractions are similar.

Diacyl-PE from spinal cord microsomes (Sun et al., 1983) is composed mainly of 16:0, 18:0, and 18:1 with significant amounts of 20:4 and 22:6. Both 18:1 and 22:6 increase with increasing age, whereas the others decrease. In myelin diacyl-PE 18:1, 18:0, and 22:6 are the major fatty acids at 1 week of age. However, during development 22:6 decreases with a concomitant threefold increase in 20:1. Both 18:0 and 18:1 decrease moderately with age. The microsomal PEpl acyl group profile exhibits marked changes during development. In the young rat the major fatty acids are 22:6, 20:4, 18:1, and 16:0, but by maturity the predominant species are 18:1 and 20:1 with lesser amounts of 22:6 and 20:4. These changes are due primarily to large decreases in 16:0, 18:0, 20:4, and 22:6 with concomitant increases in 18:1 and 20:1. The acyl group profile of PEpl in myelin is entirely different. The predominant fatty acid is 18:1, which increases from 37 to 55%, with moderate amounts of 20:1 (15%), 20:4 (10%), 22:4 (10%), and 22:6 (20%). All of the polyunsaturated fatty acids decrease with increasing age.

In both membrane fractions nearly 80% of the acyl groups of PS are composed of 18:0 and 18:1. In the microsomal fraction an increase in 18:1 and 20:1 and a decrease in 16:0, 18:0, and 22:6 occurs between 7 and 17 days of age. Few changes are observed in the myelin.

3.5 COMPOSITION OF PHOSPHOLIPIDS AND THEIR ACYL GROUPS IN PERIPHERAL NERVE

Nearly all of the studies on phospholipid composition in peripheral nerve of mammals have been limited to adult material. However, some information on developmental changes in peripheral nerve phospholipids is available. Portman et al. (1972) compared the concentration of total phospholipids in rhesus monkey sciatic nerve with three central nervous system regions during development. The adult level (50 mg/g wet wt.) is reached at 9 months of age. This amount is less than pons or spinal cord, but more than cerebral gray matter. Phospholipid accumulates most rapidly shortly before birth in all four tissues.

Hofteig et al. (1982) reported that total lipid phosphorus in rabbit sciatic nerve increases 13-fold from 2 to 14 weeks of age, at which time the adult level is reached. Thus, the absolute content of each phospholipid increases over this period of development, although the proportions of individual phospholipids change dramatically. PC and PE each decline by 40% (from 28 to 16% and from 9 to 5%, respectively). At 2 weeks of age the proportions of PEpl, PS + PI, and sphingomyelin are 27, 11, and 23%, respectively, and these increase 21–27% during development. These findings are consistent with the myelin accretion that occurs in rabbit sciatic nerve during this age period (Yates et al., 1976).

Important changes in phospholipid fatty acyl composition of myelin-enriched endoneurium from rat sciatic nerve were reported by Yao (1982). Polyunsaturated fatty acids are the major component of PE in newborn rats, and all decrease steadily from day 10 until 1 year. However, $20:4(n - 6)$, the most abundant polyene at birth (23%), declines rapidly after 3 days and then at a much slower rate after 21 days. The period of sharp decline corresponds to the period of general myelination. Concomitantly, the monounsaturated fatty acids increase from day 10 to 1 month and then decline. The proportion of $18:1$ increases most dramatically from 23 to 70%. The saturated fatty acids also decline after 1 month. In PC the major fatty acids in the newborn are $16:0$ (38%) and $18:1$ (31%). A decrease of $16:0$, $18:2$, and $20:4(n - 6)$ and an increase of $18:1$ are observed.

3.6   DIETARY EFFECTS ON BRAIN PHOSPHOLIPIDS

3.6.1   Essential Fatty Acid (EFA) Deficiency

3.6.1.1   *Linoleic Acid Deficiency*

Linoleic ($18:2$) and linolenic ($18:3$) acids are considered essential fatty acids because they are not synthesized in the body and are therefore derived mainly from dietary sources. EFA deficiency is known to affect the acyl composition of phospholipids in brain as well as in other body organs (Holman, 1968). In order to compensate for the loss of $18:2(n - 6)$ and other $n - 6$ fatty acids, body organs are able to utilize $18:1$ for the synthesis of $20:3(n - 9)$ as well as other $n - 9$ fatty acids. Mohrhauer and Holman (1963) studied changes in fatty acid composition of brain lipids by varying the levels of dietary EFA. Since the brain is more protected from external influences, phospholipid acyl group changes in brain due to EFA deficiency are usually not as extensive as in nonneural organs. However, if an EFA deficiency is developed in brain, supplementing the deficient diet with EFA can cause a reversal of the deficiency symptoms and reduction of the $20:3(n - 9)$ fatty acids. Galli et al. (1970, 1971a) fed a fatty acid–free diet to female rats during pregnancy and nursing. There was a decrease in brain weight, total lipid, and phospholipid content in the offspring. Among the phosphoglycerides, the deficient diet resulted in a decrease in the proportion of fatty acids belonging to the $n - 6$ and $n - 3$ families and an increase in the $n - 9$ fatty acids. These changes corresponded to an increase in the triene–tetraene ratio, mainly $20:3(n - 9)/20:4(n - 6)$. In pups from mothers in which an EFA-deficient diet was initiated during the mid-pregnant stage, an increase in triene/tetraene ratio in brain PE could be detected as early as 10 days of age, but the decrease in $22:6(n - 3)$ was not obvious until after 6 months of age (Galli et al., 1971a). The decrease in $22:6(n - 3)$ was more obvious in PE than PS, although the acyl groups of PS are highly enriched in this fatty acid (Sun, 1972). When the EFA-deficient diet was initiated at different ages in mice during development and maturation, the most dramatic change in membrane lipids occurred during the early postnatal period and when the deficient diet was given to pregnant mice shortly after conception (Sun et al., 1974). On the other hand, if the deficient diet was administered to 12-month-old mice for a period of 6 months, only small changes in brain acyl group composition were observed (Sun et al., 1974). When pregnant rats were fed diets supplemented with either safflower oil, which is high in $n - 6$ fatty acids, or with fish oil, which is high in $n - 3$ fatty acids, and the dietary regime was continued in the offspring up to 90 days, brain fatty acids of the $n - 6$ and $n - 3$ families underwent reciprocal replacement according to the type of diet implemented (Galli et al., 1971b). The fish oil diet led to an increase in $n - 3$ fatty acids, whereas the safflower oil diet produced an increase in the $n - 6$ fatty acids. However, the total level of unsaturated fatty acids in PE due to the two types of diets remained relatively constant.

Since the brain phosphoglycerides are highly enriched in polyunsaturated fatty acids, especially those belonging to the $n - 3$ series (Crawford et al., 1982), agents causing peroxidation of the lipids may exert an adverse effect on CNS membrane functions. Eddy and Harman (1977) fed immature rats with diets enriched in 18:3, supplemented with $22:6(n - 3)$ alone or supplemented with menhaden oil, which is high in $22:6(n - 3)$, for various periods of time. All of these dietary supplements caused a linear increase in brain $22:6(n - 3)$ level with time. The effects were less apparent if adult or aged rats were maintained on these diets.

Alling et al. (1973) suspected that the EFA present in the fat depots of pregnant rats are not so readily depleted upon feeding an EFA-deficient diet; thus, a longer induction time might be needed for the deficiency symptoms to develop. To examine this possibility, a dietary scheme consisting of three levels of a mixture of linoleic acid and linolenic acid (4:1 by wt.) in 3.0, 0.75, and 0.14 calorie percent were given to rats for two generations. Rats from the second generation which were on the 0.14 calorie percent diet had lower $n - 3$ fatty acids, especially $22:6(n - 3)$, at all ages. The proportion of $20:3(n - 9)$ in PE of cerebrum also increased most dramatically with the lowest calorie percent group, and with this dietary scheme the appearance of the $n - 9$ fatty acids was detectable in the newborn rats after the first generation. In spite of an obvious change in the acyl group profile, the amounts of brain phospholipids were not apparently altered by the deficient diets (Alling et al., 1974).

3.6.1.2 Linolenic Acid Deficiency

In general, the brain seems to be more vulnerable to dietary alteration from the linolenic-derived fatty acids as compared to the linoleic acid series of fatty acids. Since linolenic acid is not normally as abundant in the diet, there must be a special mechanism for concentrating this type of fatty acid for brain membrane synthesis during the early developmental period. Tinoco et al. (1978) studied the effects of linolenic acid deficiency on rats fed a linolenic acid–deficient diet for two generations. Although the growth rate and organ weights of control and deficient rats were not different, there was a dramatic reduction of $22:6(n - 3)$ in the membrane phosphoglycerides from all body organs including the brain. The decrease in $22:6(n - 3)$ in the phospholipids was mainly compensated for by an increase in the $n - 6$ fatty acids such as $22:5(n - 6)$, $22:4(n - 6)$, and $20:4(n - 6)$. However, in spite of the substantial replacement of one polyunsaturated fatty acid by another, the linolenic acid–deficient animals exhibited no obvious pathological symptoms.

These results suggest that while the elongated and desaturated products of linolenic acid play a structural role in membrane phospholipids, one can further conclude from these experiments that brain membrane functions can be maintained even if $22:6(n - 3)$ is replaced by other structurally similar fatty acids. Therefore, even though brain phosphoglycerides are especially enriched in $n - 3$ fatty acids, the dietary effects due to linolenic acid deficiency are comparable to those due to linoleic acid deficiency (Tinoco et al., 1971). In fact, this raises the question of whether linolenic acid is indeed essential to the body organs.

The essential role of dietary linolenic acid in developing rats was also studied by Lamptey and Walker (1976), who showed that rats fed soybean oil (high in linolenate) had a higher level of $22:6(n - 3)$ and lower level of $22:5(n - 6)$ in the brain PE. However, the nature of the dietary lipid seemed to exert no effect on the physical development and onset of neuromotor coordination in the pups. On the other hand, the performance of adult rats fed the soybean oil diet seemed to be superior to those fed a safflower oil diet.

In the retina, in which the photoreceptor membranes are also highly enriched in $22:6(n - 3)$, Benolken et al. (1973) reported changes in the physiological response of these membranes with respect to a depletion of the $22:6(n - 3)$ due to feeding an EFA-deficient diet. Apparently, linolenic acid deficiency may give rise to deleterious effects in membranes highly enriched with phospholipids containing the $n - 3$ fatty acids.

3.6.1.3   EFA Deficiency in Cells and Brain Subcellular Membranes

The endothelial cells isolated from developing rat brain showed compositional changes in response to dietary lipids which were similar to those in brain tissue (Matheson et al., 1981b). When rats were fed a corn oil diet with a high $18:2/18:3$ ratio, the $n - 3$ fatty acids were decreased and the $n - 6$ fatty acids were increased in the cells. Animals fed a fatty acid–free diet displayed an increase in $n - 9$ fatty acids in the cells, but the $(n - 6)/(n - 3)$ ratios were not changed. These results tend to indicate that cell fractions obtained from developing brain are more responsive to dietary influences than those from adult rats.

The fatty acid changes due to EFA deficiency are also manifested in the brain subcellular membranes (Galli et al., 1972; Sun, 1972; Sun et al., 1974; Karlsson, 1975). Since myelin has an especially high content of monoenoic fatty acids (i.e., $18:1$ and $20:1$), the rate of accretion for these fatty acids is closely correlated to the period of myelin synthesis. In contrast, a drop in $20:1$ level in the EFA-deficient rats is a good indication of a delay in myelin synthesis (Sun, 1972). Using the triene/tetraene ratio as an index for the degree of EFA deficiency, Galli et al. (1972) showed that the myelin membrane attained the highest and the synaptosomal membrane the lowest ratios when rats were fed an EFA deficient diet from birth to 140 days of age. Nevertheless, in Karlsson's (1975) experiment in which rats were fed three dietary levels of EFA-deficient diet (which they described as 3.0, 0.75, and 0.07 calorie percent) for two generations, no obvious differences in lipid composition of brain subcellular fractions were observed among the dietary groups. However, myelin isolated from rats fed the 0.07 calorie percent EFA-deficient diet contained lower proportions of $20:4(n - 6)$ and $22:6(n - 3)$ in the phosphoglycerides as compared to those fed a 3.0 calorie percent diet.

In the synaptic plasma membrane fraction, the group fed the same deficient diet underwent little decrease in $20:4(n - 6)$, although the proportion of $22:6(n - 3)$ was decreased considerably. These results were somewhat different from those obtained by Trapp and Bernsohn (1978) who supplied an EFA-deficient diet to pregnant rats and their offspring up to 120 days of age and found that not only was there a marked alteration of the fatty acid composition of PE, but also morphological changes in the myelin from optic nerve similar to that seen in Wallerian degeneration.

3.6.1.4 *Reversal of EFA Deficiency*

The $n - 9$ fatty acids incorporated into brain membrane phosphoglycerides due to EFA deficiency may be eliminated after replacing the deficient diet by an adequate one. The rate of disappearance of the $n - 9$ fatty acids is more rapid when a replacement is made during brain development than after maturation (Sun et al., 1975). The elimination process actually reflects a constant turnover of the acyl groups of brain membrane phosphoglycerides. The half-lives of $n - 9$ fatty acids in PE of brain microsomal, synaptosomal, and myelin fractions were shown to be respectively, 3, 10, and 15 days in the developing brain and 8–10, 10, and 22 days in the mature brain. The $n - 9$ fatty acids in PEpl showed a slower turnover of 8–12, 28, and 35–40 days, respectively. In general, the turnover of $20:3(n - 9)$ is faster in PC and PI than in PE and PS, whereas PEpl had the slowest turnover rate among the phospholipids examined.

After rats were maintained on a fat-free diet for 120 days, Trapp and Bernsohn (1977) showed that supplementation with either 18:2 or 18:3 for 10 or 30 days could completely reverse the changes in $n - 6$ and $n - 3$ fatty acids. It is worth noting that both linoleic and linolenic acids were equally effective in reducing the $n - 9$ fatty acids. The reversal of the $n - 6$ and $n - 3$ fatty acids seemed to occur prior to an observable decrease in $n - 9$ fatty acids. White et al. (1971b) showed that upon refeeding the EFA-deficient rats with a diet supplemented with corn oil, the $n - 6$ fatty acids could rebound to a level higher than the controls. After feeding a 5% corn oil diet to EFA-deficient rats for 5 weeks, animals attained normal brain weight and lost most of the deficiency symptoms (Odutuga, 1977). Nevertheless, the reduced level of 20:1 in PE and PC, which is an indication of delayed myelin synthesis, did not return completely to the control level. Odutuga (1979) further showed that when rats were maintained on the deficient diet for 37 weeks, a regimen that caused a 33% decrease in brain weight, a 10-week dietary rehabilitation program could restore neither the brain weight nor the changes in brain membrane lipids to normal. Therefore, prolonged feeding of EFA-deficient diets can retard brain maturation and cause irreversible changes in lipid acyl group composition.

3.6.1.5   Metabolism of Brain Phospholipids in EFA Deficiency

In EFA deficiency there is a delay in neuronal maturation and myelin synthesis is reduced. Although myelin synthesis is characterized by an increase in the levels of myelin lipids, especially galactolipids (Karlsson and Svennerholm, 1978; McKenna and Campagnoni, 1979), and hence may be easily followed, a delay in neuronal maturation is often difficult to define biochemically. Studies with labeled precursors indicated differences in isotopic incorporation into myelin phospholipids between controls and EFA-deficient rats (Miller et al., 1981). These investigators further showed that phospholipids containing the $n - 9$ fatty acids actually belong to the long-lived pool. Studies with [^{14}C]acetate indicated that some of the $n - 9$ fatty acids were synthesized in brain in situ, probably via recycling of other acyl groups.

Lyles et al. (1975) showed that EFA-deficient rats were more active in uptake of labeled oleic or arachidonic acids into brain than controls. Furthermore, the fatty acids taken up into the brain of the EFA-deficient rat were retained in the brain for a longer period than the controls. When labeled linolenic acid was injected intracerebrally into control and EFA-deficient rats, the latter were more active in metabolizing and converting the label to the polyunsaturated fatty acids (Dwyer and Bernsohn, 1979a). Labeled linolenic acid was incorporated into neutral lipids as well as phospholipids, but incorporation of label into phospholipids was higher in EFA-deficient rats than in controls (Dwyer and Bernsohn, 1979b). Among the phospholipids, PC was most highly labeled initially, but with increasing time PE and PS + PI also became increasingly labeled. In any case, specific radioactivity of the brain phospholipids in EFA-deprived rats was 2–3 times higher than in controls.

3.6.2   Effects of Perinatal Undernutrition and Protein Malnutrition

Perinatal undernutrition is known to give rise to a striking reduction in body weight, brain weight, and brain lipids (Geison and Waisman, 1970;

Rajalakshmi and Nakhasi, 1974). Ghittoni and Faryna de Raveglia (1972) showed that under these conditions, cerebrosides, cholesterol, and gangliosides in cerebral cortex were significantly reduced, but the levels of PC and PE were only slightly decreased. Rehabilitation from 10 to 20 days could return some of the lipids to their normal values, but the cerebroside level remained low (Ghittoni and Faryna de Raveglia, 1973). The amount of myelin in undernourished rats was lower, but the only consistent change in composition was a reduction in the PEpl content (Fishman et al., 1971). Morphological evidence suggests that the reduction of myelin in undernutrition is a result of delay in the initiation process and a retardation of the biosynthesis of the membrane components (Krigman and Hogan, 1976). Therefore, myelin from the undernourished group exhibited a lipid composition characteristic of immature brain.

As compared to undernutrition, protein malnutrition seems to exert a more direct effect on myelin (Reddy et al., 1979). Myelin reduction due to protein malnutrition (5 versus 25%) was more drastic in the developing brain, and 2′,3′-cyclic nucleotide-3′-phosphohydrolase activity was greatly reduced in gray and white matter (Reddy and Horrocks, 1982). Furthermore, total brain phospholipid was 15% lower than control, and PE and PEpl appeared to be affected most. A lack of phospholipid changes in gray matter suggests that the development of phospholipids in these areas is probably spared from the effects of undernutrition, whereas the lipids in myelin and white matter are obviously affected.

Incorporation of labeled precursor into myelin was depressed 60% in rats undernourished by maternal deprivation (Wiggins et al., 1976). The depressed activity was still obvious after 6 days of a rehabilitation program. Consequently, when rats are subjected to malnutrition during the early stage of life, which is regarded as the critical period of brain development by Dobbing (1968), the brain damage incurred may be irreversible (Pasquini et al., 1981). Wiggins et al. (1976) also showed that malnutrition can result in pronounced reduction in myelin lipids, especially the PEpl, but the nerve endings are relatively unaffected. Yusuf et al. (1981) showed that mice malnourished from birth to 30 days of age formed myelin with an "immature" phospholipid profile, as indicated by a higher proportion of PC and sphingomyelin and a lower proportion of PE. Although rehabilitation from 30 to 60 days could correct the abnormal ganglioside pattern, the cerebroside and phospholipid profiles remained unchanged.

In chronically malnourished infants a reduction in myelin lipids was observed (Fishman et al., 1969). Among these, the reduction of cerebrosides and PEpl was most obvious. When specific brain regions (forebrain, brain stem, and cerebellum) from children who died of severe malnutrition within the first 2 years of life were analyzed (Yusuf et al., 1979), a higher phospholipid–DNA ratio was found in the group of undernourished children under 1 year of age as compared to controls. Sphingomyelin was selectively decreased in all brain regions. However, in the forebrain the level of PS + PI in malnourished children was higher than in controls. These authors suspected that the increase in PS + PI in this brain region may be related to the hyperexcitability of the malnourished children.

Although the content of brain phospholipids was 7–9% less than controls in undernourished rats, there was a 28% increase in ^{32}P incorporation into phospholipids of brain homogenates (Reddy and Sastry, 1978). The increase in labeling was thought to be related to the behavioral alterations resulting from the nutritional deficiency.

The effect of postnatal undernutrition on activity of phosphocholine and phosphoethanolamine transferases in rat brain was investigated (Horrocks and Reddy, 1980). Undernourished suckling rats displayed a 15% reduction of the phospholipids in brain white matter, the reduction in PEpl being most severe. Surprisingly, the phospholipids in gray matter were elevated by 8%. In general, the V_{max} values for the phosphotransferases were higher in the white matter microsomes than in gray matter, and enzyme activity was lower in the undernourished suckling rats than in controls. These investigators attributed the difference in enzymic activity to a decrease in diradylglycerols, which is a rate-limiting substrate for the reaction. In spite of an increase in the amount of phospholipids in the gray matter, activity of the phosphotransferases was lower in the malnourished group as compared to controls. Therefore, the increase in phospholipid in gray matter of the malnourished rats was regarded to be a result of retardation in the phospholipid turnover.

3.6.3   Effects of Other Dietary Abnormalities

Many other dietary changes may influence brain development and directly or indirectly affect brain membrane lipid composition. Hirono and Wada (1978) showed that folic acid deficiency could lead to a decrease in brain weight and myelin yield. Although there was no difference in gross composition among the major lipid components (i.e., cholesterol, glycolipids and phospholipids), the proportions of polyunsaturated fatty acids in myelin phospholipids were lower in the folic acid–deficient group. The results suggest that folic acid may play a role in mediating the fatty acid desaturation and/or chain elongation processes in the developing brain.

Hyperphenylalaninemia can also exert an effect on the lipids of developing brain (Shah and Johnson, 1978). When young (21-day-old) rats were fed phenylalanine and p-chlorophenylalanine daily for 30 days, a significantly lower brain weight and lower myelin yield were observed. The myelin phospholipids also showed a marked reduction in monoenes.

3.7 PHOSPHOLIPID METABOLISM IN BRAIN

3.7.1 Enzymes for Phospholipid Biosynthesis

In contrast to the voluminous amount of information available regarding the compositional changes in brain phospholipids and their acyl groups during development under normal and deficient conditions, descriptions of metabolic changes and enzymes responsible for phospholipid biosynthesis and degradation in the developing and aging brain are still limited. Furthermore, information is scattered and incomplete due to differences in the objectives of the studies.

Carey (1975a) examined the enzymic acylation of glycerol-3-phosphate in microsomes of rabbit brain throughout maturation. The specific activity of glycerol-3-phosphate acyltransferase in brain microsomes increased at the onset of myelination (i.e., around 20 days), reached a high during the active myelination period, and was reduced about 20% from the highest level after reaching maturation. Activity of palmitoyl-CoA synthetase, which activates free fatty acids to their acyl-CoA derivatives, showed a similar developmental profile. However, a different pattern was observed when incorporation *in vitro* of labeled palmitate into phospholipids (mainly phosphatidate) was examined with respect to the different stages of postnatal development. In this study the highest level of incorporation was measured in the fetal and 5-day-old brain. The fatty acid synthetase, which is responsible for *de novo* biosynthesis of fatty acid from acetate, was found most active in the soluble fraction of brain homogenates at 5 days of age (Cantrill and Carey, 1975). The accessibility of lipid substrates to different membrane enzymes may have been a problem in these studies. Indeed, this should always be taken into account in investigations *in vitro* of enzyme activity.

In the brain excess acyl-CoA is readily hydrolyzed by acyl-CoA hydrolase, which is highly active in the cytosolic fraction (Srere et al., 1959; Anderson and Erwin, 1971). The specific activity of this enzyme in rat brain cytosol increases with age, reaches a peak around 15–20 days, and then decreases by 20–30% in the adult (Smith and Sun, 1981). When labeled oleoyl-CoA was used as substrate, activity of the oleoyl-CoA: 1-acyl-GP acyltransferase and oleoyl-CoA: 1-acyl-GPC acyltransferase in brain microsomes showed similar developmental changes. Specific activity remained constant from birth to 20 days and then increased to a peak at 30 days before declining to a lower level (70% of maximum) at 3 months of age (Smith and Sun, 1981). It is concluded from this study that enzymes involved in acyl-CoA metabolism (i.e., hydrolysis and transfer) are most active in the period of active myelination. Enzyme activity normally declines somewhat after this period and remains constant after maturation.

The activity of CDP-ethanolamine: 1,2-diacylglycerol ethanolamine phosphotransferase of rat brain increased from birth to the 16th day and then decreased (Ansell and Metcalfe, 1971). The developmental profile appeared to reflect the availability of diacylglycerols for the reaction. In the chick brain the specific activity of CDP-choline: 1,2-diacylglycerol choline phosphotransferase increased from the 10th day of embryonic life to reach a maximum at hatching and then decreased thereafter (Freysz et al., 1972). These investigators believe that several isozymes catalyze the reaction, one of which is induced at the onset of myelination. Specific activity of the ethanolamine phosphotransferase in chick brain doubled around hatching, which is a period of intense myelination, and reached adult level at 4 days of age (Freysz et al., 1980). The change in apparent K_m of the enzyme with respect to development also suggests that a new isozyme may appear during the initiation of myelination. Similar elevation of choline phosphotransferase and ethanolamine phosphotransferase activities were observed in rabbit cerebrum from 19 days gestation to 2 months of postnatal development (Fimbres et al., 1980). The specific activity of the choline phosphotransferase is normally three- to fourfold higher than that of the ethanolamine phosphotransferase, and diacyl, alkenylacyl, and alkylacylglycerols are substrates for both enzymes.

When the biosynthesis of PE and PC via CDP-choline or CDP-ethanolamine: diacylglycerol phosphotransferase was compared in young (2-month-old) and older (18-month-old) rats, enzymic activity was lower in the older age group (Brunetti et al., 1979). The decrease in enzymic activity in the older animals could be restored by addition of exogenous diacylglycerols. Their results again indicate that a limitation in available substrate may be the major reason for the apparent age-related change in enzymic activity.

When neuronal- and glial-rich cells were isolated from rat brain, the rate of PC biosynthesis in neuronal cell homogenates decreased with increasing age of the animals, but no such age change in activity was found for the glial enzyme system (Gaiti et al., 1981). The decrease in neuronal PC biosynthesis with age was again correlated with a decrease in endogenous diacylglycerols in the neurons but not the glial cells. The investigators concluded that the availability of endogenous diacylglycerols is an important rate-determining factor in the biosynthesis of choline and ethanolamine phosphoglycerides during brain development and aging.

In addition to the *de novo* pathway for phospholipid biosynthesis with phosphatidate and diacylglycerol as intermediates, other reactions of phospholipid metabolism have been investigated with respect to development-related changes. Natarajan and Sastry (1974) studied the activities of brain acyltransferases as a function of age. Using ^{32}P-labeled 1-acyl, 1-alkyl, and 1-alkenylglycerophosphorylethanolamine (GPE), these investigators showed that enzymes for transferring acyl groups to these substrates in brain microsomes increased in activity with age. In the 22-day-old rat brain the order of activity toward the three types of substrates is 1-acyl-GPE > 1-alkenyl-GPE > 1-alkyl-GPE in crude mitochondria and 1-acyl-GPE > 1-alkyl-GPE > 1-alkenyl-GPE in the microsomes.

The biosynthesis *in vivo* of choline and ethanolamine phosphoglycerides in different brain regions was examined in rats of different age groups (Gaiti et al., 1982). In this study mixtures of labeled lipid precursors were injected into the lateral ventricles of rat brain. A significant decrease in the biosynthesis of phospholipids in cerebral cortex and striatum with aging was observed, but no significant change was detected in the cerebellum. The decrease in activity was apparent at 9 months of age but did not change thereafter. These age-related changes were more obvious for PC than for PE.

3.7.2 Turnover of Brain Membrane Phospholipids during Development

Previous studies of phospholipid metabolism during brain development have been largely centered on the mechanism of myelination. In rodents myelination occurs during early postnatal development. Using various radioactive precursors injected into the lateral ventricles of rat brain, label was found to be incorporated into both myelin and microsomal phospholipids, although labeling of the microsomal lipids was much higher (Sun and Horrocks, 1973). When ^{32}P$_i$ was injected into 10-day-old rat brain, specific radioactivity of the phospholipids in microsomes reached a peak shortly after injection, but the rate of incorporation into myelin lipids tended to follow a slower course (Jungalwala and Dawson, 1971). Nevertheless, after reaching a maximum, both types of membranes showed turnover of the acid-soluble phosphorus-containing compounds at comparable rates. The results suggest that a substantial portion of the phospholipid molecules in adult myelin membranes is readily exchangeable, although a small pool of more slowly exchangeable material also exists.

Miller and Morell (1978) compared the turnover of myelin lipid components of 3-month-old and 17-day-old rats using [^{3}H]glycerol, [methyl-^{14}C]choline, and [U-^{14}C]glucose as precursors. Their results, especially those using labeled glycerol as precursor, also supported the presence of phospholipids with slow and fast turnover pools in myelin of the 17-day-old rats. Although lipid turnover in myelin was, in general, slower than in microsomes, the difference was not so obvious in developing as compared to adult rats. The findings in this investigation also indicated that different moieties of the phospholipid molecule could have different turnover rates.

Pasquini et al. (1979) showed that both myelin and myelinlike fractions from rat brain undergo changes in chemical composition, enzymic activity, and PC turnover during maturation. These authors believe that although a precursor–product relationship exists between these two fractions, they are undergoing metabolic changes independently during the developmental period. The study of labeled choline injected intracranially into 5-day-old brain indicated that myelin PC displayed a more rapid turnover during the developmental period than after maturation (Pasquini et al., 1979).

3.7.3 Incorporation of Fatty Acids into Brain Phosphoglycerides

Since a large proportion of the fatty acids in brain phospholipids are polyunsaturated, especially in the early postnatal period, metabolism of those phospholipid species possessing unsaturated acyl group species must be of special significance to the developmental process. Most of the polyunsaturated fatty acids are 20 and 22 carbon chain lengths, and only trace amounts of the EFA (18:2 and 18:3) are present in brain phosphoglycerides (see previous sections). Much evidence has accumulated to show that the brain is capable of converting essential fatty acids to long-chain polyunsaturated fatty acids after uptake from the circulation (see Naughton, 1981, for a review). Crawford et al. (1982) suggested that as fatty acids are transported from liver to the placenta, there is a selective concentration of the long-chain polyunsaturated fatty acids with resultant exclusion of the EFA. Another explanation for the low level of EFA in brain is the existence of an active desaturation and elongation system so that the EFA are rapidly converted to the longer-chain polyunsaturated fatty acids.

When labeled linolenic acid was injected intraperitoneally into young rats (12–13 days old), the fatty acid was maximally taken up by brain 8 h after injection (Dhopeshwarkar and Subramanian, 1975). These investigators further showed that considerable amounts of the labeled phospholipids were undergoing turnover between 48 h and 15 days after injection of the precursor. The results indicate that brain phospholipid acyl groups are undergoing active turnover even at a time when lipid biosynthesis is maximal. Stearic acid subcutaneously injected into developing rats was shown to be partially taken up by the brain and then metabolized either by elongation, desaturation, or resynthesis (Gozlan-Devillierre et al., 1978). The transformed fatty acids were subsequently incorporated into phospholipids of brain subcellular membranes. The uptake of stearate into rat brain phospholipids increased during development up to 18 days of age and then decreased thereafter. Stearic acid was preferentially incorporated into PC (30%) and PE (22%), but some of the label also appeared in cholesterol (8–15%), indicating that fatty acid degradation and reincorporation of label occurred (Gozlan-Devillierre et al., 1978). The pattern of distribution among phospholipids, however, seemed to vary somewhat with age. Thus, peak incorporation of the fatty acid into PC took place at 15 days, that into PE at 18 days, and that into PS + PI at 21 days. When labeled linolenic acid was fed to rats, this fatty acid was transported to brain and was directly elongated and desaturated to $22:6(n - 3)$ without appreciable breakdown and resynthesis (Dhopeshwarkar et al., 1971). These results show that the saturated fatty acids in brain are primarily utilized in breakdown and resynthesis processes, whereas the EFA may be largely elongated and desaturated to furnish the necessary content of polyunsaturated fatty acids of brain membranes.

When labeled stearic acid was injected intracerebrally into the developing mouse brain, a large portion of the precursor fatty acid was incorporated into membrane phospholipids within 1 h after injection (Wise et al., 1979). During this time a portion of the stearic acid was desaturated to oleate, and the newly formed oleate was rapidly incorporated into the membrane phosphoglycerides. The rate of conversion of stearate to oleate decreased steadily with age (4–45 days). Although these studies again indicate that enzymes for desaturation and elongation of fatty acids are active in brain (Brenner, 1971; Cook, 1978a), attempts to study this enzymic process have met with problems because most enzymes for metabolic conversion of the fatty acids are membrane bound and the entire conversion sequence occurs within the membrane matrix itself (Aeberhard et al., 1981). Consequently, studies using exogenous lipid substrates may give results different from those in which endogenous substrates are employed. It should be noted that mechanisms also exist whereby brain can utilize acetate derived from breakdown of glucose for *de novo* biosynthesis of fatty acids (Carey, 1975b). Such fatty acids synthesized *de novo* seemed to be more readily elongated, desaturated, and incorporated into the membrane phospholipids (Dhopeshwarkar and Subramanian, 1977). However, an age relationship of the fatty acid metabolism *de novo* has not been studied.

After intracerebral injection the rate of incorporation of arachidonate into brain membrane phospholipids was more rapid than the saturated

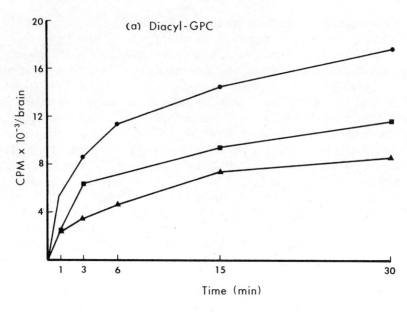

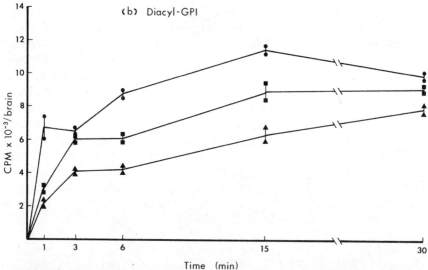

FIGURE 3.1 Incorporation of [1-^{14}C]arachidonate into (*a*) PC, (*b*) PI and (*c*) diacylglycerols of mouse brain during development. Groups of mice at 1 day (bottom), 1 week (middle), and 4 weeks (top) of age were injected intracerebrally with [1-^{14}C]arachidonate (1 μCi each). Animals were sacrificed at the time indicated and brain lipids were analyzed by two-dimensional TLC and radioactivity of individual lipids in the three age groups at various times after injection was measured.

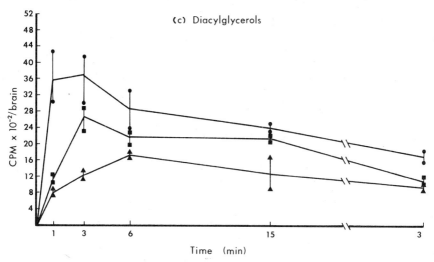

FIGURE 3.1   (*continued*)

fatty acids such as stearate (Sun, 1977). Both saturated and unsaturated fatty acids were incorporated into the phospholipids of brain subcellular fractions, including myelin (Sun, 1973; Sun and Horrocks, 1973; Sun and Yau, 1976b), although a more rapid turnover of the phospholipids with an arachidonoyl group was found in the microsomal and synaptosomal fractions (Sun and Su, 1979). Arachidonate was preferentially taken up into PC and PI in all subcellular membranes (Yau and Sun, 1974). We have also examined the metabolism of [^{14}C]arachidonate injected intracerebrally into mouse brain during the developmental period (Su and Sun, unpublished data).

As shown in Figure 3.1, arachidonate uptake by PC resulted in a smooth curve which increased with time up to 30 min after injection. The gradual increase in uptake was similar at all ages. The uptake of label by PI indicated two rates, a rapid uptake, which occurred between 1 and 3 min, and a less rapid uptake similar to that by PC. By 4 weeks of age the biphasic uptake of arachidonate into PI was apparent. The initial phase of incorporation was extremely rapid, and significant label was found in PI within 1 min after injection of the precursor. The incorporation of arachidonate into diacylglycerols (DG) during development followed a course similar to that for PI. In fact, the appearance of a rapid-uptake phenomenon was apparent at 1 week of age, and at 4 weeks of age peak labeling was observed at 1 and 3 min after injection.

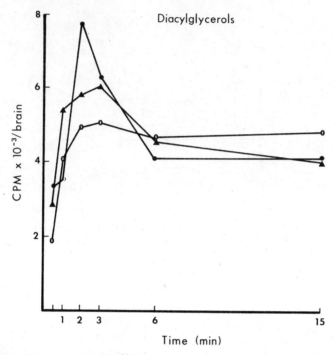

FIGURE 3.2 Incorporation of [1-¹⁴C]arachidonate into diacylglycerols of mouse brain at 16, 20, and 24 days of age. Experimental procedure was the same as described in Figure 3.1.

Unlike the PI, radioactivity in DG started to decline after 6 min, and this metabolism occurred in all three age groups. When the rapid uptake of labeled arachidonate by PI and DG was further examined in mice at 16, 20, and 24 days of age, which is a period corresponding to rapid myelination and synaptogenesis, similar metabolic profiles were found. The DG from all three age groups displayed peak uptake activity around 3 min after intracerebral injection of labeled arachidonate (Fig. 3.2).

The biphasic uptake of arachidonate into PI reflects the presence of two metabolic pathways for labeling of PI, namely the acylation via lysophospholipid: acyl-CoA acyltransferase and *de novo* biosynthesis via PA and CDP-diacylglycerol. Apparently, the uptake via acyltransferase is the more rapid of the two. The results have also provided evidence for a metabolic relationship *in vivo* between the arachidonoyl groups in PI and DG. The appearance of this metabolic relationship seems to coincide with the time of synaptogenesis. The conversion of PI to DG is known to be mediated by the PI-dependent phospholipase C, which is highly active in brain (see Chapter 2). Results of the *in vivo* study suggest that the metabolic relationship results from an increase in activity of this enzyme during brain development.

There is not much information regarding the metabolic turnover of brain membrane phospholipids during aging. In our laboratory we showed that there is a 20% decrease in the relative specific radioactivity of the lysophospholipid: acyl-CoA acyltransferase in brain synaptosomes in the 24-month-old group as compared to the 8-month-old group (Sun, unpublished data). This result reflects a retardation of phospholipid turnover. In another study labeled palmitate was injected intracerebrally, and its incorporation into mouse brain phospholipids was examined in animals 3, 10, and 28 months of age (Sun, 1971). In each age group mice were sacrificed at 1–40 min after injection. The extent of uptake of fatty acid by the phospholipids was highest in the 3-month-old group and lowest in the 28-month-old group. However, the rate of labeled palmitate incorporation into phospholipids was similar among the three age groups. Results from this study again demonstrated the decrease in enzyme activity with respect to aging. A better understanding of the mechanisms involved in membrane phospholipid turnover may help to elucidate some aspects of the pathological conditions associated with the aged brain, since most of these conditions result from disturbances of metabolic processes.

3.7.4   Incorporation of *Trans*-unsaturated Fatty Acids into Brain Phosphoglycerides

Cook (1978b) compared the incorporation of elaidic acid (*trans*) and oleic acid (*cis*) into phospholipids of 10-day-old and adult rat brain. He found that the rates and extent of incorporation of the *trans*-unsaturated fatty acids into complex lipids were similar to the *cis*-unsaturated ones. A large proportion of both types of labels was incorporated into brain PC at 4–8 h after injection. However, elaidic acid was mainly incorporated into the 1-position of phospholipids, whereas oleate was incorporated into both. The phospholipids containing the elaidate also underwent a substantial turnover. These results indicate that although the developing brain does not exclude the incorporation of *trans*-unsaturated fatty acids into the phospholipids, the metabolic machinery may treat the nonnaturally occurring fatty acids differently after they enter the membrane.

When incorporation and metabolism of the *trans*-isomers of 18-carbon dienoic fatty acids by the developing rat brain were examined, Cook (1980) found that the incorporation of *trans,trans*-18:2 acid into phosphoglycerides and triacylglycerols was slower than the *cis,cis*-18:2 acid. In ad-

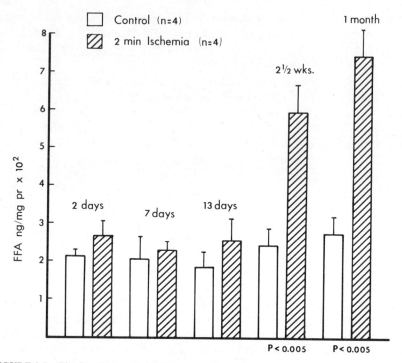

FIGURE 3.3 The free fatty acid (FFA) content in rat cerebral cortex and the FFA released due to a 2-min postdecapitative ischemia treatment with respect to age during brain development. For each age group ($n = 8$), four animals were subjected to the ischemia treatment. Results are means $\pm$ SD of the FFA expressed as ng/mg protein from the cerebral cortex. Analysis of variance indicates that FFA values in ischemic brain samples from the 2.5-week-old and 1-month-old rats are significantly different from the matched-age controls, $p < 0.005$.

dition, desaturation and elongation *in vivo* of the *trans,trans*-18:2 by brain enzymes were less extensive than for the *cis,cis*-diene acid. The *trans,trans*-18:2 was preferentially esterified to the 1-position of the phosphoglycerides, whereas the *cis,cis*-18:2 was incorporated exclusively in the 2-position. These results, plus the fact that more *trans,trans*-18:2 was incorporated into triacylglycerols and less into PC, suggest that the *trans,trans*-acid is metabolized similarly to saturated fatty acids by brain tissue.

3.7.5   Release of Free Fatty Acids from Membrane Phospholipids

Stimulation such as that induced by ischemia, edema, and electroconvulsive shock is known to elicit a release of free fatty acids (FFA) from brain phosphoglycerides (Bazan, 1970, 1971; De Medio et al., 1980; Tang and Sun, 1982). The FFA in brain are maintained in a dynamic equilibrium with the phosphoglycerides, the metabolism of which in turn are mediated by a number of enzymic pathways (Sun et al., 1979). Many factors affecting the equilibrium can result in an increase in FFA. However, the increase in brain FFA due to postdecapitative ischemia is not found in the early postnatal period (Bazan, 1976). Instead, the FFA release phenomenon starts to develop in the rat brain between 2–3 weeks of age (Fig. 3.3) (Tang and Sun, unpublished data). After this period the brain becomes highly susceptible to the ischemic insult. We conclude that the appearance of the FFA release phenomenon is a biochemical event associated with synaptogenesis. Experiments with labeled linoleate also showed that exposure of 4-day-old rats to hypoxic and ischemic conditions does not apparently alter the incorporation of the fatty acid into brain phospholipids, whereas an obvious decrease in incorporation was manifested in older animals subjected to similar treatments (Strosznajder, 1980).

Relatively little is known about phospholipid degradative enzymes with respect to brain development and aging, although it is becoming obvious that the degradative enzymes play an important role in metabolic turnover of membrane lipid components. Since brain phospholipids are undergoing turnover even during the period of active lipid synthesis, the enzymes responsible for breakdown may follow the same course as the biosynthetic enzymes during development and aging. An example of this is the lysoplasmalogenase, a microsomal enzyme that liberates aldehydes from lysoplasmalogens. This enzyme was shown to be active in developing brain and exhibited a peak activity at 21 days (Gunawan and Debuch, 1982).

3.8   CONCLUSIONS

1.   Although nearly all of the phospholipids are increasing in absolute concentration during development of the nervous tissue, the proportions of individual phospholipids change characteristically during development due to differences in the rate of accretion. The deposition of specific phospholipids may be associated with specific neurochemical events. For example, sphingomyelin and PEpl, which are highly enriched in the myelin, increase dramatically relative to the other phospholipids during the period of rapid myelination.

2.   The age at which specific phospholipid changes occur among animal species is a function of the degree of development at the time of birth. Thus, the myelin lipids of rat brain increase most rapidly between

10 and 20 days after birth, whereas in guinea pig brain this increase is obvious immediately after birth.

3. In whole brain the proportion of PC decreases, PE increases moderately, while PS and PI remain relatively constant. Sphingomyelin, PEpl, and polyphosphoinositides increase several-fold in a relatively short period of time. The pattern for rabbit brain seems to be different from human and rodents. In general, the proportions of individual phospholipids remain constant or decline slightly after maturation and during aging.

4. The concentration of total lipid phosphorus is highest in brain stem, intermediate in cerebrum, and lowest in cerebellum. The pattern of change in individual phosphoglycerides during fetal development is similar in all three brain regions, but the pattern for brain stem differs during postnatal development. The general trends of whole brain are found in the individual brain regions. Cerebral white matter shows relatively larger changes in PC, PS, and sphingomyelin as compared to gray matter.

5. The phospholipid compositions of neurons and glial cells are similar and remain relatively unchanged throughout development and aging. Capillary endothelial cell phospholipids reflect the changes found in total brain.

6. The myelin lipids seem to vary among species more than other subcellular fractions. The amount of human myelin decreases during aging, whereas rat myelin continues to increase beyond maturity. Phospholipids comprise 40–57% of the total lipid in myelin. The main constituent is PE, and a large proportion of that is in the plasmalogen form. During development in the human, PC decreases 30% and sphingomyelin increases twofold. Total PE remains relatively constant, but PEpl increases slightly. In rat PEpl increases continuously and sphingomyelin does not vary. An immature myelin fraction resembling the lipid composition of cellular membranes is found in very young rats. The composition of microsomal phospholipids in brain does not seem to vary much with age.

7. The ratios of different fatty acids from total phosphoglycerides can be used as an index of maturation. Each phospholipid class has a specific acyl group profile that undergoes distinct changes during maturation according to species and brain region. These changes during development may affect membrane properties and fluidity and therefore enzyme and receptor functions.

8. The concentration of phospholipid in spinal cord is higher than in brain at all ages and increases throughout maturation. Spinal cord is enriched in PEpl, which increases significantly during development (as does sphingomyelin) to become the predominant phospholipid. The acyl groups of PC, PE, and PEpl in both myelin and microsomes of rat spinal cord show marked changes in proportions during development.

9.   Rabbit peripheral nerve (sciatic nerve) has nearly equal proportions of PC, PEpl, and sphingomyelin (27% each). The latter two lipids increase during development, while PC and diacyl-PE decrease. Significant changes in the fatty acyl composition of PC and PE have been observed.

10.   An EFA-deficient diet imposed on pregnant rats can result in a change in phospholipids and their acyl group composition in brain of the developing pups. Dietary deficiency is induced more readily when initiated at the early postnatal age than after maturation. Brain lipid changes produced by the EFA-deficient diet are also more readily reversible during the developmental period than after maturation.

11.   Both undernutrition and protein malnutrition affect brain development and synthesis of the myelin lipids. Under these conditions, the compositions of PE and PEpl are most altered.

12.   Enzymes for fatty acid synthesis *de novo* and fatty acid desaturation and elongation are most active at birth. Enzymes for acyl-CoA hydrolysis and acyl transfer to phospholipids are most active during the period of active myelination and synaptogenesis.

13.   Activity of CDP-ethanolamine(choline): 1,2-diacylglycerol ethanolamine(choline) phosphotransferase in rat brain increases from birth to 3 weeks of age and then decreases. These enzymes are thought to be present in the form of isozymes, one of which is induced at the onset of myelination. The availability of endogenous diacylglycerols is a rate-determining factor in the biosynthesis of choline and ethanolamine phosphoglycerides during development and aging.

14.   Regional differences exist in the biosynthesis of phospholipids in brain. The age-related changes are more obvious for PC than for PE.

15.   During brain development myelin phospholipids are present in pools with slow and fast turnover rates. The phosphatidylcholines in myelin seem to display a more rapid turnover during brain development than after maturation.

16.   Fatty acids injected intracerebrally into the rodent brain are rapidly taken up by the phospholipids. Incorporation of fatty acids into phospholipids in rat brain increases during development up to 18 days of age before declining to a steady level at adult age.

17.   Although the developing brain does not exclude the incorporation of *trans*-unsaturated fatty acids into phospholipids, differences in metabolism exist after these fatty acids are incorporated into the membrane lipids.

18.   Labeled arachidonate is incorporated into phospholipids of all subcellular fractions in mouse brain. A metabolic relationship is observed

between the arachidonoyl groups of PI and DG. Appearance of this relationship seems to coincide with the time of synaptogenesis.

19.   Most phospholipid-metabolizing enzymes decrease in activity during aging.

20.   Free fatty acids are released from brain phosphoglycerides, and the release process is affected by many pathophysiological factors. However, newborn rats up to 17 days of age are more resistant to FFA release due to ischemic insult than the mature rats. The FFA release phenomenon is therefore regarded as another event associated with synaptogenesis.

3.9   SUMMARY

Development of the central nervous system can be categorized into three broad stages: (1) establishment of cell populations and neuronal multiplication; (2) axonal and dendritic growth, glial multiplication; and (3) myelination and general brain growth (Davison and Dobbing, 1968). These developmental processes are accompanied by biochemical changes, including alterations of the lipid composition of the nervous system. The membrane phospholipids undergo distinct changes in both absolute quantity and relative proportion throughout maturation and even during aging. The acyl group profiles of the individual phospholipids also show large changes throughout development. The patterns of change may vary according to the time of birth in relation to brain growth in different animal species and also according to the regions of the nervous system studied.

The phospholipid developmental patterns can be influenced by many factors, particularly dietary alterations. The effects of EFA deficiency, perinatal undernutrition, protein malnutrition, and other nutritional factors on lipid composition during development have been reviewed. Some of the compositional alterations can be reversed by dietary rehabilitation, but apparently others are not. Both induction of deficiency symptoms and reversal of the changes are affected by the age during which these events are imposed.

The biochemical events leading to lipid compositional changes during development and aging are complex and difficult to dissociate from each other. We have reviewed the available data on enzymes of phospholipid metabolism and metabolic changes occurring during development and aging. This is an area of developmental neurochemistry that should be investigated more fully.

ACKNOWLEDGMENT

The authors thank Diane Torres for her expert secretarial assistance in the preparation of the manuscript.

REFERENCES

Aeberhard, E.E., Gan-Elepano, M., and Mead, J.F., *Lipids, 16*, 705–713 (1981).

Alling, C., and Karlsson, I., *J. Neurochem., 21*, 1051–1057 (1973).

Alling, C., Bruce, A., Karlsson, I., and Svennerholm, L., in C. Galli, G. Jacini, and A. Pecile, Eds., *Dietary Lipids and Postnatal Development*, Raven Press, New York, 1973, pp. 203–214.

Alling, C., Bruce, A., Karlsson, I., and Svennerholm, L., *J. Neurochem., 23*, 1263–1270 (1974).

Altrock, K., and Debuch, H., *J. Neurochem., 15*, 1351–1359 (1968).

Anderson, A.D., and Erwin, V.G., *J. Neurochem., 18*, 1179–1186 (1971).

Ansell, G.B., and Metcalfe, R.F., *J. Neurochem., 18*, 647–665 (1971).

Ansell, G.B., and Spanner, S., *Biochem. J., 79*, 176–184 (1961).

Baker, R.R., *Can. J. Biochem., 57*, 378–384 (1979).

Balakrishnan, S., Goodwin, H., and Cumings, J.N., *J. Neurochem., 8*, 276–284 (1961).

Ballabriga, A., and Martinez, M., *Brain Res., 159*, 363–370 (1978).

Banik, N.L., and Davison, A.N., *Biochem. J., 115*, 1051–1062 (1969).

Bazan, N.G., *Biochim. Biophys. Acta, 218*, 1–10 (1970).

Bazan, N.G., *Acta Physiol. Latinoam., 21*, 15–20 (1971).

Bazan, N.G., in G. Porcellati, L. Amaducci, and C. Galli, Eds., *Function and Metabolism of Phospholipids in the Central and Peripheral Nervous Systems*, Plenum Press, New York, 1976, pp. 317–335.

Benolken, R.M., Anderson, R.E., and Wheeler, T.G., *Science, 182*, 1253–1254 (1973).

Berlet, H.H., and Volk, B., in L. Amaducci, A.N. Davison, and P. Antuono, Eds., *Aging of the Brain and Dementia*, Raven Press, New York, 1980, pp. 81–90.

Biran, L.A., and Bartley, W., *Biochem. J., 79*, 159–176 (1961).

Brante, G., *Acta Physiol. Scand. (Suppl. 63), 18*, 1–189 (1949).

Brenner, R.R., *Lipids, 6*, 567–575 (1971).

Brunetti, M., Gaiti, A., and Porcellati, G., *Lipids, 14*, 925–931 (1979).

Cantrill, R.C., and Carey, E.M., *Biochim. Biophys. Acta, 380*, 165–175 (1975).

Carey, E.M., *Biochim. Biophys. Acta, 398*, 231–243 (1975a).

Carey, E.M., *J. Neurochem., 24*, 237–244 (1975b).

Clausen, J., Christensen, L.H.O., and Anderson, H., *J. Neurochem., 12*, 599–606 (1965).

Cook, H.W., *J. Neurochem., 30*, 1327–1334 (1978a).

Cook, H.W., *Biochim. Biophys. Acta, 531*, 245–256 (1978b).

Cook, H.W., *Can. J. Biochem., 58*, 121–127 (1980).

Crawford, C.G., and Wells, M.A., *Lipids, 14*, 757–762 (1979).

Crawford, M.A., Hassam, A.G., and Stevens, P.A., *Prog. Lipid Res., 20*, 31–40 (1982).

Crawford, M.A., Hassam, A.G., Williams, G., and Whitehouse, W., in N.G. Bazan, R.R. Brenner, and N.M. Giusto, Eds., *Advances in Experimental Medicine and Biology*, Vol. 83, *Function and Biosynthesis of Lipids*, Plenum Press, New York, 1977, pp. 135–143.

Cumings, J.N., Goodwin, H., Woodward, E.M., and Curzon, G., *J. Neurochem., 2*, 289–294 (1958).

Cuzner, M.L., and Davison, A.N., *Biochem. J., 106*, 29–34 (1968).

Dalal, K.B., and Einstein, E.R., *Brain Res., 16*, 441–451 (1969).

Davison, A.N., and Dobbing, J., in A.N. Davison and J. Dobbing, Eds., *Applied Neurochemistry*, Blackwell Scientific Publications, Oxford, 1968, pp. 253–286.

Davison, A.N., and Wajda, M., *J. Neurochem., 4*, 353–359 (1959).

Davison, A.N., Cuzner, M.L., Banik, N.L., and Oxberry, J.M., *Nature, 212*, 1373–1374 (1966).

Dekaban, A.S., Patton, V.M., and Cain, D.F., *J. Neurochem., 18*, 2451–2459 (1971).

De Medio, G.E., Gorracci, G., Horrocks, L.A., Lazarewicz, J.W., Mazzari, S., Porcellati, G., Strosznajder, J., and Trovarelli, G., *Ital. J. Biochem., 29*, 412–432 (1980).

De Sousa, B.N., and Horrocks, L.A., *Dev. Neurosci., 2*, 122–128 (1979).

Dhopeshwarkar, G.A., and Subramanian, C., *Lipids, 10*, 242–247 (1975).

Dhopeshwarkar, G.A., and Subramanian, C., *Lipids, 12*, 762–764 (1977).

Dhopeshwarkar, G.A., Subramanian, C., and Mead, J.F., *Biochim. Biophys. Acta, 239*, 162–167 (1971).

Dobbing, J., in A.N. Davison and J. Dobbing, Eds., *Applied Neurochemistry*, Blackwell Scientific Publications, Oxford, 1968, pp. 287–316.

Dwyer, B.E., and Bernsohn, J., *Biochim. Biophys. Acta, 575*, 309–317 (1979a).

Dwyer, B.E., and Bernsohn, J., *J. Neurochem., 32*, 833–838 (1979b).

Eddy, D.E., and Harman, D., *J. Amer. Gerontol. Soc., 25*, 220–229 (1977).

Eichberg, J., and Hauser, G., *Biochim. Biophys. Acta, 144*, 415–422 (1967).

Eichberg, J., and Hauser, G., *Biochim. Biophys. Acta, 326*, 210–223 (1973).

Eng, L.F., and Noble, E.P., *Lipids, 3*, 157–162 (1968).

Eng, L.F., Chao, F.C., Gerstl, B., Pratt, D., and Tavaststjerna, M.G., *Biochemistry, 7*, 4455–4464 (1968).

Erickson, N.E., and Lands, W.E., *Proc. Soc. Expt. Biol. Med., 102*, 512–514 (1959).

Fillerup, D.L., and Mead, J.F., *Lipids, 2*, 295–298 (1967).

Fimbres, E., Saenz, R., Smith, N., and Percy, A.K., *J. Neurosci. Res., 5*, 431–438 (1980).

Fishman, M.A., Agrawal, H.C., Alexander, A., Golterman, J., Martenson, R.E., and Mitchell, R.F., *J. Neurochem., 24*, 689–694 (1975).

Fishman, M.A., Madyastha, P., and Prensky, A.L., *Lipids, 6*, 458–465 (1971).

Fishman, M.A., Prensky, A.L., and Dodge, P.R., *Nature, 221*, 552–553 (1969).

Folch-Pi, J., in H. Waelsch, Ed., *Biochemistry of the Developing Nervous System*, Academic Press, New York, 1955, pp. 121–136.

Freysz, L., Horrocks, L.A., and Mandel, P., *J. Neurochem., 34*, 963–969 (1980).

Freysz, L., Lastennet, A., and Mandel, P., *J. Neurochem., 19*, 2599–2605 (1972).

Gaiti, A., Brunetti, M., Piccinin, G.L., Woelk, H., and Porcellati, G., *Lipids, 17,* 291–296 (1982).

Gaiti, A., Sitkievicz, D., Brunetti, M., and Porcellati, G., *Neurochem. Res., 6,* 13–22 (1981).

Galli, C., and Cecconi, D., *Lipids, 2,* 76–82 (1967).

Galli, C., Trzeciak, H.E., and Paoletti, R., *Biochim. Biophys. Acta, 248,* 449–454 (1971b).

Galli, C., Trzeciak, H.I., and Paoletti, R., *J. Neurochem., 19,* 1863–1867 (1972).

Galli, C., White, H.B., and Paoletti, R., *J. Neurochem., 17,* 347–355 (1970).

Galli, C., White, H.B., and Paoletti, R., *Lipids, 6,* 378–387 (1971a).

Geison, R.L., and Waisman, H.A., *J. Nutr., 100,* 315–324 (1970).

Gerstl, B., Eng, L.F., Hayman, R.B., Tavaststjerna, M.G., and Bond, P.R., *J. Neurochem., 14,* 661–670 (1967).

Ghittoni, N.E., and Faryna de Raveglia, I.A., *Neurobiology, 2,* 41–51 (1972).

Ghittoni, N.E., and Faryna de Raveglia, I.A., *J. Neurochem., 21,* 983–987 (1973).

Gozlan-Devillierre, N., Baumann, N., and Bourre, J.M., *Dev. Neurosci., 1,* 153–158 (1978).

Gunawan, J., and Debuch, H., *J. Neurochem., 39,* 693–699 (1982).

Hauser, G., and Eichberg, J., *Biochim. Biophys. Acta, 326,* 201–209 (1973).

Heipertz, R., Pilz, H., and Scholz, W., *J. Neurol., 216,* 57–65 (1977).

Hirono, H., and Wada, Y., *J. Nutr., 108,* 766–772 (1978).

Hofteig, J.H., Phung, N.V., Yates, A.J., Leon, K.S., *J. Neurochem., 39,* 401–408 (1982).

Holman, R.T., in R.T. Holman, Ed., *Progress in Chemistry of Fats and Other Lipids,* Vol. 9, Part 2, Pergamon Press, Oxford, 1968, pp. 279–348.

Horrocks, L.A., *J. Neurochem., 15,* 483–488 (1968).

Horrocks, L.A., in D.H. Ford, Ed., *Progress in Brain Research,* Vol. 40, *Neurobiological Aspects of Maturation and Aging,* Elsevier Scientific, Amsterdam, 1973, pp. 383–395.

Horrocks, L.A., and Reddy, T.S., in C. Di Benedetta, R. Balasz, G. Gombos, and G. Porcellati, Eds., *Multidisciplinary Approach to Brain Development,* Elsevier/North Holland Biomedical Press, Amsterdam, 1980, pp. 343–345.

Horrocks, L.A., Sun, G.Y., and D'Amato, R.A., in J.M. Ordy and K.R. Brizzee, Eds., *Neurobiology of Aging,* Plenum Press, New York, 1975, pp. 359–367.

Horrocks, L.A., Van Rollins, M., and Yates, A.J., in A.N. Davison and R.H.S. Thompson, Eds., *The Molecular Basis of Neuropathology,* Edward Arnold Publishers, London, 1982, pp. 601–630.

Jacobson, S., *J. Compar. Neurol., 121,* 5–29 (1963).

Joffe, S., *J. Neurochem., 16,* 715–723 (1969).

Jungalwala, F.B., and Dawson, R.M.C., *Biochem. J., 123,* 683–693 (1971).

Karlsson, I., *J. Neurochem., 25,* 101–107 (1975).

Karlsson, I., and Svennerholm, L., *J. Neurochem., 31,* 657–662 (1978).

Kishimoto, Y., Davies, W.E., and Radin, N.S., *J. Lipid Res., 6,* 532–536 (1965).

Korey, S.R., and Orchen, M., *Arch. Biochem. Biophys., 83,* 381–389 (1959).

Krigman, M.R., and Hogan, E.L., *Brain Res., 107,* 239–255 (1976).

Lamptey, M.S., and Walker, B.L., *J. Nutr., 106,* 86–93 (1976).

Levi, G., in A. Lajtha, Ed., *Handbook of Neurochemistry,* Vol. 2, Plenum Press, New York, 1969, pp. 71–101.

Lyles, D.S., Sulya, L.L., and White, H.B., Jr., *Biochim. Biophys. Acta, 388,* 331–338 (1975).

Manukyan, K.G., Smirnov, A.A., and Chirkovskaya, E.V., *Biokhimiya, 27*, 859–865 (1962) (trans.).

Marshall, E., Fumagalli, R., Niemiro, R., and Paoletti, R., *J. Neurochem., 13*, 857–862 (1966).

Martinez, M., *J. Neurochem., 39*, 1684–1692 (1982).

Martinez, M., and Ballabriga, A., *Brain Res., 159*, 351–362 (1978).

Martinez, M., Conde, C., and Ballabriga, A., *Pediatr. Res., 8*, 93–102 (1974).

Matheson, D.F., Oei, R., and Roots, B.I., *Neurochem. Res., 5*, 683–695 (1980).

Matheson, D.F., Oei, R., and Roots, B.I., *Dev. Neurosci., 4*, 201–210 (1981a).

Matheson, D.F., Oei, R., and Roots, B.I., *J. Neurochem., 36*, 2073–2079 (1981b).

Matthieu, J.-M., Widmer, S., and Herschkowitz, N., *Brain Res., 55*, 391–402 (1973).

McKenna, M.C., and Campagnoni, A.T., *J. Nutr., 109*, 1195–1204 (1979).

Miller, S.L., and Morell, P., *J. Neurochem., 31*, 771–777 (1978).

Miller, S.L., Klurfeld, D.M., Weinsweig, D., and Kritchevsky, D., *J. Neurosci. Res., 6*, 203–210 (1981).

Mohrhauer, H., and Holman, R.T., *J. Neurochem., 10*, 523–530 (1963).

Natarajan, V., and Sastry, P.S., *J. Neurochem., 23*, 187–192 (1974).

Naughton, J.M., *Int. J. Biochem., 13*, 21–32 (1981).

Norton, W.T., in R. Paoletti and A.N. Davison, Eds., *Advances in Experimental Medicine and Biology*, Vol. 13, *Chemistry and Brain Development*, Plenum Press, New York, 1971, pp. 327–337.

Norton, W.T., and Poduslo, S.E., *J. Lipid Res., 12*, 84–90 (1971).

Norton, W.T., and Poduslo, S.E., *J. Neurochem., 21*, 759–773 (1973).

O'Brien, J.S., and Sampson, E.L., *J. Lipid Res., 6*, 537–544 (1965a).

O'Brien, J.S., and Sampson, E.L., *J. Lipid Res., 6*, 545–551 (1965b).

Odutuga, A.A., *Biochim. Biophys. Acta, 487*, 1–9 (1977).

Odutuga, A.A., *Clin. Expt. Pharmacol. Physiol., 6*, 361–366 (1979).

Odutuga, A.A., Carey, E.M., and Prout, R.E.S., *Biochim. Biophys. Acta, 316*, 115–123 (1973).

Ogino, H., Matsumura, T., Satouchi, K., and Saito, K., *Biochim. Biophys. Acta, 574*, 57–63 (1979).

Pasquini, J.M., Bizzozero, O., Sato, C., Oteiza, P., and Soto, E.F., in N.G. Bazan, R. Paoletti, J.M. Iacono, Eds., *New Trends in Nutrition, Lipid Research and Cardiovascular Diseases*, Alan R. Liss, New York, 1981, pp. 73–89.

Pasquini, J.M., Najle, R., and Soto, E.F., *Brain Res., 171*, 295–306 (1979).

Portman, O.W., Alexander, M., and Illingworth, D.R., *Brain Res., 43*, 197–213 (1972).

Rajalakshmi, R., and Nakhasi, H.L., *Expt. Neurol., 44*, 103–113 (1974).

Ramsey, R.B., and Nicholas, H.J., in R. Paoletti and D. Kritchevsky, Eds., *Advances in Lipid Research*, Vol. 10, Academic Press, New York, 1972, pp. 143–232.

Rawlins, F.A., and Smith, M.E., *J. Neurochem., 18*, 1861–1870 (1971).

Reddy, P.V., and Sastry, P.S., *Brit. J. Nutr., 40*, 403–410 (1978).

Reddy, P.V., Anasuya, D., and Sastry, P.S., *Brain Res., 161*, 227–235 (1979).

Reddy, T.S., and Horrocks, L.A., *J. Neurochem., 38*, 601–605 (1982).

Rouser, G., and Yamamoto, A., *Lipids, 3*, 284–287 (1968).

Rouser, G., and Yamamoto, A., in A. Lajtha, Ed., *Handbook of Neurochemistry*, Vol. 1, Plenum Press, New York, 1969, pp. 121–169.

Rouser, G., Kritchevsky, G., Yamamoto, A., and Baxter, C.F., in R. Paoletti and D. Kritchevsky, Eds., *Advances in Lipid Research*, Vol. 10, Academic Press, New York, 1972, pp. 261–360.

Rouser, G., Yamamoto, A., and Kritchevsky, G., in R. Paoletti and A.N. Davison, Eds., *Advances in Experimental Medicine and Biology*, Vol. 13, *Chemistry and Brain Development*, Plenum Press, New York, 1971, pp. 91–109.

Samorajski, T., and Rolsten, C., in D.H. Ford, Ed., *Progress in Brain Research*, Vol. 40, *Neurobiological Aspects of Maturation and Aging*, Elsevier, Amsterdam, 1973, pp. 253–265.

Shah, S.N., and Johnson, R.C., *Expt. Neurol.*, *61*, 370–379 (1978).

Sheltawy, A., and Dawson, R.M.C., *Biochem. J.*, *111*, 147–155 (1969).

Sinclair, A.J., and Crawford, M.A., *J. Neurochem.*, *19*, 1753–1758 (1972).

Skrbic, T.R., and Cumings, J.N., *J. Neurochem.*, *17*, 85–90 (1970).

Smith, M.E., *J. Lipid Res.*, *14*, 541–551 (1973).

Smith, R.E., and Sun, G.Y., *Dev. Neurosci.*, *4*, 337–344 (1981).

Spence, M.W., and Wolf, L.S., *Can. J. Biochem.*, *45*, 671–688 (1967).

Sperry, W.M., in H. Waelsch, Ed., *Biochemistry of the Developing Nervous System*, Academic Press, New York, 1955, pp. 261–265.

Srere, P.A., Seubert, W., and Lynen, F., *Biochim. Biophys. Acta*, *33*, 313–319 (1959).

Srinivasa Rao, P., and Subba Rao, K., *Lipids*, *8*, 374–377 (1973).

Ställberg-Stenhagen, S.K., and Svennerholm, L., *J. Lipid Res.*, *6*, 146–155 (1965).

Strosznajder, J., *Neurochem. Res.*, *15*, 1265–1277 (1980).

Su, K.L., and Sun, G.Y., *J. Neurochem.*, *31*, 1043–1047 (1978).

Sun, G.Y., *Neurobiology*, *1*, 232–238 (1971).

Sun, G.Y., *J. Lipid Res.*, *13*, 56–62 (1972).

Sun, G.Y., *Lipids*, *12*, 661–665 (1977).

Sun, G.Y., and Horrocks, L.A., *Lipids*, *5*, 1006–1012 (1970).

Sun, G.Y., and Horrocks, L.A., *Fed. Proc.*, *30*, 1248 (1971) (abstr.).

Sun, G.Y., and Horrocks, L.A., *J. Lipid Res.*, *14*, 206–214 (1973).

Sun, G.Y., and Samorajski, T., *J. Gerontol.*, *27*, 10–17 (1972).

Sun, G.Y., and Samorajski, T., *Biochim. Biophys. Acta*, *316*, 19–27 (1973).

Sun, G.Y., and Su, K.L., *J. Neurochem.*, *32*, 1053–1059 (1979).

Sun, G.Y., and Yau, T.M., *J. Neurochem.*, *26*, 291–295 (1976a).

Sun, G.Y., and Yau, T.M., *J. Neurochem.*, *27*, 87–92 (1976b).

Sun, G.Y., de Sousa, B.N., Danopoulos, V., and Horrocks, L.A., *Int. J. Devl. Neurosci.*, *1*, 59–64 (1983).

Sun, G.Y., Go, J., and Sun, A.Y., *Lipids*, *9*, 450–454 (1974).

Sun, G.Y., Su, K.L., Der, O.M., and Tang, W., *Lipids*, *14*, 229–235 (1979).

Sun, G.Y., Tang, W., Majewska, M.D., Hallett, D.W., Foudin, L., and Huang, S., in G.Y. Sun, N.G. Bazan, J.Y. Wu, G. Porcellati, and A.Y. Sun, Eds., *Neural Membranes*, Humana Press, Clifton, N.J., 1983, pp. 67–95.

Sun, G.Y., Winniczek, H., Go, J., and Sheng, S.L., *Lipids*, *10*, 365–373 (1975).

Svennerholm, L., in J. Folch-Pi and H. Bauer, Eds., *Brain Lipids and Lipoproteins, and the Leucodystrophies*, Elsevier, Amsterdam, 1963, pp. 104–119.

Svennerholm, L., *J. Neurochem.*, *11*, 839–853 (1964).

Svennerholm, L., *J. Lipid Res.*, *9*, 570–579 (1968).

Svennerholm, L., and Vanier, M.T., *Brain Res.*, *47*, 457–468 (1972).

Svennerholm, L., and Vanier, M.T., *Brain Res.*, *50*, 341–351 (1973a).

Svennerholm, L., and Vanier, M.T., *Brain Res.*, *55*, 413–423 (1973b).

Svennerholm, L., and Vanier, M.T., in J. Palo, Ed., *Advances in Experimental Medicine and Biology*, Vol. 99, *Myelination and Demyelination*, Plenum Press, New York, 1977, pp. 27–41.

Svennerholm, L., Vanier, M.T., and Jungbjer, B., *J. Neurochem.*, *30*, 1383–1390 (1978).

Tang, W., and Sun, G.Y., *Neurochem. Int.*, *4*, 269–273 (1982).

Tinoco, J., Babcock, B., Hincenbergs, I., Medwadowski, B., and Miljanich, P., *Lipids, 13*, 6–17 (1978).

Tinoco, J., Williams, M.A., Hincenbergs, I., and Lyman, R.L., *J. Nutr.*, *101*, 937–945 (1971).

Trapp, B.D., and Bernsohn, J., *J. Neurochem.*, *28*, 1009–1013 (1977).

Trapp, B.D., and Bernsohn, J., *J. Neurol. Sci.*, *37*, 249–266 (1978).

Uma, S., and Ramakrishnan, C.V., *J. Neurochem.*, *40*, 914–916 (1983).

Vanier, M.T., Holm, M., Ohman, R., and Svennerholm, L., *J. Neurochem.*, *18*, 581–592 (1971).

Wells, M.A., and Dittmer, J.C., *Biochemistry, 6*, 3169–3174 (1967).

Wender, M., *Folia Biol.* (*Krakow*), *13*, 323–332 (1965).

White, H.B., Jr., Galli, C., and Paoletti, R., *J. Neurochem.*, *18*, 1337–1339 (1971a).

White, H.B., Jr., Galli, C., and Paoletti, R., *J. Neurochem.*, *18*, 869–882 (1971b).

Wiggins, R.C., Miller, S.L., Benjamins, J.A., Krigman, M.R., and Morell, P., *Brain Res.*, *107*, 257–273 (1976).

Wise, R.W., MacQuarrie, R., and Sun, G.Y., *J. Neurochem.*, *33*, 351–354 (1979).

Yao, J.K., *Biochim. Biophys. Acta, 712*, 542–546 (1982).

Yates, A.J., Bouchard, J.-P., and Wherrett, J.R., *Brain Res.*, *104*, 261–271 (1976).

Yau, T.M., and Sun, G.Y., *J. Neurochem.*, *23*, 99–104 (1974).

Yusef, H.K.M., and Dickerson, J.W.T., *J. Neurochem.*, *28*, 783–788 (1977).

Yusef, H.K.M., Dickerson, J.W.T., and Waterlow, J.C., *Amer. J. Clin. Nutr.*, *32*, 2227–2232 (1979).

Yusef, H.K.M., Haque, Z., and Mozaffar, Z., *J. Neurochem.*, *36*, 924–930 (1981).

four

TRANSPORT, EXCHANGE, AND TRANSFER OF PHOSPHOLIPIDS IN THE NERVOUS SYSTEM

ROBERT W. LEDEEN

Departments of Biochemistry and Neurology
Albert Einstein College of Medicine
Bronx, New York

CONTENTS

4.1   INTRODUCTION   136

4.2   GENERAL CONSIDERATIONS   137

4.3   AXONAL TRANSPORT   140

    4.3.1.   Historical, 140
    4.3.2.   Central Nervous System, 141
    4.3.3.   Peripheral Nerve, 149
    4.3.4.   Phospholipid Transport in Regenerating Nerve, 150
    4.3.5.   Extra-Axonal Diffusion, 150
    4.3.6.   Retrograde Transport, 151
    4.3.7.   Mechanisms of Phospholipid Transport, 151

4.4.   AXON–MYELIN TRANSFER   153

    4.4.1.   Central Nervous System, 154
    4.4.2.   Peripheral Nervous System, 155
    4.4.3.   Mechanism and Function, 159

4.5.   INTRACELLULAR PHOSPHOLIPID TRANSFER   161

    4.5.1.   Historical, 161
    4.5.2.   General Properties, 162
    4.5.3.   Transfer Proteins of the Nervous System, 163
    4.5.4.   Mechanism and Physiological Role, 165

    REFERENCES   167

4.1   INTRODUCTION

Phospholipids comprise the matrix of the diverse membranes that exist in the highly compartmentalized nervous system. Both neurons and glial cells are characterized by extensive processes, the neuronal ones being especially remarkable for the fact that they extend over distances which are often thousands of times greater than the diameter of the cell body. Exchange and transport of phospholipids are important aspects of membrane renewal made necessary by the fact that the site of synthesis generally differs from the site of utilization. When one considers that virtually all the phospholipids needed for renewal of this vast array of membranes originate in the cell body, the need for efficient transport and exchange of these substances becomes evident.

A number of pathways exist for transporting phospholipids from their synthetic sites to the cell surface and to the various intracellular compartments. Such transport may occur in concert with proteins, as for example in membrane flow and recycling, or independently through specific exchange reactions in which proteins play a catalytic role. The latter process causes the well-known flux of phospholipids between cellular compartments. Within the membrane itself, phospholipids often appear to have the capacity for transbilayer movement in addition to the more usual lateral movement proteins also display. Transfer of phospholipids from one cell to another, such as occurs between the axon and its surrounding myelin sheath, is another phenomenon pointing up the distinctive mobility that characterizes these substances.

Axonal transport is a specific type of intracellular movement adapted to the requirements of the neuron. Movement of phospholipids by this pathway is now well documented, although the details of mechanism remain to be elucidated. One might anticipate similar movement of phospholipids in dendrites, analogous to dendritic transport of macromolecules (Kreutzberg et al., 1973); some evidence for this has come from the apparent labeling of dendritic phospholipids after intracellular injection of [^{3}H]choline (Kreutzberg and Schubert, 1973; Schubert et al., 1971).

This chapter will deal with three of the above-mentioned aspects of phospholipid movement: axonal transport, transcellular axon–myelin transfer, and intracellular protein-catalyzed transfer. These are among the more extensively studied areas but do not of course exhaust the possible modes of phospholipid movement within and between cells.

4.2   GENERAL CONSIDERATIONS

Considerable effort has gone into elucidating the mechanism and site of phospholipid synthesis within the cell, and indeed such information is essential for a full understanding of phospholipid movement. Eukaryotic cells in general are considered to carry out *de novo* phospholipid synthesis in the endoplasmic reticulum (Thompson, 1980; Bell et al., 1981; Ansell and Spanner, 1982) and there is no evidence that neural cells depart from this pattern. Autoradiographic studies of glycerol incorporation in perikarya suggest that the rough endoplasmic reticulum in particular is the major locus of phospholipid synthesis (Boyenvel and Droz, 1976). Brain mitochondria resemble mitochondria generally in having limited synthetic ability (Miller and Dawson, 1972a), although they are capable of *de novo* synthesis of phosphatidic acid and diphosphatidylglycerol (Miller and Dawson, 1972a) and decarboxylative conversion of phosphatidylserine† to phosphatidylethanolamine (Percy et al. 1983; Butler and Morell, 1983. Neural plasma membranes are generally considered incapable of *de novo* synthesis (Miller and Dawson, 1972a) but are known to effect a number of interconversions, such as base-exchange (Goracci et al., 1973) and phospholipid methylation (Hirata and Axelrod, 1980). Plasma membrane preparations from liver also lack the phosphotransferase required for *de novo* synthesis of phosphoglycerides (Stahl and Trams, 1968; Victoria et al., 1971), while containing those for transacylation (Wright and Green, 1971; Victoria et al., 1971) and the above interconversions, so the pattern may be general. An apparent exception is myelin, the modified plasma membrane of glial cells, which contains a number of enzymes for *de novo* synthesis of phosphatidylcholine and phosphatidylethanolamine (see below).

Since protein synthesis in neurons is confined to the perikaryon and initial segments of dendritic trunks (Schultze et al., 1959; Droz and Leblond, 1963), it has been of interest to ascertain whether the same applies to phospholipids or whether these are capable of being synthesized in processes and nerve endings as well. Extruded squid axoplasm was in fact shown to incorporate a number of precursors into phospholipids: $^{32}P_i$, [^{3}H]choline, [^{3}H]serine, [^{3}H]ethanolamine, and [^{3}H]*myo*-inositol (Larrabee and Brinley, 1968; Brunetti et al., 1979; Gould et al., 1983a). The fact that [^{3}H]glycerol was incorporated into a few lipids suggested some degree of *de novo* synthesis (Gould et al., 1983a); however, the slow rate and limited diversity indicated this was probably not a general pathway in the axon.

Phosphatidylinositol is a phospholipid shown to be synthesized at an appreciable rate in both mammalian (Gould, 1976; Kumara-Siri and Gould, 1980) and squid (Gould et al., 1983a,b) axoplasm. Furthermore, the terminal synthetic enzyme for this substance, CDP-diacylglycerol: inositol phosphatidyltransferase, was shown to undergo axonal transport in mouse sciatic nerve (Kumara-Siri and Gould, 1980). The same study could find no evidence for the axonal transport of cholinephosphotransferase, the terminal enzyme in the synthesis of phosphatidylcholine, and this was consistent with other results, indicating no synthesis of this lipid

---

† The nomenclature designations phosphatidylserine, phosphatidylethanolamine, phosphatidylcholine, and so on, are used to denote the entire class of lipid irrespective of aliphatic chain.

in sciatic nerve axoplasm (Gould and Dawson 1976). Aside from phosphatidylinositol, the evidence to date thus suggests primary dependence on axonal transport for the bulk of axonal phospholipid.

With regard to nerve endings, Miller and Dawson (1972a) found low activity of cholinephosphotransferase in synaptosome fractions, as compared to microsomes, some if not all of the synaptosomal activity being ascribed to microsomal contamination. The more recent study of Strosznajder et al. (1979) reported substantial activities of cholinephosphotransferase and ethanolaminephosphotransferase in lysed synaptosomes, but not intact synaptosomes, from adult rat brains. Despite the presence of the microsomal marker, NADPH–cytochrome c reductase, the authors considered the relatively high activities in synaptosomes and the large increase due to lysis to rule out microsomal contamination as an explanation for all of the transferase activities in synaptosomes. Thus, while nerve endings undoubtedly rely on axonal transport for renewal of a large portion of their membrane phospholipids (see below), contribution by local synthesis remains a possibility that requires further assessment.

As mentioned above, diffusion of phospholipids within the membrane is another motional vector available to phospholipids, although the distances encompassed are relatively short compared to axonal flow. Lateral diffusion studies of phospholipids in the plane of the bilayer (Kornberg and McConnell, 1971a) have indicated velocities greater than 0.05 μm/s. Using diffusion constants of 2–20×10^{-8} cm^2/s (Scandella et al., 1972; Devaux and McConnell, 1973) and the Einstein diffusion equation (Einstein, 1926), one can estimate the time required for diffusion over a distance of 5 mm between several days and several weeks, depending on the diffusion constant employed. This was the mechanism invoked by Gould and Dawson (1976) to explain the relatively slow movement of radioactive choline-labeled lipid from the Schwann cell cytoplasm into the myelin sheaths of the sciatic nerve. Such diffusion might account for equilibration of phospholipids over portions of the neuronal membrane, but it clearly cannot provide a mechanism for distributing phospholipids to distal portions of the longer processes.

Transbilayer movement, termed *flip-flop* by Kornberg and McConnell (1971b), might account for the presence of certain phospholipids in both halves of membrane bilayers despite their apparently exclusive synthesis on the cytoplasmic side of the endoplasmic reticulum (Bell et al., 1981). Some reports have suggested rapid flip-flop in this membrane (Zilversmit and Hughes, 1977; Van den Besselaar et al., 1978) while at least one (Higgins, 1979) indicated a slower transition. Transbilayer movement of phosphatidylcholine in the erythrocyte membrane was reported to be very slow (Van Meer et al., 1980), as it was in artificial membranes (Bloj and

Zilversmit, 1981a). It may be noted that transbilayer movement accompanies the stepwise methylation of phosphatidylethanolamine to phosphatidylcholine (Hirata and Axelrod, 1980).

The concept of membrane flow, according to which "the biogenesis of certain membranes is accomplished by the physical transfer of membrane material from one cell component to another in the course of their formation or normal functioning" (Franke et al., 1971), has proved useful in understanding the movement of phospholipids throughout the cell. This pictures the plasma membrane as supplied by structural lipids and proteins assembled in the endoplasmic reticulum and transported to the cell periphery via the Golgi apparatus (Morré and Outracht, 1977). In this bulk transport process, membrane movement is postulated to result from vesicles budding off of one membrane and fusing with another (Palade, 1975; Holtzman and Mercurio, 1980). A key role for the Golgi apparatus has also been postulated in the processing of phospholipids for axonal transport (Hammerschlag and Stone, 1982; see also below). Cells economize their membranes by reutilizing them while carrying out these transport processes (Holtzman and Mercurio, 1980; Lentz, 1983). Several reviews on the origin, circulation, and fate of membranes in neurons have appeared in recent years (Grafstein, 1977; Heuser and Reese, 1977; Boyne, 1978; Schwartz, 1979; Holtzman and Mercurio, 1980).

4.3   AXONAL TRANSPORT

4.3.1   Historical

The first evidence for axonal transport of phospholipids came from the work of Miani (1963). Using $^{32}P_i$ to label phospholipids in the cell bodies of the medulla oblongata in the rabbit, he observed transport into the vagus and hypoglossal nerves at rates of 72 and 40 mm/day, respectively. Comparing his own findings with those of Weiss and Hiscoe (1948), which had first established the phenomenon of slow axoplasmic flow, Miani concluded that "the swift phospholipids do not move *with* the axoplasm, but *in* the axoplasm."

Although this was one of the first demonstrations of faster movement in the axon, in retrospect it is clear that the "intermediate" rates reported in that study underestimated the true rate of phospholipid movement. They were well below the velocity of fast transport of protein reported subsequently by Sjostrand (1969) in the same system. Later Abe et al. (1973) were to demonstrate close correspondence in the transport velocities of phospholipids and the fast wave of protein transport in this system (see below). The general characteristics of phospholipid transport have now been defined in both the central nervous system (CNS) and the peripheral nervous system (PNS).

4.3.2 Central Nervous System

The vertebrate optic system has been widely used for the study of axonal transport in the CNS. Employed originally by Taylor and Weiss (1965) for the study of proteins, this paradigm has since shown its usefulness for phospholipids as well. In their work with the goldfish optic system, Grafstein et al. (1975) followed the movement of labeled phospholipid into the optic nerve and optic tectum after intraocular injection of [^{3}H]glycerol. The first radioactively labeled phospholipids appeared in these structures within 1 day, this corresponding in rate to the fast component of protein transport. Of special significance was the fact that inhibition of protein synthesis in the retina reduced the amount of transported phospholipid appearing in the tectum about as much as the transported protein. This indicated linkage between the rapidly transported protein and phospholipid and suggested that whereas the protein in the transported lipid–protein complex is newly synthesized, the lipid component need not be.

An apparent difference between protein and phospholipid was noted in their respective time course of appearance, namely that phospholipid continued to increase in optic nerve and tectum over a period of 4–8 days while the fast component of protein peaked within 1 day. The prolonged period of accumulation for the phospholipid was interpreted as reflecting a prolonged period of release from the cell body into the axon, followed by its transport at the rapid rate. This was supported by the observation that accumulation of phospholipid in the optic tectum was rapidly terminated after the optic axons were separated from their cell bodies. The prolonged time course of release was explained by assuming that most of the transportable phospholipid was not immediately transported after synthesis but entered a pool in the cell body from which the material to be transported would subsequently be drawn. Presumably, the phospholipid entering the axon at any given time would consist of a mixture of newly synthesized molecules and those synthesized earlier. It was pointed out that since phospholipids are readily exchanged between cellular components, it is possible that the pool from which the transported portion is drawn may actually comprise a considerable part of total phospholipid of the nerve cell body. Supporting that notion was the recent finding that [^{14}C]dipalmitoyl phosphatidylcholine, injected intravitreally into rabbits,

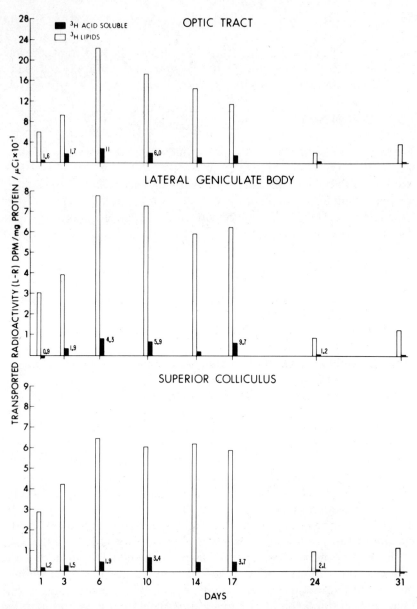

FIGURE 4.1 Transported radioactivity of lipids in the rabbit optic system labeled with [2-³H]glycerol. Ten microcuries of [3-¹⁴C]serine and 20 μCi of [2-³H]glycerol were injected into the right eyes of adult rabbits, and the animals sacrificed at the times shown. Trichloracetic acid-phosphotungstic acid (TCA-PTA) precipitates were obtained for the three sets of tissues, left (L) and right (R), at each time point and the lipids removed by chloroform-methanol extraction. L/R ratios for TCA-PTA-soluble fractions are indicated next to bars. Lipids had high L/R ratios (>15) in virtually all cases. The average variation (S.E.M.) of L-R values was 30% of the mean for ³H-labeled lipids and 46% for the acid-soluble fraction. (From Haley et al., 1979a. Reproduced with permission of Pergamon Press.)

142

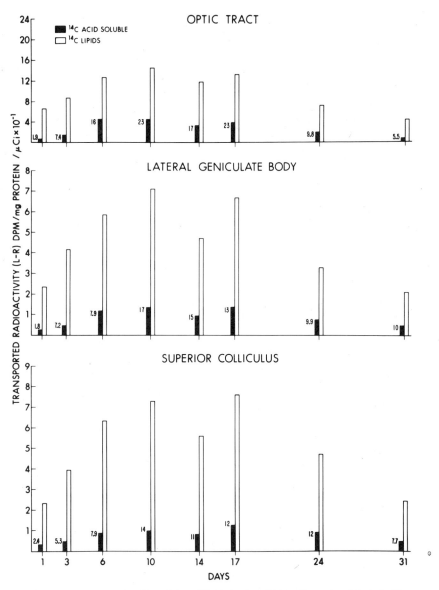

FIGURE 4.2 Transported radioactivity of lipids in the rabbit optic system labeled with DL-[3-¹⁴C]serine. Procedure as described in Figure 4.1. L/R ratios from TCA-PTA-soluble fractions are indicated next to bars; those without values had undetectable radioactivity on the control side. Lipids had high L/R ratios (>15) in all cases. The average variation (S.E.M.) of L–R values was 21% of the mean for ¹⁴C-labeled lipids and 23% for the acid-soluble fraction. (From Haley et al., 1979a. Reproduced with permission of Pergamon Press.)

143

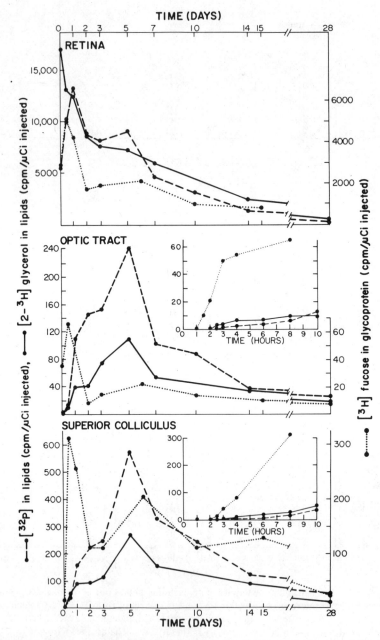

FIGURE 4.3 Time course of synthesis (retina) and axonal transport and accumulation (optic tract and superior colliculus) of lipids and of glycoproteins in the rat visual system. Rats were killed at various times following intraocular injection of [2-³H]glycerol and

144

was transported to the superior colliculus in a manner analogous to endogenously synthesized phospholipid (Lee et al., 1982).

Three subsequent reports appearing more or less simultaneously utilized the optic systems of the goldfish (Currie et al., 1978), rat (Toews et al., 1979), and rabbit (Haley et al., 1979a) to compare various radiolabeled lipid precursors. These were glycerol, choline, serine, and inorganic phosphate, all of which proved effective in labeling phospholipids (and in some cases other lipids) undergoing transport. In each study radiolabeled lipid first appeared in 1 day or less in the optic tract and nerve ending structure (optic tectum of goldfish; superior colliculus and/or lateral geniculate body of rat and rabbit). The conclusion that this corresponded to fast transport was supported by the near-simultaneous appearance of label in optic nerve/tract and nerve-ending structure(s), so that there was little evidence for a phase difference of the kind one would expect for a slow or intermediate transport rate. This finding did not preclude the possibility of a small pool of slower-moving phospholipids that might have been masked.

The phenomenon of prolonged build-up of transported labeled lipid was consistently observed in these studies, although details varied. With [2-^{3}H]glycerol as precursor, accumulation peaked at 4–7 days in all three animals (Figs. 4.1, 4.3, and 4.4). Choline label, on the other hand, did not peak until 14 days, at least in the goldfish (Fig. 4.5). Serine injected into the rabbit eye labeled lipids whose transport pattern (Fig. 4.2) resembled that of [2-^{3}H]glycerol-labeled lipids (Fig. 4.1): accumulation peaked over a broad plateau between 6 and 17 days and then declined in a parallel manner in all three anatomical regions. The same precursor injected into the goldfish eye, however, produced a different pattern in which transported lipid peaked in the optic nerve over a broad plateau between 7 and 35 days but rose continually in the optic tectum over the same period (Fig. 4.6). In the rat, transported lipids peaked abruptly at 5 days followed by rapid decline; this pattern was the same in all three

---

[^{32}P]phosphate (to label lipids) or [^{3}H]fucose (to label glycoproteins), and the visual structures dissected. In the lipid experiments radioactivity was determined on a portion of the washed lipid extracts (modified Folch extraction procedure). In the glycoprotein experiments values were determined as trichloroacetic acid–phosphotungstic acid-insoluble radioactivity. All data have been corrected for systemic background labeling by subtraction of radioactivity in corresponding contralateral structures. Values plotted are means of at least two separate experiments (three to four values at most time points). Early time points are plotted in the insets (left and right ordinates have the same scales). Although the rapid accumulation of transported glycoproteins contrasts with the more gradual accumulation of transported lipids, correction for the biphasic decay of fucose label gives transport kinetics for the peptide backbone similar to phospholipids (see text). (From Toews and Morell, 1985. Reproduced with permission of authors and Raven Press.)

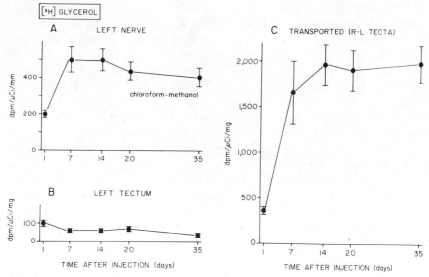

FIGURE 4.4 Distribution of labeled lipid (chloroform/methanol-soluble material) after injection of [³H]glycerol into left eye. A, axonally transported in left nerve; B, "background" (locally synthesized) in left tectum; C, axonally transported to right tectum (difference between right and left tecta). Values are given in dpm/μCi injected per millimeter of nerve or per milligram of dry weight of tectum, and each point represents the mean plus or minus the standard error of the mean for six fish. The values for the labeled TCA-soluble and protein fractions were negligible. (From Currie et al., 1978. Reproduced with permission of authors and Plenum Publishing Co.)

anatomical structures irrespective of whether the precursor was $^{32}P_i$ or [2-³H]glycerol (Fig. 4.3).

These differences in accumulation curves observed between species and precursors probably reflected differences in metabolic conservation rather than intrinsic differences in the transport process itself. To some extent such conservation involves retention by myelin of substances leaving the axon. The phenomenon of axon–myelin transfer has been reported by a number of laboratories and is discussed below. For the nerve-ending structures the same process could occur accompanied by reincorporation in postsynaptic neurons, as described by Heacock and Agranoff (1977). The unique patterns in the goldfish (Figs. 4.4–4.6) would thus correspond to highly efficient conservation of the three precursors tested, while rat, showing rapid decline after a sharp peak at 4 days, would have the least capacity for conservation according to this model. Comparing the three precursors employed in the goldfish, it might be concluded that the radiolabel in [2-³H]glycerol is recycled somewhat less efficiently than the

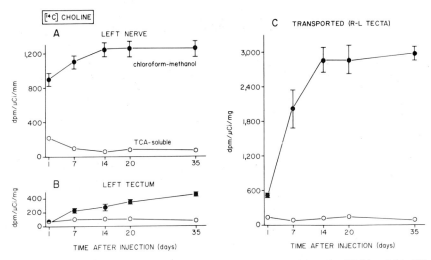

FIGURE 4.5 Distribution of labeled chloroform/methanol-soluble (●) and TCA-soluble (○) material after injection of [^{14}C]choline into left eye. Ordinates and data expression as in Figure 4. The values for the labeled protein fraction were negligible. (From Currie et al., 1978. Reproduced with permission of authors and Plenum Publishing Co.)

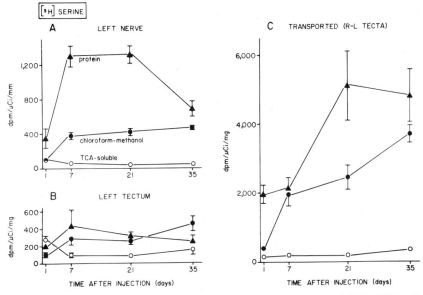

FIGURE 4.6 Distribution of labeled chloroform/methanol-soluble material (●), TCA-soluble material (○), and insoluble material, i.e., protein ▲, after injection of [^{3}H]serine into left eye. Ordinates and data expression as in Figure 4. (From Currie et al., 1978. Reproduced with permission of authors and Plenum Publishing Co.)

147

labels in [^{14}C]choline or [^{3}H]serine. This would be consistent with the generally accepted view that reutilization of glycerol results in substantial loss of ^{3}H at the 2-position due to involvement of the dihydroxyacetone phosphate pathway (Benjamins and McKhann, 1973; Miller et al., 1977). It should be recognized, however, that reutilization of glycerol by pathways not involving this keto intermediate would lead to retention of ^{3}H. While such pathways are well known, their importance in these optic systems has not been assessed. The problem of metabolic conservation, or reutilization, was further considered in a study of the turnover of axonally transported phospholipids in nerve endings of retinal ganglion cells (Toews and Morell, 1981).

Two additional CNS systems have been used to study axonal transport of phospholipids; the nigrostriatal tract and the lateral geniculovisual cortical tract (Toews et al., 1980). Following injection of [^{3}H]glycerol into the substantia nigra or lateral geniculate body, labeled phospholipids began to appear 2 h later in the ipsilateral corpus striatum or visual cortex, respectively. This indicated transport at a rapid rate for at least some of the lipid. As in the previous studies, radiolabeled lipid continued to accumulate in the projection sites reaching a maximum at 3 days in both systems. In comparison to glycerol, ^{32}P$_i$ proved less satisfactory as precursor as evidenced by the presence of considerable amounts of ^{32}P-soluble label at the projection sites and the fact that colchicine only partially blocked the accumulation of ^{32}P-labeled lipid. A possible explanation for this finding is extra-axonal diffusion of injected precursor (see below).

Axonal transport of individual phospholipids in the CNS has been studied by use of either specific or general precursors, the latter requiring subsequent fractionation of the transported phospholipids. Radiolabeled choline is an example of the former, having been used in the optic system (Currie et al., 1978; Toews and Morell, 1981) and in several peripheral nerve studies (see below). It labels primarily phosphatidylcholine and only a minor amount of sphingomyelin. For the latter, as well as sphingolipids in general, serine proved a useful precursor (Currie et al., 1978; Haley et al., 1979a). Its use in conjunction with glycerol, a superior precursor for glycerophospholipids, led to demonstration of fast transport of nearly all lipids in the rabbit optic system (Haley et al., 1979a). Transported ethanolamine phosphoglycerides were well labeled by both precursors. When [^{3}H]glycerol and ^{32}P$_i$ were used in the rat optic system, all phosphoglycerides were labeled by both precursors and rapidly transported (Toews et al., 1979). Phosphatidylcholine and phosphatidylethanolamine together accounted for over 80% of the total transported lipid radioactivity. Phosphatidylcholine appeared to be committed to transport somewhat sooner than phosphatidylethanolamine, as indicated by the fact that at early time points the ratio of radioactivity in the former to that in the latter increased in structures progressively farther removed from the site of synthesis in the retina. By 2 days, however, a constant ratio was reached. A study of inositol phosphoglycerides employing [^{3}H]inositol as precursor in the rabbit optic system revealed fast transport of phosphatidylinositol along with small quantities of the 5-phosphate and 4,5-bisphosphate derivatives (Alberghina et al., 1982a).

4.3.3   Peripheral Nerve

As mentioned above, the first systematic study of phospholipid transport (Miani, 1963) utilized peripheral nerve, and in subsequent studies the long axons of sciatic nerve have been used to advantage. Using bullfrog sciatic nerve, Abe et al. (1973) carefully defined the transport characteristics of one type of phospholipid (phosphatidylcholine) and deduced the existence of a close relationship to protein transport. After injecting [^{3}H]choline into the dorsal root ganglion, labeled phosphatidylcholine was shown to move anterogradely at 152 mm/day (25°), corresponding to the fast wave of protein transport. That study also demonstrated that the rates of phospholipid and protein showed the same temperature dependence, with a Q_{10} of 2.6, and that both were simultaneously blocked in their movement by colchicine. These substances showed parallel subcellular distributions with highest specific radioactivities in the microsomal subfractions. The authors concluded that transported phosphatidylcholine and certain membrane proteins reside in the same structural entity, believed to be a precursor material of axonal and synaptic membranes.

Toews et al. (1983) compared the transport patterns of individual phospholipids in sensory neurons of rat sciatic nerve following injection of [2-^{3}H]glycerol in the dorsal root ganglion. Phosphatidylcholine moved as a sharply defined front at an estimated rate of 300 mm/day, the wave front being evident only during the first few hours after injection. The fastest portion of phosphatidylethanolamine migrated at the same rate but without a well-defined leading edge. This lipid required from 1 to 4 days to equilibrate along the 60-mm length of nerve. Accumulation continued for both lipids over a period of days, as also reported by Gould et al. (1982) for the motor neurons of rat sciatic nerve. To explain the discrepant patterns of these two lipids, it was proposed (Toews et al., 1983) that phosphatidylethanolamine, presumably present in migrating membranous particles, exchanged extensively with unlabeled molecules in stationary axonal structures, thereby causing the initial moving crest to be continually attenuated. Phosphatidylcholine, on the other hand, was presumed to exchange at a slower rate and thus retain a stable front. Diphosphatidylglycerol, a mitochondrial marker that does not exchange, exhibited a discrete crest similar to phosphatidylcholine but moved at about half the rate. This accords with what is currently known about the rate of mitochondrial transport (Grafstein and Forman, 1980).

4.3.4   Phospholipid Transport in Regenerating Nerve

Regeneration studies have demonstrated enhanced flow of phospholipids into the axon following nerve injury. Dziegelewska et al. (1980) utilized [^{3}H]choline to label phospholipids (primarily phosphatidylcholine) in the anterior horn region of the lumbosacral spinal cord in rats. Transport velocity, reported to be about 20 mm/h in normal sciatic nerve, apparently did not increase following nerve crush. Labeled phospholipid accumulated rapidly at a site immediately proximal to the crush, and in all the segments between the ganglion and crush site as well. This finding of a general increase in the level of phospholipid radioactivity over the entire proximal nerve was not duplicated with labeled proteins in the sciatic nerve.

Alberghina and co-workers illustrated a similar phenomenon in the rat sciatic (Alberghina et al., 1983a) and rabbit hypoglossal (Alberghina et al., 1983b) nerves. They studied regeneration in both proximal and distal segments following cutting and fascicular repair by surgical sutures. After injecting a mixture of radiolabeled choline and glycerol in spinal motor neurons, labeled phospholipids were first seen to accumulate in the transected sciatic nerve in the region immediately proximal to the suture and later, about 9 days after suture, in the distal segments. Similar results were obtained with regenerating hypoglossal nerve of the rabbit, where incorporation was again elevated along the entire length of the nerve containing both regenerating axons and the postcrush sprouting terminals. Against this background of overall enhancement of phospholipid transport, it was noted that the incorporation of radiolabel into phosphatidylcholine greatly exceeded that of other phosphoglycerides in the nerve segments distal to the crush, suggesting that this lipid class may be preferentially assembled into the regenerating tips. Transport of phospholipids into regenerating axons has also been observed by light and electron microscopic autoradiography (Gould et al., 1982).

4.3.5   Extra-Axonal Diffusion

The above-mentioned behavior of ^{32}P$_i$ in the nigrostriatal tract was suggestive of extra-axonal diffusion, a problem previously highlighted in the rabbit optic nerve (Chihara, 1979; Haley et al., 1979b). In the latter system diffusion of lipid precursors in the periaxonal space was observed following blockage of transport by colchicine; this extended for several millimeters down the optic nerve but did not pass beyond the chiasm into the optic tract. Hence, it was suggested that the latter structure be used in preference to the optic nerve when studying transport down the axons of retinal ganglion cells; at the very least the first several millimeters of optic nerve must be rejected. The phenomenon applies to peripheral nerve as well since various precursors were observed to diffuse over considerable distances (10–20 mm) along the sciatic nerve (Gould et al., 1982; Toews et al., 1983). The extent of such diffusion varies according to the nature of the precursor, the volume in which it is injected, and the intrinsic properties of the system itself.

4.3.6 Retrograde Transport

Evidence for retrograde transport of phospholipids was recently reported by Bisby and Guy (1983) from studies with rat peripheral nerve. Mobile material was trapped at two ligatures spaced several millimeters apart, that collecting on the distal side of the distal ligature representing retrograde transported material (Bisby and Bulger, 1977). Following injection of [^{3}H]glycerol and [^{35}S]methionine, it was observed that anterograde and retrograde transports were synchronous for both proteins and phospholipids in this system. In injured axons premature reversal of transport occurred. These results were interpreted as supporting the concept that retrograde transported materials are derived from axonal membranes.

4.3.7 Mechanisms of Phospholipid Transport

As outlined in the preceding sections, the results of several studies indicate that phospholipids are associated primarily with the fast component of transport in both the central and peripheral nervous systems. Their estimated rate of 300–480 mm/day in mammalian sciatic nerve approximates that of rapidly transported proteins in similar systems (Ochs, 1972). Transported proteins have been grouped into at least five classes based on flow velocity, each class reflecting delivery of a distinct population of molecules in specific organelles (Lorenz and Willard, 1978; Black and Lasek, 1979; Lasek, 1980). Group I of Lorenz and Willard (1978) contains the bulk of phospholipids along with glycoproteins and some nonglycosylated proteins. Phospholipids are not generally found in the other groups, with the exception of the small intermediate wave of velocity 34–68 mm/day (group II of Lorenz and Willard), which includes mitochondria.

Virtual restriction to the fast-transport mode is consistent with the emerging view that this is the membrane wave carrying preassembled lipid–protein aggregates destined for renewal of axonal and nerve-ending membranes. Close association of lipid and protein during transport was first suggested by the above-mentioned discovery of Abe et al. (1973) that phospholipids have a rate, subcellular distribution and colchicine sensitivity similar to those of fast-transported proteins. Additional evidence came from the observation that both lipid and protein transport are reduced following inhibition of protein synthesis in the neuronal perikaryon (Grafstein et al., 1975). Equally relevant was the demonstration that inhibition of somal synthesis of either phospholipid or cholesterol resulted in a proportional depression of fast-transported protein (Longo and Hammerschlag, 1980). The latter study suggested that the lipid–protein complex forms during the initiation phase of transport and persists throughout the journey down the axon.

The above-described phenomenon of prolonged phospholipid buildup in axons, observed in virtually every study designed to reveal it, has until recently been considered a property of transported lipids but not of proteins. That such a conclusion runs counter to the prevailing model of coordinated lipid and protein movement in preassembled membrane entities is evident. However, some recent studies have indicated that those earlier conclusions about the transport kinetics of membrane proteins may have been erroneous. One was a study of glycoconjugate transport in the rabbit optic system (Ledeen et al., 1981), which revealed similar prolonged build-up of labeled gangliosides and sialoglycoproteins in the optic tract and superior colliculus. The peak of accumulation (ca. 8 days) corresponded to that previously reported for phospholipids in the same system (Haley et al., 1979a). In another study of fucose-labeled glycoproteins in the rat optic system (Morell and Goodrum, 1983), the data indicated that the previously reported (Goodrum and Morell, 1982) biphasic turnover of these substances was due to the presence of multiple fucose moieties with independent turnover rates. Correcting for this biphasic decay of fucose label, the transport kinetics of the peptide backbones showed the same gradual accumulation over 6 days as did phospholipids. Careful examination of the transport kinetics of other axonal/nerve-ending membrane components might reveal whether all such substances share a common pattern of movement.

Axonal transport has been considered an example of endomembrane flow involving mechanisms of plasma membrane renewal common to all cells. Hammerschlag and co-workers have emphasized the similarities between transport in the neuron and mechanisms employed by nonneural cells for delivering membrane and secretory products to the surface of the cell (Hammerschlag and Lavoie, 1979; Hammerschlag, 1980; Hammerschlag and Stone, 1982). They ascribe a key role to the Golgi apparatus in the processing of all membrane proteins (including the expected glycoproteins) prior to beginning transport in the axon; if such is the case, concurrent processing of membrane lipids destined for the axon would also be expected. This model postulates the existence of Golgi-derived vesicles, formed as vesiculotubular structures that act as transport vectors within the axon.

However, a different view expressed by Droz and co-workers (Rambourg and Droz, 1980) postulates that most proteins bypass the Golgi apparatus. Similarly, for phospholipids, they have proposed that following synthesis in the rough endoplasmic reticulum, these are directly transferred to the smooth endoplasmic reticulum which retains structural continuity with the former and runs through the perikaryon and axon. This interconnected agranular network of tubules was proposed by these workers to be a major (but not necessarily exclusive) anatomical pathway for fast axonal transport. In electron microscope autoradiographs labeled phospholipids were seen to be preferentially associated with these structures at early times, followed by transfer to axolemma and axonal mitochondria. Rambourg and Droz (1980), in agreement with suggestions by Schwartz (1979) and earlier calculations of their own (Droz et al., 1973), stated that "the visualization of labeled macromolecules in subaxolemmal profiles of smooth endoplasmic reticulum probably results from their slackening down prior to their subsequent integration in the axolemma." Rambourg and Droz (1980) proposed that this structure is not necessarily rigid but may constitute a dynamic system of membrane in permanent remodeling. It is clearly too early to draw any final conclusions regarding the role of the smooth endoplasmic reticulum or the above Golgi-derived transport vectors in regard to phospholipid transport.

4.4   AXON–MYELIN TRANSFER

The view of the neuronal cell body as an "axoplasmic fountain" supplying the principal requirements of its own processes through axonal and dendritic flow is now widely accepted, and attention has turned to the possibility that supporting glial cells may receive a portion of their required nutrients from this source as well. Singer (1966) pictured the axon as an open system, permitting flow to and from adjacent glia, and proposed that the facts of Wallerian degeneration reflected a trophic contribution of the axon to the integrity of the myelin sheath. Ramon y Cajal (1928) had earlier attributed Wallerian degeneration to loss of trophic substances produced by catabolism within the axon.

The idea of transcellular transport to and from the axon has gained strong support from the recent demonstration of protein transfer into the axoplasm of the squid giant axon from adaxonal glia (Lasek et al., 1977; Gainer et al., 1977). Recent work has suggested that phospholipids may undergo similar transfer into the squid giant axon (R. Gould, personal communication). Movement in the reverse direction, from axon to glia, was observed by Alvarez and Chen (1972) upon injection of [^{3}H]choline into the giant mauthner axon of the goldfish. This was most probably an example of substrate movement, the choline being incorporated into myelin phospholipids after entering the glial cell. Further examples of such transfer have been reported in mammals, along with the companion phenomenon, axon-to-myelin transfer of intact phospholipids (see below).

4.4.1   Central Nervous System

The optic system of young rabbits proved a useful paradigm for studying transcellular movement of lipids and lipid precursors (Haley and Ledeen 1978; 1979, Ledeen and Haley 1983). Intraocular injection of both [^{3}H]glycerol and [^{14}C]serine provided a double label for transported lipids and a single label for transported proteins, all of which were measured over time in myelin isolated from the contralateral optic tracts. The key observation was that the ^{14}C label in myelin lipids increased over a 21-day period while the ^{3}H label declined, albeit more slowly than ^{3}H in axolemma- and axon-enriched fractions obtained from the same source. The data indicated two mechanisms by which myelin lipids became labeled: (1) transfer of intact lipid from the axon revealed especially by the [^{3}H]glycerol label which was not extensively recycled; (2) transfer of lipid precursor (serine or derivative thereof) into the glia–myelin compartment followed by enzymatic incorporation into myelin lipids. The latter (reutilization) process was tracked by lipid-bound ^{14}C. The protein ^{14}C label found in myelin did not increase with time, and the evidence suggested this represented contamination by residual axonal membranes.

The precise nature and origin of the metabolite(s) entering myelin to become reincorporated were not determined. Two possibilities were serine itself, released by proteolysis in the axon, or ethanolamine released from ethanolamine phosphoglycerides by lipolysis. The fact that such ^{14}C labeling in myelin was restricted to certain lipids and appeared to exclude incorporation into myelin proteins suggested that reutilization did not occur in the glial cell body where such selectivity would not be expected. The possibility that myelin itself was the locus of reincorporation was given credence by the discovery of phospholipid-synthesizing enzymes in highly purified preparations of this membrane. Thus far, three enzymes involved in *de novo* synthesis of phosphatidylethanolamine have been detected (Wu and Ledeen, 1980; Kunishita and Ledeen, 1984; Kunishita et al., 1984), consistent with the *in vivo* observation that this myelin lipid showed increasing ^{14}C radioactivity over the 21-day period. Preliminary evidence was also reported for a parallel set of enzymes that synthesize phosphatidylcholine (Ledeen and Wu, 1979; Kunishita and Ledeen, 1982; Kunishita et al., 1984).

Subsequent reports have demonstrated that serine is not unique in its ability to label CNS myelin phospholipid through transcellular migration from the axon. Intravitreally injected inorganic phosphate, for example, labeled phosphatidylcholine in myelin of the rabbit optic system, radioactivity increasing between 7 and 21 days analogous to the behavior of serine (Fig. 4.7). Phosphatidylethanolamine of myelin was similarly labeled (Ledeen and Haley, 1983). An experiment of the same type with [^{14}C]palmitate (Alberghina et al., 1982b) gave similar results, ^{14}C radioactivity in myelin of the rabbit optic system increasing over a 10-day period during which time ^3H label from [2-^3H]glycerol declined. Further support for efficient reutilization by glial myelin enzymes of acyl chains originating in the axon was suggested in the study of Toews and Morell (1981) employing radiolabeled acetate in the rat optic system.

4.4.2 Peripheral Nervous System

Axon to myelin transfer of phospholipids in peripheral nerve has been well documented by Droz and co-workers (Droz, 1979; Droz et al., 1979). They applied a combination of biochemical and radioautographic techniques to the ciliary ganglion of the chicken, [^3H]glycerol and [^3H]choline being injected into the cerebral aqueduct to label phospholipids which then migrated into the oculomotor axons and caliciform nerve endings. One ganglion was processed to locate phospholipids by radioautography and the other was processed biochemically.

Electron microscope radioautographs revealed numerous silver grains over the myelin sheath for both precursors (Figs. 4.8 and 4.9), these peaking in intensity at about 40–72 h after injection (Droz et al., 1978). The time course of radioactivity accumulation in myelin thus differed from that observed with the rabbit optic system (Haley and Ledeen, 1979; Alberghina et al., 1982b), peak radioactivity occurring sooner and dropping off faster than for the latter. The rapid appearance (6 h) of grains over myelin following [^3H]glycerol injection and the subsequent 3-day buildup was attributed to transfer of intact phospholipid. With [^3H]choline

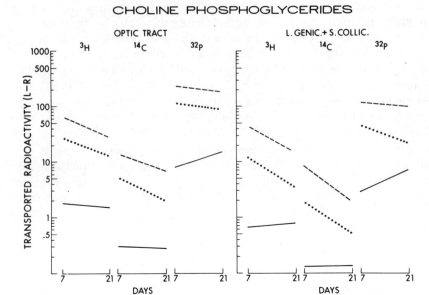

FIGURE 4.7 Transported radioactivity of choline phosphoglycerides. Young rabbits were given intraocular injections (right eye) of mixture of [2-^{3}H]glycerol, [^{14}C]glycerol, and ^{32}PO$_4$ in saline. Two groups were sacrificed after 7 days and 21 days, respectively. Left and right superior colliculi and lateral geniculates were pooled separately, and fractionated into myelin, axolemma-enriched, and axon-enriched fractions. Left and right optic tracts were similarly treated. Transported radioactivity represents normalized left minus right values. Data are presented in dpm/mg phospholipid $\times$ 10^{-3}. L/R ratios were >10 in all cases. Designations: ____, myelin; . . . . ., axolemma; -----, axons. To be noted are the selective increases in ^{32}P radioactivity over time of phosphatidylcholine in myelin. (From Ledeen and Haley, 1983; reproduced with permission of Elsevier Science Publishers.)

as precursor, however, the data suggested that in addition to phospholipid transfer, free choline also diffused from the axon into adjacent myelin and Schwann cell cytoplasm to become reincorporated into myelin lipids. The free choline was believed to be released from transported choline phosphoglycerides either by base-exchange reaction or the action of phospholipase D. This possibility was made plausible by recent demonstration of phospholipase D activity in an axolemma-enriched fraction from brain (DeVries et al., 1983).

A more detailed study of this problem with quantitative radioautography (Droz et al., 1981) reinforced the initial conclusion that [^{3}H]choline label detected in myelin could originate from both direct transfer of intact lipid and local biosynthesis. Early detection of radioactive choline in the

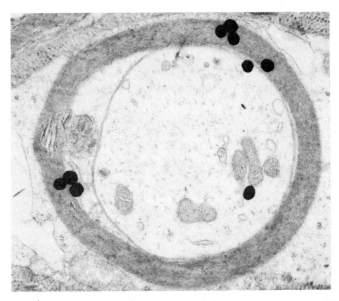

FIGURE 4.8 Electron microscope radioautograph of a preganglionic nerve fiber in the chicken ciliary ganglion 3 days after an intracerebral injection of [2-^{3}H]glycerol. Silver grains located over the axon are produced by labeled glycerophospholipids transported by fast axonal flow in close association with membranous structures. The silver grains superimposed to the myelin sheath reveal that part of the transported lipids are transferred from the axon to adjacent myelin. (From Droz et al., 1981. Reproduced with permission of authors and Elseiver Science Publishers.)

outer Schwann cell cytoplasm close to the Schmidt–Lanterman incisures suggested to these workers that such channels provided a principal diffusion route from the axon into myelin and Schwann cell. Grain distribution with this precursor differed from that with [^{3}H]glycerol in its presence over outer Schwann cell cytoplasm, as well as in satellite cells and perikarya of the postsynaptic ganglion cells. This difference was attributed to the inability of the glycerol label to undergo the same kind of reutilization as choline in extra-axonal compartments. Quantification revealed that the label moved from inner to outer layers of myelin. Gould et al. (1982) obtained similar results with rat sciatic nerve, employing radioautography with [^{3}H]choline as precursor. Grains were seen over myelin as early as 6 h, and the labeling of myelin relative to axon increased with time; at 12 days most of the labeled lipid was localized in myelin. This study also demonstrated movement of the choline label from axon to glia in regenerating nerve.

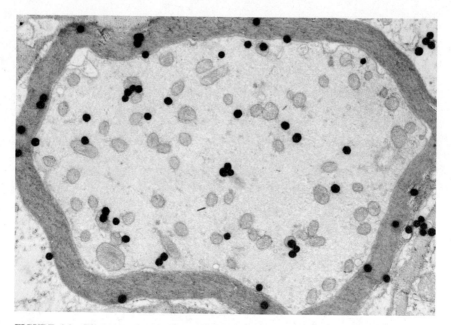

FIGURE 4.9 Electron microscope radioautograph of a preganglionic nerve fiber in the chicken ciliary ganglion 3 days after an intracerebral injection of [methyl-³H]choline. The axon is overlaid with silver grains frequently related to mitochondria. Many silver grains are seen over the myelin sheath. As distinct from Figure 4.8, numerous silver grains are found over the outer Schwann cell cytoplasm. Thus, with [methyl-³H]choline, the tracer reveals both a transfer of choline-glycerophospholipid and a reincorporation of labeled choline into choline-glycerophospholipids and sphingomyelin synthesized by Schwann cells. (From Droz et al., 1978. Reproduced with permission of authors and Elsevier Science Publishers.)

The above study of Droz et al. (1981) demonstrated sharp contrast between lipids and proteins, the latter remaining largely confined to the neuron while in transit down the axon. Thus, use of either [³H]fucose or [³H]lysine as precursor resulted in no grain detection over myelin. A similar conclusion was reached in the use of serine with the rabbit optic system (Haley and Ledeen, 1979), this precursor causing significant labeling of myelin lipids but not of myelin proteins. In this regard Gould et al. (1982) have cautioned that since protein diffusion within myelin would be slower than that of lipid, its occurrence might not be observed under the conditions of the experiment.

Biochemical analysis of individual lipids from the oculomotor nerve of the chicken (Brunetti et al., 1981) revealed labeling of the major classes by [^{3}H]glycerol, with phosphatidylcholine predominating. Radioactivity peaked in all cases at 40 h and then declined by 7 days. In contrast, [^{14}C]choline labeling of sphingomyelin and phosphatidylcholine in myelin continued to rise over 7 days. This result, pointing up an efficient mechanism of choline reutilization in myelin/Schwann cells, resembles the findings with serine (Haley and Ledeen, 1979) and palmitate (Alberghina et al., 1982b) in the rabbit optic system. In regard to other lipids, Droz et al. (1979) reported preliminary findings that axonally transported phosphatidylinositol, resulting from intracerebral injection of [^{3}H]*myo*-inositol, did not pass into myelin in appreciable quantities. With respect to phosphatidylethanolamine, a recent study (Brunetti et al., 1983) revealed the interesting fact that whereas the diacyl form of this phospholipid is transported to the axolemma and nerve ending, the plasmalogen form is preferentially transferred to myelin in which it accumulates (Fig. 4.10). This followed intracerebral injection of [^{3}H]ethanolamine.

4.4.3 Mechanism and Function

Neither the mechanism of the transfer nor its physiological significance are well understood at present. The flow of axonal lipids and lipid precursors into the myelin–glial compartment may eventually be shown to represent a form of metabolic dependence of the latter on the neuron, although it is too early to assert that these are the long-sought trophic substances. The transfer of axonal choline into Schwann cells has been specifically cited (Brunetti et al., 1981) as a potentially important contribution of the neuron to myelin maintenance, considering that the entry of choline into peripheral nerve is limited by the blood–nerve barrier and the perineurial sheath (Gould and Dawson, 1976; Hendelman and Bunge, 1969). However, such contribution need not be restricted to choline and could well encompass a variety of metabolites required for renewal of specific myelin components. It has been suggested that although the translocation of phospholipids into myelin may be quantitatively minor compared with the larger amount synthesized by Schwann cells, the axon's contribution may exert significant influence on a limited pool of myelin phospholipid (Haley and Ledeen, 1979; Brunetti et al., 1981; Ledeen and Haley, 1983).

Brunetti et al., (1981) proposed that axon–myelin transfer of phospholipid could correspond to a series of equilibration processes with reversible exchanges occurring between several membrane structures:

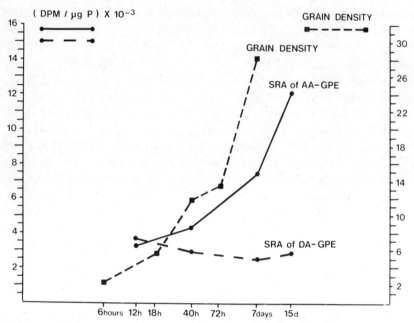

FIGURE 4.10   Comparison of the kinetics of the specific radioactivity of alkenylacyl-(AA)-GPE (●—●) and of the silver grain density (■-----■) in myelin of the chicken ciliary ganglion at different time intervals after the intracerebral injection of [1-³H]ethanolamine. Note that the kinetics of the silver grain accumulation fits the kinetics of labeled alkenylacyl-GPE but not of diacyl-(DA)-GPE (●-----●). (SRA: specific radioactivity.) (From Droz et al., 1984. Reproduced with permission of authors and Raven Press.)

Axonal smooth endoplasmic reticulum ⇄ axolemma

⇄ glial plasmalemma ⇄ loose myelin of the

Schmidt–Lanterman clefts ⇄ compact myelin

They point out that exchange with the inner myelin layers would permit rapid equilibration of phospholipids in that structure, a considerably faster result than arrival of new lipids synthesized by the Schwann cell, which requires a number of days (Gould and Dawson, 1976). The more facile exchange of choline phosphoglycerides over ethanolamine phosphoglycerides (Droz et al., 1979) was proposed as due to the former being present in the outer leaflet and the latter the inner leaflet of the axolemma (Brunetti et al., 1981). These ideas are in keeping with the ability of phospholipids to undergo transfer as a result of membrane contact and membrane fusion (Pagano and Weinstein, 1978). A possible role for phospholipid exchange proteins in this process seems worth exploring in view of the recent *in vitro* demonstration that myelin is an effective recipient of such transfer (see below).

4.5 INTRACELLULAR PHOSPHOLIPID TRANSFER

4.5.1 Historical

The discovery of phospholipid transfer proteins is generally credited to Wirtz and Zilversmit (1968), who observed that a postmicrosomal supernatant from rat liver stimulated the transfer of phospholipids between microsomes and mitochondria. Little phospholipid redistribution was found in the absence of the cytosolic factor, a result subsequently confirmed with phospholipid vesicles (Kornberg and McConnel, 1971b; Ehnholm and Zilversmit, 1972). The results are consistent with bidirectional exchange of phospholipids between the two fractions, and the proteins eventually identified as the causative agents were called *phospholipid exchange proteins*. Later, when it was realized that such proteins can under some circumstances catalyze a true net transfer, the generic term *phospholipid transfer protein* was adopted. This is now the preferred terminology, but it should not obscure the fact that the large majority of *in vitro* studies involve exchange and that special conditions are required to reveal net transfer of phospholipid mass.

The exchange phenomenon was soon confirmed by many other workers, and phospholipid transfer proteins are now regarded as ubiquitous in eucaryotic cells. A few reports have documented their presence in procaryotic sources as well (Bureau and Mazliak, 1974; Cohen et al., 1979; Lemaresquier et al., 1982). The animal tissues most widely studied have been liver, brain, and heart, with some attention also to intestine, lung, retina, plasma, and others. Beef heart cytosol was the source of the first phospholipid transfer protein to be isolated in pure form (Wirtz and Zilversmit, 1970). Since then additional transfer proteins have been purified and characterized from bovine liver (Kamp et al., 1973; Demel et al., 1973; Crain and Zilversmit, 1980a), rat liver (Bloj and Zilversmit, 1977), and rat hepatoma (Dyatlovitskaya et al., 1978).

The presence of such activity in brain was demonstrated by Wirtz (1970) using rat brain cytosol and by Miller and Dawson (1972b) using a guinea pig brain-soluble fraction. The large number of reviews that have appeared on this topic over the past decade (Dawson, 1973; Wirtz, 1974; Zilversmit and Hughes, 1976; Kader, 1977; Wirtz and van Deenan, 1977;

Brammer, 1981; Kader et al., 1982) attest to the growing interest in this phenomenon.

4.5.2 General Properties

Phospholipid transfer proteins mediate the exchange of phospholipids between a large variety of natural and artificial membranes. While the original studies employed microsomes and mitochondria, later variations utilized among other things the inner and outer mitochondrial membranes, lung lamellar bodies, plasma membranes, and lipoproteins. In addition to such natural membranes, the discovery that transfer proteins can function with liposomes, monolayers, and other artificial membranes led to systems with controlled lipid compositions. Such systems have proved highly beneficial in elucidating the nature and mechanism of the transfer reaction. Liposomes have been used in conjunction with natural membranes of the above types as well as myelin, synaptic membranes, rod outer segments, and others. Some studies have employed liposomes entirely, depending on such techniques as immunoprecipitation (Ehnholm and Zilversmit, 1973), lectin agglutination (Sasaki and Sakagami, 1978), and ion-exchange chromatography (Hellings et al., 1974) to separate donor and acceptor populations. The liposomes employed in most studies have been unilamellar vesicles obtained by sonication, but the larger multilamellar vesicles prepared by handshaking of the lipids in buffer have also found use in some instances (Dicorleto and Zilversmit, 1977, 1979).

The principal subcellular localization is the cytosol, consistent with the fact that these are soluble proteins assayed in and isolated from the postmicrosomal supernatant. A common procedure is to bring the postmicrosomal supernatant to pH 5.1 and remove the precipitated proteins by centrifugation. A radioimmunoassay for the phosphatidylcholine-transfer protein from rat liver revealed that approximately 60% of this protein was present in the 105,000g supernatant from liver homogenate, the remainder being distributed over the particulate fractions (Teerlink et al., 1982). Since the particle-bound activity was almost completely removed by a single washing step, the authors proposed a dynamic equilibrium between the membrane-bound and soluble pools. However, in view of the hydrophobic character of most transfer proteins, it needs to be demonstrated that such binding has functional significance. Applying the same radioimmunoassay to tissue homogenates, the highest levels of the transfer protein were found in liver and intestinal mucosa with lower levels in kidney, spleen, and lung. Heart and brain contained very little of this particular transfer protein (see below).

Most of the transfer proteins from animal sources have M_r values ranging from 11,000 to 33,000, the majority being around 22,000. The list compiled by Kader et al. (1982) includes proteins with both acidic and basic isoelectric points. It was pointed out (Kader et al., 1982) that no special correlation exists between the isoelectric point and other properties (e.g., specificity). The complete amino acid sequence for the phosphatidylcholine-specific transfer protein of beef liver has been determined (Moonen et al., 1980; Akeroyd et al., 1981) and its average hydrophobicity found to be high.

In relation to molecular specificity, two broad categories of transfer protein have been observed: monospecific and nonspecific. They have also been classified as phosphatidylcholine-transfer, phosphatidylinositol-transfer, sphingomyelin-transfer, and nonspecific phospholipid-transfer proteins (Teerlink et al., 1982). Transfer proteins specific for phosphatidylcholine have been isolated from such sources as beef liver (Kamp et al., 1973) and rat liver (Lumb et al., 1976; Poorthius et al., 1980). Other proteins obtained from beef and rat tissues preferentially catalyzed the transfer of phosphatidylinositol (Dicorleto et al., 1979; Helmkamp et al., 1974; Lumb et al., 1976; Wirtz et al., 1976a), but these invariably showed some activity toward phosphatidylcholine or sphingomyelin as well. A transfer protein specific for the latter lipid has been reported (Dyatlovitskaya et al., 1982). Nonspecific transfer proteins have been isolated from such sources as rat liver (Bloj and Zilversmit, 1977), bovine liver (Crain and Zilversmit, 1980a), rat lung (Read and Funkhouser, 1983), and rat hepatoma (Dyatlovitskaya et al., 1978). These are believed to be important in the net transfer of phospholipids (see below). The nonspecific protein of liver is capable of transferring all major types of phospholipid and also cholesterol. Recent evidence suggests that it (or a closely related species in the pH 5.1 supernatant) is able to transfer glycolipids as well (Bloj and Zilversmit, 1981b).

The phospholipid exchange proteins are apparently nonspecific toward different types of membranes (Zilversmit, 1971; Helmkamp et al., 1974; Brammer and Sheltawy, 1975; Dicorleto et al., 1977). Adding to the complexity of the transfer picture is the fact that multiple transfer proteins for a single phospholipid may exist in the same tissue (e.g., brain, see below). The possible physiological significance of these multiple transfer proteins has been discussed by Helmkamp et al. (1976).

4.5.3   Transfer Proteins of the Nervous System

The early studies of Miller and Dawson (1972b) demonstrating the existence of a soluble, nondialyzable, heat-labile fraction that stimulated transfer of phospholipid between brain subfractions led to the isolation of specific phospholipid-transfer proteins from bovine cerebral cortex (Helmkamp et al., 1974). Two such proteins were obtained with very similar M_r values, phospholipid specificities, amino acid compositions, and immunochemical properties but different isoelectric points. They showed highest transfer activity toward phosphatidylinositol and about one-eighth as much toward phosphatidylcholine (Demel et al., 1977). This was in contrast to the beef liver enzyme, which showed very high transfer activity for phosphatidylcholine and only minor activity toward phosphatidylinositol. These data were consistent with binding studies, the latter protein containing one molecule of non-covalently bound phosphatidylcholine upon isolation and the brain protein binding both phospholipids with 12-fold higher affinity for phosphatidylinositol. No proteins entirely specific for phosphatidylinositol have been isolated to date.

According to immunological criteria these were the major phospholipid transfer proteins in brain, accounting for more than 85% and 60% of the phosphatidylinositol- and phosphatidylcholine-transfer activities, respectively (Helmkamp et al., 1976). Similar activities have been observed in sheep (Brammer and Sheltawy, 1975) and rat brain (Wirtz et al., 1976a). The specificity of the bovine enzyme was further emphasized by the finding that it was incapable of transferring phosphatidylinositol 4-phosphate between vesicles (Schermoly and Helmkamp, 1983). It has been reported that the postmicrosomal supernatant of rat brain does not have any phosphatidylethanolamine-transfer activity (Wirtz, 1974). This implies that rat brain lacks the nonspecific transfer protein that presumably is responsible for this activity (Bloj and Zilversmit, 1977). It thus appears that the large majority of all phospholipid-transfer activity in rat brain is due to the phosphatidylinositol-transfer protein.

In their study of brain subcellular fractions Miller and Dawson (1972b) found that in the presence of supernatant, ^{32}P-labeled microsomes could donate phospholipids to the isolated synaptosomal fraction but more slowly than to mitochondria. Phospholipids of the myelin fraction did not exchange. Brammer and Sheltawy (1976) also observed no exchange between phosphatidylcholine in liposomes and that in a whole myelin fraction from guinea pig brain, although liposomes prepared from total lipids of myelin in the Ca^{2+} form could exchange to some extent with brain mitochondria. Carey and Foster (1977), on the other hand, found that myelin phosphatidylcholine was able to exchange at a low but measurable rate with phosphatidylcholine in other membranes. This was reinforced by Brammer (1978) who observed transfer to myelin subfractions in the presence of rat brain pH 5.1 supernatant, phosphatidylcholine going more rapidly into the dense myelin subfraction than the lighter ones. However, possible contamination of this subfraction by other membranes (e.g., microsomes) requires caution in interpretation of these results.

The detailed study of Ruenwongsa et al. (1979) revealed that the rate of exchange of myelin phospholipids depended on the pH and temperature, optima being observed at pH 7 and 50°C. The extent of catalyzed exchange increased dramatically on using sonicated or heat-treated myelin as the acceptor membrane. In the presence of pH 5.1 supernatant from brain the principal lipid exchanged was phosphatidylinositol and, to a lesser extent, phosphatidylcholine. In developing rat brain the catalytic activity increased after birth and reached a maximum around 21 days of age, corresponding to the process of myelination. The authors proposed that the transfer proteins may have a physiological role in facilitating *in vivo* transfer or exchange of phospholipids from their site of synthesis in the endoplasmic reticulum to myelin.

The presence of phospholipid transfer proteins in myelin itself was inferred from detection of such activity in aqueous extracts of this membrane (Wirtz et al., 1976a). Compared with the crude 105,000g supernatant from total rat brain, the phosphatidylinositol- and phosphatidylcholine-transfer activities per milligram of soluble protein were enriched seven- and twofold, respectively, in the myelin extract. Similar results were obtained with synaptosomes, enrichments in this case being eight- and four-fold, respectively. Based on electrophoretic behavior and activity ratios, the two major phospholipid-exchange proteins in the synaptosomes appeared identical to those in the total brain cytosol.

4.5.4 Mechanism and Physiological Role

From numerous studies with model systems a comprehensive picture of the mode of action of transfer proteins has begun to emerge (reviewed by Kader et al., 1982). Correlations have been observed between transfer activity and such factors as acyl chain structure, temperature, and membrane fluidity (Helmkamp, 1980; Kaspar and Helmkamp, 1981). Hydrophobic interactions, although important, do not seem to be highly specific with respect to the nature of the acyl chains. The amino acid sequence of the hydrophobic binding site was determined by binding of phosphatidylcholine with a photosensitive group and study of the proteolytic digestion products (Moonen et al., 1979).

Electrostatic interactions also play an important role in binding of phospholipid to transfer proteins. Alteration of binding was induced through changes in the polar group (Kamp et al., 1977) as well as by ionic strength manipulation (Johnson and Zilversmit, 1975) and introduction of various cations (Wirtz et al. 1976b). A molecular model based on these and other observations has been proposed (Kader et al., 1982) that places the phospholipid in a crevice on the transfer protein with separate binding sites for the hydrophobic and polar moieties. This accords with the observation that bound phospholipid is well protected from phospholipase action until dislodged from the protein by detergent or organic solvent (Kamp et al., 1975). It is not known whether nonspecific transfer proteins have one multispecific site or several sites for phospholipid binding.

Many studies have shown that the lipid composition of both donor and acceptor membranes exert a profound effect on the transfer process. Membrane properties such as charge, fluidity, and curvature not only govern the activity of the transfer proteins but also control the relative contribution of net transfer as compared to exchange. Details of the various steps involved in the exchange process have been summarized (Kader et al., 1982).

Despite these advances in the understanding of mechanism, the physiological role(s) of transfer proteins still require(s) elucidation. Renewal of membrane lipid and maintenance of desired phospholipid compositions are putative functions of these proteins acting as catalytic agents for exchange. One could envision this as a mechanism for replacement of "altered" lipids (e.g., oxidized), for example, or as a device for the rapid turnover of phospholipids before extensive alteration occurs. The exchange phenomenon highlights the fact that membrane lipids are not necessarily coupled to membrane proteins in terms of metabolic behavior but can "turn over" independently.

The facilitated transfer of phospholipids between mitochondria and microsomes observed *in vitro* suggests similar transfer *in vivo*, although only indirect evidence has supported this idea to date (Abdelkader and Mazliak, 1970; Eggens et al., 1979). In more general terms, transfer proteins have been proposed to participate in membrane biogenesis by inserting newly formed phospholipids (e.g., from the endoplasmic reticulum) into membranes unable to synthesize their own. A potential problem with this hypothesis is that the types of exchange usually catalyzed by these proteins would only mediate renewal or modification of existing membranes rather than creation of new ones. However, the recent demonstration that a nonspecific phospholipid-transfer protein is able to catalyze net transfer of phospholipids (Crain and Zilversmit, 1980b) makes the concept of membrane biogenesis more credible. This property together with their lack of specificity and absence of "bound" phospholipid (Crain and Zilversmit, 1980a) may indicate a different mechanism of transfer and a different physiological role than the previously studied exchange proteins.

The special properties of neural cells, in particular their possession of long processes with little capacity for *de novo* lipid synthesis, would suggest an important role for phospholipid-transfer proteins in neural membrane renewal. Phospholipids undergoing axonal transport, for example, presumably require a vehicle for exchanging with phospholipids of the axonal membrane, and it may therefore be significant that transfer activity was recently detected in the axoplasm of the squid giant axon (Gould et al., 1983b). A role in myelination and myelin renewal can be inferred from the studies described previously. In addition to the above modes of intracellular transfer, the possibility that phospholipid transfer proteins mediate intercellular movement, as in the above-described transfer from axon to myelin, may be another area worth exploring in the future.

ACKNOWLEDGMENTS

This study was supported by PHS grants NS-03356, NS-04834, and NS-11853. I wish to thank Drs. Bernard Droz and Pierre Morell for sharing their results prior to publication and for providing Figures 4.3 and 4.8–4.10. Thanks are also due to Dr. Bernice Grafstein for providing Figures 4.4–4.6.

REFERENCES

Abdelkader, A.B., and Mazliak, P., *Eur. J. Biochem., 15*, 250–262 (1970).

Abe, T., Haga, T., and Kurokawa, M., *Biochem. J., 136*, 731–740 (1973).

Akeroyd, R., Moonen, P., Westerman, J., Puyk, W.C., and Wirtz, K.W.A., *Eur. J. Biochem., 114*, 385–391 (1981).

Alberghina, M., Karlsson, J.O., and Giuffrida, A.M., *J. Neurochem., 39*, 223–227 (1982a).

Alberghina, M., Viola, M., and Giuffrida, A.M., *Neurochem. Res., 7*, 139–149 (1982b).

Alberghina, M., Moschella, F., Viola, M., Brancoti, V., Micali, G., and Giuffrida, A.M., *J. Neurochem., 40*, 32–38 (1983a).

Alberghina, M., Viola, M., and Giuffrida, A.M., *J. Neurochem., 40*, 25–31 (1983b).

Alvarez, J., and Chen, W.Y., *Acta Physiol. Lat. Amer., 22*, 270–273 (1972).

Ansell, G.B., and Spanner, S., in J.N. Hawthorne and G.B. Ansell, Eds., *Phospholipids, New Comprehensive Biochemistry*, Vol. 4, Elsevier Biomedical Press, Amsterdam, 1982, pp. 23–28.

Bell, R.M., Ballas, L.M., and Coleman, R.A., *J. Lipid Res., 22*, 391–403 (1981).

Benjamins, J.A., and McKhann, G., *J. Neurochem., 20*, 1111–1120 (1973).

Bisby, M.A., and Bulger, V.T., *J. Neurochem., 29*, 313–320 (1977).

Bisby, M.A., and Guy, J.R., *Can. J. Physiol. and Pharmacol., 61*, III (1983).

Black, M.M., and Lasek, R.J., *Brain Res., 171*, 401–413 (1979).

Bloj, B., and Zilversmit, D.B., *J. Biol. Chem., 252*, 1613–1619 (1977).

Bloj, B., and Zilversmit, D.B., *Mol. & Cell Biochem., 40*, 163–172 (1981a).

Bloj, B., and Zilversmit, D.B., *J. Biol. Chem., 256*, 5988–5991 (1981b).

Boyenval, J., and Droz, B., *J. Microsc., 27*, 129–132 (1976).

Boyne, A.F., *Life Sci., 22*, 2057–2066 (1978).

Brammer, M.J., *J. Neurochem., 31*, 1435–1440 (1978).

Brammer, M.J., *Res. Methods in Neurochem., 5*, 179–200 (1981).

Brammer, M.J., and Sheltawy, A., *J. Neurochem., 25*, 699–705 (1975).

Brammer, M.J., and Sheltawy, A., *J. Neurochem., 27*, 937–942 (1976).

Brunetti, M., Giudetta, A., and Porcellati, G., *J. Neurochem., 32*, 319–324 (1979).

Brunetti, M., Di Giamberardino, L., Porcellati, G., and Droz, B., *Brain Res., 219*, 73–84 (1981).

Brunetti, M., Droz, B., Di Giamberardino, L., Koenig, H.L., Carretero, F., and Porcellati, G., *Neurochem. Pathol., 1*, 59–80 (1983).

Bureau, G., and Mazliak, P., *FEBS Lett., 39*, 332–336 (1974).

Butler, M., and Morell, P., *J. Neurochem., 41*, 1445–1454 (1983).

Carey, E.M., and Foster, P.C., *Biochem. Soc. Trans., 5*, 1412–1414 (1977).

Chihara, E., *Invest. Ophthalmol. Vis. Sci., 18*, 339–345 (1979).

Cohen, L.K., Lueking, D.R., and Kaplan, S., *J. Biol. Chem., 254*, 721–728 (1979).

Crain, R.C., and Zilversmit, D.B., *Biochemistry, 19*, 1433–1439 (1980a).

Crain, R.C., and Zilversmit, D.B., *Biochim. Biophys. Acta, 620*, 37–48 (1980b).

Currie, J.R., Grafstein, B., Whitwall, M.H., and Alpert, R., *Neurochem. Res., 3*, 479–492 (1978).

Dawson, R.M.C., *Sub-Cell. Biochem., 2*, 68–89 (1973).

Demel, R.A., Wirtz, K.W.A., Kamp, H.H., Geurts van Kessel, W.S.M., and van Deenen, L.L.M., *Nature New Biol., 246*, 102–105 (1973).

Demel, R.A., Kalsbeek, R., Wirtz, K.W.A., and van Deenen, L.L.M., *Biochim. Biophys. Acta, 466*, 10–22 (1977).

Devaux, P., and McConnell, H.M., *Ann. N.Y. Acad. Sci., 222*, 489–498 (1973).

DeVries, G.H., Chalifour, R.J., and Kanfer, J.N., *J. Neurochem., 40*, 1189–1191 (1983).

Dicorleto, P.E., and Zilversmit, D.B., *Biochemistry, 16*, 2145–2150 (1977).

Dicorleto, P.E., and Zilversmit, D.B., *Biochim. Biophys. Acta, 552*, 114–119 (1979).

Dicorleto, P.E., Fakharzadeh, F. F., Searles, L.L., and Zilversmit, D.B., *Biochim. Biophys. Acta, 468*, 296–304 (1977).

Dicorleto, P.E., Warach, J.B., and Zilversmit, D.B., *J. Biol. Chem., 254*, 7795–7802 (1979).

Droz, B., *Trends in Neurosci., 2*, 146–148 (1979).

Droz, B., and Leblond, C.P., *J. Comp. Neurol., 121*, 325–337 (1963).

Droz, B., Koenig, H.L., and Di Giamberardino, L., *Brain Res., 60*, 93–127 (1973).

Droz, B., Di Giamberardino, L., Koenig, H.L., Boyenval, J., and Hassig, R., *Brain Res., 155*, 347–353 (1978).

Droz, B., Brunetti, M., Di Giamberardino, L., Koenig, H. L., and Porcellati, G., *Soc. Neurosci. Symp., 4*, 344–360 (1979).

Droz, B., Di Giamberardino, L., and Koenig, H.L., *Brain Res., 219*, 57–71 (1981).

Dyatlovitskaya, E.V., Timofeeva, N.G., and Bergelson, L.D., *Eur. J. Biochem., 82*, 463–471 (1978).

Dyatlovitskaya, E.V., Timofeeva, N.G., Yakimenko, E.F., Barsukov, L.I., Muzya, G.I., and Bergelson, L.D., *Eur. J. Biochem., 123,* 311–315 (1982).

Dziegielewska, K.M., Evans, C.A.N., and Saunders, N.R., *J. Physiol., 304,* 83–98 (1980).

Eggens, I., Valtersson, C., Dallner, G., and Ernster, L., *Biochem. Biophys. Res. Commun., 91,* 709–714 (1979).

Ehnholm, C., and Zilversmit, D.B., *Biochim. Biophys. Acta, 274,* 652–657 (1972).

Ehnholm, C., and Zilversmit, D.B., *J. Biol. Chem., 248,* 1719–1724 (1973).

Einstein, A., in A. Furth, Ed., A.D. Cowper, Trans., *Investigations on the Theory of the Brownian Movement,* Methuen, London, p. 39, 1926.

Franke, W.W., Morre, D.J., Deumling, B., Cheetham, R.D., Kartenbeck, J., Jarasch, E.D., and Zentgraf, H.-W., *Z. Naturforsch., 26,* 1031–1039 (1971).

Gainer, H., Tasaki, I., and Lasek, R.J., *J. Cell Biol., 74,* 524–530 (1977).

Goodrum, J.F., and Morell, P., *J. Neurochem., 38,* 696–704 (1982).

Goracci, G., Blomstrand, C., Arienti, G., Hamberger, A., and Porcellati, G., *J. Neurochem., 20,* 1167–1180 (1973).

Gould, R.M., *Brain Res., 117,* 169–174 (1976).

Gould, R.M., and Dawson, R.M.C., *J. Cell Biol., 68,* 480–496 (1976).

Gould, R.M., Spivack, W.D., Sinatra, R.S., Lindquist, T.D., and Ingoglia, N.A., *J. Neurochem., 39,* 1569–1578 (1982).

Gould, R.M., Pant, H., Gainer, H., and Tytell, M., *J. Neurochem., 40,* 1293–1299 (1983a).

Gould, R.M., Spivack, W.D., Robertson, D., and Poznansky, M.J., *J. Neurochem., 40,* 1300–1306 (1983b).

Grafstein, B., in E. Kandel, Ed., *Handbook of Physiology, Section 1, The Nervous System,* Waverly Press, Bethesda, Md., 1977, pp. 691–717.

Grafstein, B., and Forman, D.S., *Physiol. Revs., 60,* 1167–1283 (1980).

Grafstein, B., Miller, J.A., Ledeen, R.W., Haley, J., and Specht, S.C., *Exp. Neurol., 46,* 261–281 (1975).

Haley, J.E., and Ledeen, R.W., *Trans. Amer. Soc. Neurochem., Abstr., 9,* 202 (1978).

Haley, J.E., and Ledeen, R.W., *J. Neurochem., 32,* 735–742 (1979).

Haley, J.E., Tirri, L.J., and Ledeen, R.W., *J. Neurochem., 32,* 727–734 (1979a).

Haley, J.E., Wisniewski, H.M., and Ledeen, R.W., *Brain Res., 179,* 69–76 (1979b).

Hammerschlag, R., *Fed. Proc., 39,* 2809–2814 (1980).

Hammerschlag, R., and Lavoie, P.-A., *Neuroscience, 4,* 1195–1201 (1979).

Hammerschlag, R., and Stone, G.C., *Trends in Neurosci., 5,* 12–15 (1982).

Heacock, A.M., and Agranoff, B., *Brain Res., 122,* 243–254 (1977).

Hellings, J.A., Kamp, H.H., Wirtz, K.W.A., and van Deenen, L.L.M., *Eur. J. Biochem., 47,* 601–605 (1974).

Helmkamp, G.M., Jr., *Biochem., 19,* 2050–2056 (1980).

Helmkamp, G.M., Jr., Harvey, M.S., Wirtz, K.W.A., and van Deenen, L.L.M., *J. Biol. Chem., 249,* 6382–6389 (1974).

Helmkamp, G.M., Jr., Nelemans, S.A., and Wirtz, K.W.A., *Biochim. Biophys. Acta, 424,* 168–182 (1976).

Hendelman, W., and Bunge, R.P., *J. Cell Biol., 40,* 190–208 (1969).

Heuser, J.E., and Reese, T.S., in E. Kandel, Ed., *Handbook of Physiology, Section 1, The Nervous System,* Waverly Press, Baltimore, Md., 1977, pp. 261–294.

Higgins, J.A., *Biochim. Biophys. Acta, 558,* 48–57 (1979).

Hirata, F., and Axelrod, J., *Science, 209,* 1082–1090 (1980).

Holtzman, E., and Mercurio, A.M., *Int. Rev. Cytol., 67,* 1–67 (1980).

Johnson, L.W., and Zilversmit, D.B., *Biochim. Biophys. Acta, 375,* 165–175 (1975).

Kader, J.-C., in G. Poste and G.L. Nicolson, Eds., *Cell Surface Reviews,* Vol. 3, Elsevier, Amsterdam, 1977, pp. 127–204.

Kader, J.-C., Douady, D., and Mazliak, P., in J.N. Hawthorne and G.B. Ansell, Eds., *Phospholipids, New Comprehensive Biochemistry* Vol. 4, Elsevier Biomedical Press, Amsterdam, 1982, pp. 279–312.

Kamp, H.H., Wirtz, K.W.A., and van Deenen, L.L.M., *Biochim. Biophys. Acta, 318,* 313–325 (1973).

Kamp, H.H., Springers, E.D., Westerman, J., Wirtz, K.W.A., and van Deenen, L.L.M., *Biochim. Biophys. Acta, 398,* 415–423 (1975).

Kamp, H.H., Wirtz, K.W.A., Baer, P.R., Slotboom, A.J., Rosenthal, A.F., Paltauf, F., and van Deenen, L.L.M., *Biochemistry, 16,* 1310–1316 (1977).

Kaspar, A.M., and Helmkamp, G.M., *Biochemistry, 20,* 146–151 (1981).

Kornberg, R.D., and McConnell, H.M., *Proc. Natl. Acad. Sci. U.S.A., 68,* 2564–2568 (1971a).

Kornberg, R.D., and McConnell, H.M., *Biochemistry, 10,* 1111–1120 (1971b).

Kreutzberg, G.W., and Schubert, P., in E. Genazzani and H. Herken, Eds., *Central Nervous System—Studies on Metabolic Regulation and Function,* Springer-Verlag, Berlin, 1973, pp. 84–93.

Kreutzberg, G.W., Schubert, P., Toth, L., and Rieske, E., *Brain Res., 62,* 399–404 (1973).

Kumara-Siri, M.H., and Gould, R.M., *Brain Res., 186,* 315–330 (1980).

Kunishita, T., and Ledeen, R.W., *Trans. Amer. Soc. Neurochem.,* (Abstr.), *13,* 192 (1982).

Kunishita, T., and Ledeen, R.W., *J. Neurochem., 42,* 326–333 (1984).

Kunishita, T., Novak, J., Morrow, C.R., and Ledeen, R.W. (in press).

Larrabee, M.G., and Brinley, F.J., *J. Neurochem., 15,* 533–545 (1968).

Lasek, R.J., *Trends in Neurosci. 3,* 87–91 (1980).

Lasek, R.J., Gainer, H., and Barker, J.L., *J. Cell Biol., 74,* 501–523 (1977).

Ledeen, R.W., and Haley, J.E., *Brain Res., 269,* 267–275 (1983).

Ledeen, R.W., and Wu, P.-S., *7th Int. Meet. Int. Soc. Neurochem.,* (Abstr.), Jerusalem, 117 (1979).

Ledeen, R.W., Skrivanek, J.A., Nunez, J., Sclafani, J.R., Norton, W.T., and Farooq, M., in M.M. Rapport and A. Gorio, Eds., *Gangliosides in Neurological and Neuromuscular Function, Development, and Repair,* Raven Press, New York, 1981, pp. 211–224.

Lee, P.K., Deshmukh, D.S., Wisniewski, H.M., and Brockerhoff, H., *Neurochem. Intern., 4,* 355–359 (1982).

Lemaresquier, H., Bureau, G., Mazliak, P., and Kader, J.-C., *Int. J. Biochem., 14,* 71–74 (1982).

Lentz, T.L., *Trends in Neurosci., 6,* 48–53 (1983).

Longo, F.M., and Hammerschlag, R., *Brain Res., 193,* 471–485 (1980).

Lorenz, T., and Willard, M., *Proc. Natl. Acad. Sci. U.S.A., 75,* 505–509 (1978).

Lumb, R.H., Kloosterman, A.D., Wirtz, K.W.A., and van Deenen, L.L.M., *Eur. J. Biochem., 69,* 15–22 (1976).

Miani, N., *J. Neurochem.*, *10*, 859–874 (1963).

Miller, E.K., and Dawson, R.M.C., *Biochem. J.*, *126*, 805–821 (1972a).

Miller, E.K., and Dawson, R.M.C., *Biochem. J.*, *126*, 823–835 (1972b).

Miller, S.L., Benjamins, J.A., and Morell, P., *J. Biol. Chem.*, *252*, 4025–4037 (1977).

Moonen, P., Haagsman, H.P., van Deenen, L.L.M., and Wirtz, K.W.A., *Eur. J. Biochem.*, *99*, 439–445 (1979).

Moonen, P., Akeroyd, R., Westerman, J., Puyk, W.C., Smits, P., and Wirtz, K.W.A., *Eur. J. Biochem.*, *106*, 279–290 (1980).

Morell, P., and Goodrum, J.F., *J. Neurochem.*, *41*, Suppl. (Abstrs.), 569C (1983).

Morre, D.J., and Outracht, L., *Int. Rev. Cytol.*, (*Suppl. 5*), 61–188 (1977).

Ochs, S., *Science*, *176*, 252–260 (1972).

Pagano, R.E., and Weinstein, J.N., *Ann. Rev. Biophys. Bioeng.*, *7*, 435–468 (1978).

Palade, G.E., *Science*, *189*, 347–357 (1975).

Percy, A.K., Moore, J.F., Carson, M.A., and Waechter, C.J., *Arch. Biochem. Biophys.*, *233*, 484–494 (1983).

Poorthius, B.J.H.M., Van der Krift, T.P., Teerlink, T., Akeroyd, R., Hostetler, K.Y., and Wirtz, K.W.A., *Biochim. Biophys. Acta*, *600*, 376–386 (1980).

Rambourg, A., and Droz, B., *J. Neurochem.*, *35*, 16–25 (1980).

Ramon y Cajal, S., in R.M. May, Transl. and Ed., *Degeneration and Regeneration of the Nervous System*, Vol. 1, Hafner, New York, 1928, p. 77.

Read, R.J., and Funkhouser, J.D., *Biochim. Biophys. Acta*, *752*, 118–126 (1983).

Ruenwongsa, P., Singh, H., and Jungalwala, F.B., *J. Biol. Chem.*, *254*, 9385–9393 (1979).

Sasaki, T., and Sakagami, T., *Biochim. Biophys. Acta*, *512*, 461–471 (1978).

Scandella, C.J., Devaux, P., and McConnell, H.M., *Proc. Natl. Acad. Sci. U.S.A.*, *69*, 2056–2060 (1972).

Schermoly, M.J., and Helmkamp, G.M., Jr., *Brain Res.*, *268*, 197–200 (1983).

Schubert, P., Lux, H.D., and Kreutzberg, G.W., *Acta Neuropathol.*, (*Berl.*), *5*, 179–186 (1971).

Schultze, B., Oehlert, W., and Maurer, W., *Beitr. Pathol. Anat.*, *120*, 58–65 (1959).

Schwartz, J.H., *Annu. Rev. Neurosci.*, *2*, 467–505 (1979).

Singer, M., and Salpeter, M.M., *J. Morph.*, *120*, 281–316 (1966).

Sjostrand, J., *Exp. Brain Res.*, *8*, 105–112 (1969).

Stahl, W.L., and Trams, E.G., *Biochim. Biophys. Acta*, *163*, 459–471 (1968).

Strosznajder, J., Radominska-Pyrek, A., and Horrocks, L.A., *Biochim. Biophys. Acta*, *574*, 48–56 (1979).

Taylor, A.C., and Weiss, P., *Proc. Natl. Acad. Sci.* (*USA*), *54*, 1521–1527 (1965).

Teerlink, T., Van der Krift, T.P., Post, M., and Wirtz, K.W.A., *Biochim. Biophys. Acta*, *713*, 61–67 (1982).

Thompson, G.A., Jr., *The Regulation of Membrane Lipid Metabolism*, C.R.C. Press, Boca Raton, Fla., 1980, pp. 147–158.

Toews, A.D., and Morell, P., *J. Neurochem.*, *37*, 1316–1323 (1981).

Toews, A.D., and Morell, P., in G. Porcellati, L.A. Horrocks, and J.N. Kanfer, Eds., *Phospholipids in the Nervous System. II. Physiological Roles*, Raven Press, New York, 1985, pp. 299–314.

Toews, A.D., Goodrum, J.F., and Morell, P., *J. Neurochem., 32*, 1165–1173 (1979).

Toews, A.D., Padilla, S.S., Roger, L.J., and Morell, P., *Neurochem. Res., 5*, 1175–1183 (1980).

Toews, A.D., Saunders, B.F., Blaker, W.D., and Morell, P., *J. Neurochem., 40*, 555–562 (1983).

Van den Besselaar, A.M.H.P., De Kruijff, B., Van den Bosch, H., and Van Deenen, L.L.M., *Biochim. Biophys. Acta, 510*, 242–255 (1978).

Van Meer, G., Porthius, B.J.H.M., Wirtz, K.W.A., Op den Kamp, J.A.F., and van Deenen, L.L.M., *Eur. J. Biochem., 103*, 283–288 (1980).

Victoria, E.J., van Golde, L.M.G., Hostetler, K.Y., Scherphof, G.L., and van Deenen, L.L.M., *Biochim. Biophys. Acta, 239*, 443–457 (1971).

Weiss, P., and Hiscoe, H.B., *J. Exp. Zool., 107*, 315–396 (1948).

Wirtz, K.W.A., Ph.D. Thesis, University of Utrecht, 1970.

Wirtz, K.W.A., *Biochim. Biophys. Acta, 344*, 95–117 (1974).

Wirtz, K.W.A., and van Deenen, L.L.M., *Trends in Biochem. Sci., 2*, 49–51 (1977).

Wirtz, K.W.A., and Zilversmit, D.B., *J. Biol. Chem., 243*, 3596–3602 (1968).

Wirtz, K.W.A., and Zilversmit, D.B., *FEBS Lett., 7*, 44–46 (1970).

Wirtz, K.W.A., Jolles, J., Westerman, J., and Neys, F., *Nature, 260*, 354–355 (1976a).

Wirtz, K.W.A., Geurts van Kessel, W.S.M., Kamp, H.H., and Demel, R.A., *Eur. J. Biochem., 61*, 515–523 (1976b).

Wright, J.D., and Green, C., *Biochem. J., 123*, 837–844 (1971).

Wu, P.-S., and Ledeen, R.W., *J. Neurochem. 35*, 659–666 (1980).

Zilversmit, D.B., *J. Biol. Chem., 246*, 2645–2649 (1971).

Zilversmit, D.B., and Hughes, M.E., in E.D. Korn, Ed., *Methods in Membrane Biology*, Vol. 7, Plenum, New York, 1976, pp. 211–259.

Zilversmit, D.B., and Hughes, M.E., *Biochim. Biophys. Acta, 469*, 99–110 (1977).

five

METABOLISM AND FUNCTION OF FATTY ACIDS IN BRAIN

LLOYD A. HORROCKS

Department of Physiological Chemistry
College of Medicine
The Ohio State University
Columbus, Ohio

CONTENTS

5.1   INTRODUCTION   174

    5.1.1   Techniques for Analysis, 174
    5.1.2   Content of Free Fatty Acids in Normal Brain, 175

5.2   TRANSPORT   177

5.3   OXIDATION   178

5.4   SYNTHESIS   178

    5.4.1   Synthesis from Glucose and Acetate, 178
    5.4.2   Synthesis from Ketone Bodies, 180
    5.4.3   Elongation and Desaturation, 181

5.5   RELEASE OF FREE FATTY ACIDS   186

    5.5.1   Pathological Response, 186
    5.5.2   Regulation of Free Fatty Acid Release, 189

5.6   UTILIZATION OF FATTY ACIDS   191

    5.6.1   Acylation, 191
    5.6.2   Prostaglandin Formation, 192

5.7   SUMMARY   194

    REFERENCES   195

5.1   INTRODUCTION

The topic of fatty acids in nervous tissues was reviewed very recently (Horrocks and Harder, 1983). The present discussion will emphasize newer developments with regard to transport and oxidation of fatty acids in brain, the metabolic activity of fatty acids, and the release of free fatty acids from phospholipids in pathological situations.

5.1.1   Techniques for Analysis

The extremely rapid increase in free fatty acid concentrations in brain within seconds after decapitation (Bazán et al., 1982) presents a difficulty for the assay of free fatty acid levels in normal brain tissue. Rapid dissection (Aveldano and Bazán, 1975) may be adequate but microwave irradiation (Cenedella et al., 1975) or rapid freezing in liquid nitrogen (DeMedio et al., 1980) is preferable. During dissection the tissue is subjected to ischemia, which is a potent stimulus for release of fatty acids. However, the procedure for microwave irradiation stresses the animal and thus may increase free fatty acid levels. A finite time is required for complete freezing in liquid nitrogen with ischemia occurring sooner than cessation of all metabolic activity; prior decapitation also introduces stress effects.

An example of the methodology required for the complete recovery, assay, and analysis of free fatty acids in tissues was described by Agardh et al. (1981). The tissue was extracted twice with mixtures of chloroform and methanol. The extract was washed with an acidified salt solution. The lower phase was evaporated and the residue was separated by thin-layer chromatography on silica gel with light petroleum–diethyl ether–acetic acid, 55:42:2 by volume. The silica gel with free fatty acids was treated with 0.38 M H_2SO_4 in 1:1 methanol–toluene in order to form fatty acid methyl esters which were separated and quantitated by gas–liquid chromatography.

Most methods of complete lipid extraction are adequate for extraction of free fatty acids. Either alkaline or strongly acidic conditions may cause an artefactual hydrolytic release of fatty acids. Agardh et al. (1981) acidified the wash solution in order to avoid losses of free fatty acids during the washing step. Most other investigators have not washed the extract or have not measured losses due to washing. For the thin-layer chromatographic separation of free fatty acids, Bazán advocates the use of gradient-thickness thin-layer plates with the sample spotted at the thick end (Bazán, 1970; Bazán and Bazán, 1975; Bazán and Cellik, 1972; Bazán and Joel, 1970). An internal standard is generally used for quantitation by gas–liquid chromatography. All of the above procedures were reviewed by Bazán and Bazán (1975).

5.1.2 Content of Free Fatty Acids in Normal Brain

Bazán et al. (1971) reported a free fatty acid content of 35 µg/g fresh weight for rat whole brain that was dissected and extracted within 30 s. The value was 41 for brains frozen in liquid N_2 before extraction. Somewhat lower values, about 23 and 30 µg/g fresh weight for liquid N_2 and dissection methods, respectively, were reported recently by Tang and Sun (1982). An even lower value of approximately 18 µg/g fresh weight

TABLE 5.1   Ratios of Contents of $18:0$, $20:4(n - 6)$, and $22:6(n - 3)$ to $16:0$ in Free Fatty Acids from Brain

Source	$18:0$	$20:4(n - 6)$	$22:6(n - 3)$	Reference
Mouse brain	1.91	1.11	0.14	Aveldano and Bazán (1975)
Gerbil brain	0.77	0.27	—	Yoshida et al. (1980)
Rat cerebrum	0.70	0.28	0.10	Marion and Wolfe (1978)
Rat cerebrum	0.77	0.23	0.12	Rehncrona et al. (1982)
Rat brain	0.45	<0.04	<0.04	Kuwashima et al. (1978)
Rat brain	1.44	1.10	0.12	Tang and Sun (1982)
Rat brain	0.52	<0.03	0.04	Yoshida et al. (1982)

was obtained by Yoshida et al. (1982) for rat brain that was frozen *in situ* with liquid N_2.

The only value reported after microwave irradiation is 79 µg free fatty acid per gram of fresh weight (Cenedella et al., 1975). This value is at least twofold greater than the most reliable values mentioned above. The original report (Lunt and Rowe, 1968) of 500 µg free fatty acid per gram fresh rat brain must reflect both lipolysis and contamination of the free fatty acid fraction with other lipids. Of course, at that time the lability of brain phospholipids had not been established. The composition included fairly high proportions of seven unusual components that have not been found since then.

Quite different distributions of free fatty acids in control brain have been reported by different groups (Table 5.1). As described in Section 5.5 on release of free fatty acids, arachidonate and stearate are released preferentially in pathological situations that stimulate free fatty acid release. Thus, the ratios of arachidonate and stearate to palmitate may be a sensitive measure of the degree of disturbance of normal phospholipid metabolism due to killing of the animal and removal of the brain. Yoshida et al. (1982) believe that the appearance of arachidonate is a postmortem phenomenon and thus even the ratios of 0.27 and 0.28 indicate an abnormality. The very low ratios of Yoshida et al. (1982) were obtained by freezing the brain *in situ*.

The free fatty acids have had much less study in peripheral nerve than in brain. According to Yao et al. (1981), the free fatty acids of human and rat peripheral nerves have a composition quite different from that of brain but resembling that of erythrocytes. Less than 5% of the free fatty acids are polyunsaturated and about 75% are saturated. Approximately 10–15% of free fatty acids have unusually long chain lengths. The identity of the

24:0, 26:0, 28:0, and 30:0 species was confirmed by mass spectrometry. The latter three fatty acids were not detected in brain. Also unlike brain tissue, rat sciatic nerves had no increase in free fatty acid concentration during 30 min after death.

5.2 TRANSPORT

A source for much of the fatty acid in brain phospholipids is uptake from the circulation (Bourre, 1982; Dhopeshwarkar and Mead, 1973). Dhopeshwarkar and colleagues (Dhopeshwarkar and Mead, 1973) have shown the uptake of palmitic, oleic, linoleic, and linolenic acids on the basis of metabolic requirements and turnover. Free fatty acids are taken up much faster than other lipids. The rate of uptake of free fatty acids depends in part on the strength of binding to serum albumin since transport depends on prior dissociation of the fatty acid from the binding site. Approximately 5% of plasma palmitate is unidirectionally cleared by brain on a single pass (Pardridge and Mietus, 1980) and is incorporated into phospholipids within 15 s (Dhopeshwarkar et al., 1972). In the steady state the amount of free fatty acid transported into the brain is balanced by the free fatty acid released after hydrolysis from lipids in the brain.

All essential fatty acids must be transported into the brain from the circulation. In addition, during growth there is a net uptake of a substantial proportion of the non-essential fatty acids. After transport into the brain, exogenous palmitate mixes with endogenous palmitate (Carey, 1975b) and is incorporated into mitochondrial, synaptosomal, microsomal and myelin membranes (Sun and Horrocks, 1973). The net flux of palmitate into the brain at 4 h after injection into the circulation was assessed by Kimes et al. (1983) in various regions of the rat brain by quantitative autoradiography. This flux ranged from 2.0×10^{-5} to 9.3×10^{-5} μmol/g·s for internal capsule and arcuate nucleus, respectively. The flux into gray matter exceeds the flux into white matter. A good correlation was noted for palmitate flux with the cerebral metabolic rate measured with 2-deoxyglucose. The actual flux is greater than the values above because the content of radioactivity at earlier times was twofold greater. Four hours was chosen for the study because the level of radioactivity was stable from 4 to 24 h. The flux value thus probably represents the replacement of esterified palmitate.

The uptake of fatty acids into cells of neuronal and glial origin has also been studied in culture because single-cell types can be placed in a controlled environment. Long-chain saturated (16:0, 18:0, 20:0) and unsaturated fatty acids are taken up (Cook et al., 1982; McGee, 1981). Chemically defined media must be used for these studies since fetal calf serum, which is normally used, contains fatty acids that are utilized by the cells. Hybrid cloned cells grow well in defined media with unsaturated fatty acids but saturated fatty acids as the only fatty acid are toxic (McGee, 1981). Eicosapentaenoic acid, $20:5(n - 3)$, is taken up from the vitreous humor into the retina and then elongated and desaturated to $22:6(n - 3)$, docosahexaenoic acid (H.E.P. Bazán et al., 1982).

5.3 OXIDATION

Long-chain fatty acid oxidation seems to have little importance for energy production in adult brain except in the silkmoth, *Bombyx mori* (Carey, 1975b; Wegener, 1983). Beta oxidation of fatty acids and reincorporation of acetate into other fatty acids is well known. Examples include arachidate, $20:0$, in neuroblastoma and glioma cell lines (Cook et al., 1982), stearate in neurons and astrocytes *in vivo* (Morand et al., 1979), and elaidate, $18:1t$, by intracerebral injection into brain (Cook, 1978). In the adult rat brain 21% of the recovered radioactivity had been reincorporated into palmitate and oleate at 2 days after injection of labeled elaidate. Microvessels from brain can oxidize fatty acids to CO_2 at a rate greater than the rates for liver, heart, or arterial tissue (Morisaki et al., 1982).

Very long chain fatty acids, such as lignocerate, $24:0$, may be metabolized by alpha or a unique beta oxidation (Uda et al., 1982). The primary product from the latter is glutamate. Alpha oxidation requires particulate enzyme, pyridine nucleotide, a heat-labile factor with M_r 32,700 and a heat-stable factor which in part is glucose-6-phosphate. CoA is not required, so a CoA-independent activation of very long chain fatty acids must exist (Uda et al., 1982).

This system oxidizes about 20 pmol lignocerate per milligram of protein per hour. Regular beta oxidation is capable of oxidizing 150 pmol palmitate per milligram of protein per hour. Much of the acetyl-CoA is utilized for lipogenesis rather than oxidation to CO_2 and H_2O by the tricarboxylic acid cycle. In the brain most of the acetyl-CoA from fatty acids that enters the tricarboxylic acid cycle is converted to amino acids by transamination (Kawamura and Kishimoto, 1981).

5.4 SYNTHESIS

5.4.1 Synthesis from Glucose and Acetate

The synthesis of fatty acids in brain was reviewed recently by Horrocks and Harder (1983) and by Bourre (1980). As in other tissues, fatty acid synthetase in brain utilizes 1 acetyl-CoA and 7 malonyl-CoA molecules to make 1 molecule of palmitate with 14 NADPH molecules also required (Volpe and Kishimoto, 1972). The rate-controlling enzyme is acetyl-CoA carboxylase (EC 6.4.1.2) which activates acetyl-CoA by forming malonyl-CoA utilizing energy from ATP and biotin as a cofactor. This enzyme is inhibited by low levels of long-chain acyl-CoA. Thus, the uptake of exogenous fatty acids followed by the action of fatty acid–CoA ligase to produce acyl-CoA may regulate the short-term activity for fatty acid synthesis (Volpe and Marasa, 1977).

Acetyl-CoA carboxylase and the fatty acid synthetase complex are actively turned over in brain (Patel and Tonkonow, 1974; Volpe et al., 1973). The synthesis of these enzymes is closely coordinated and is inhibited by exogenous fatty acids, hydrocortisone, dibutyryl cAMP, and theophylline (Volpe and Marasa, 1976a,b). The specific activities of these enzymes are highest during the developmental stages with cell multiplication. During the stage of myelination and dendritic arborization, the specific activities are lower, suggesting a dependence on exogenous fatty acids for lipid synthesis for myelin (Bourre et al., 1977; Cantrill and Carey, 1975; Koeppen et al., 1980). In rat cerebrum the specific activity of the enzymes for fatty acid synthesis is high throughout the fetal stage, peaks at 1 day, then declines markedly after 5 days (Yeh, 1981). The specific activity in cerebrum during early development is greater than that in cerebellum, midbrain, thalamus, and brain stem. During the third week of life the specific activities in brain stem and cerebellum are greater than those in midbrain and thalamus. In adult rat brain regions the specific activities are 17–50% of those in developing brain (Yeh, 1981). Since the rat brain is increasing in weight during development, the total activity per brain rises during the first 3 weeks of life (Volpe and Kishimoto, 1972).

During development, when fatty acid synthesis is most active, both glucose and ketone bodies are utilized by the brain. Ketone bodies are the best precursors for synthesis of brain lipids (Patel and Owen, 1977). When lipids are synthesized from ketone bodies, glucose metabolism is required for the provision of NADPH. In rats (Patel and Tonkanow, 1974) and rabbits (Carey, 1975b) the incorporation of carbon atoms from glucose into lipids correlates well with the specific activities of acetyl-CoA carboxylase and fatty acid synthetase.

Acetate is incorporated into esterified palmitate within seconds after injection into the carotid artery (Dhopeshwarkar et al., 1971; Dhopeshwarkar et al., 1972). The acetyl-CoA from glucose metabolism is produced by pyruvate dehydrogenase in the mitochondria. The acetate portion can be transported into the cytosol via citrate, N-acetylaspartate, and glutamate or 2-oxoglutarate (D'Adamo et al., 1975; Patel and Clark, 1980).

The latter can be reconverted to citrate. Much of the transport in developing brain is through citrate which is cleaved to oxaloacetate and acetyl-CoA by ATP-dependent citrate lyase. The acetyl portion of N-acetylaspartate is a good source of acetyl groups for fatty acid synthesis in developing brain (D'Adamo et al., 1968; Patel and Clark, 1979).

5.4.2   Synthesis from Ketone Bodies

The extraction of ketone bodies by brain from the blood is directly proportional to plasma saturation (Robinson and Williamson, 1980). During postnatal development concentrations in plasma and utilization by brain are several-fold higher than in adulthood. The transport mechanism for the ketone bodies is facilitated diffusion utilizing the monocarboxylic acid carrier that is used for lactate and pyruvate (Cremer et al., 1982). In 21-day rats the K_m and V_{max} values are 7- and 10-fold greater than the corresponding values in adult rats. Thus, the developing rat brains have a greater capacity with little likelihood for saturation of ketone body transport.

The pathways for utilization of ketone bodies were reviewed by Robinson and Williamson (1980). In addition to the well-known mitochondrial pathway, the ketone bodies can be converted to CoA derivatives in the cytosol for direct utilization in lipid synthesis (Fig. 5.1). This explains why ketone bodies are more efficient than glucose as precursors for lipid synthesis (Webber and Edmond, 1974; Webber and Edmond, 1979), particularly in oligodendroglia which are markedly enriched in acetoacetyl-CoA synthetase (Pleasure et al., 1979). For fatty acid synthesis the acetoacetyl-CoA must be cleaved by the thiolase to 2-acetyl-CoA, whereas for sterol synthesis the acetoacetyl-CoA can be used directly for synthesis of 3-hydroxy-3-methylglutaryl-CoA. This explains why the relative utilization for sterols is greater than for fatty acids for acetyl groups from ketone bodies or leucine as compared with acetyl groups from glucose (Dhopeshwarkar and Subramanian, 1979; Webber and Edmond, 1977; Webber and Edmond, 1979). The sterol–fatty acid ratio for radioactivity was 0.48 with D-(−)-3-hydroxybutyrate, 0.49 with acetoacetate, 0.22 with glucose, 0.30 with acetate, and 0.29 with octanoate (Webber and Edmond, 1979). This preference for sterol synthesis is greater in oligodendroglia than in whole brain (Koper et al., 1981). With a [3-^{14}C]ketone body as precursor, the sterol–fatty acid ratio of radioactivity was 0.67 in whole brain and 1.48 in myelin. Both ketone bodies, acetoacetate and D-(−)-3-hydroxybutyrate, are equivalent as lipid precursors (Koper et al., 1981).

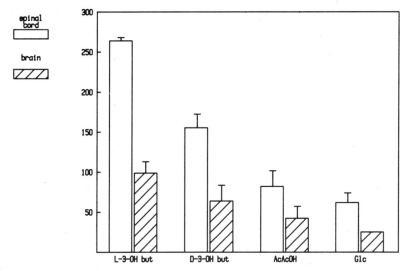

FIGURE 5.1   Relative rates of fatty acid synthesis from different precusors in brains (open bars) and spinal cords (striped bars) of 18-day-old rats. The data is from Webber and Edmond (1977). Rats were killed 3 h after injection of 10 μCi of either L(+)-3-hydroxy[3-^{14}C]butyrate, D(−)-3-hydroxy[3-^{14}C]butyrate, [3-^{14}C]acetoacetate, or D-[2-^{14}C]glucose. The ^{14}C content is expressed as disintegrations × 10^{-3}/min per gram of tissue. The D(−) isomer of 3-hydroxybutyrate is the naturally occurring ketone body. The L(+) isomer is included because it is utilized only by the cytosolic pathway, not by the mitochondrial pathway.

5.4.3   Elongation and Desaturation

After entry into the brain fatty acids may be desaturated, elongated, or oxidized to acetyl groups with resynthesis of fatty acids (Fig. 5.2). Palmitic acid, 16:0, is desaturated at the 9-position to produce palmitoleic acid, 16:1, and is also elongated to produce stearic acid, which is another substrate for the 9-desaturase with production of oleic acid. At 8 and 30 days after an intracerebral injection of [U-^{14}C]palmitic acid in 3-month old mice, only 51 and 22%, respectively, of the radioactivity in the acyl groups was in palmitic acid (Sun and Horrocks, 1973). The extent of resynthesis cannot be estimated when palmitic acid is the labeled precursor. From results in Figure 5.2 (center), it is obvious that stearic acid is extensively oxidized with resynthesis of palmitic acid and utilization of some labeled acetyl groups for elongation of polyunsaturated fatty acids. Both stearic acid and its elongation product arachidic acid, 20:0, may be desaturated. An example of the metabolism of a polyunsaturated fatty acid is shown on the right side of Figure 5.2. All of the radioactivity in 16:0, 18:0, and

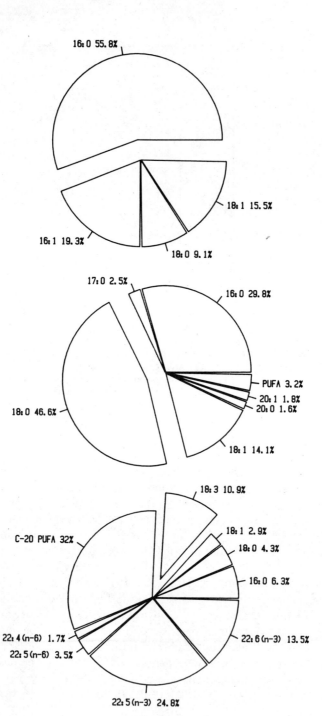

16:0 55.8%

18:1 15.5%

16:1 19.3%

18:0 9.1%

17:0 2.5%

16:0 29.8%

PUFA 3.2%

20:1 1.8%

20:0 1.6%

18:0 46.6%

18:1 14.1%

18:3 10.9%

C-20 PUFA 32%

18:1 2.9%

18:0 4.3%

16:0 6.3%

22:6 (n-3) 13.5%

22:4 (n-6) 1.7%

22:5 (n-6) 3.5%

22:5 (n-3) 24.8%

18:1 and $n - 6$ polyunsaturated fatty acids was derived from labeled acetyl groups produced by beta oxidation. Since the levels of linolenate in the brain are very low, it is not surprising that very little of the radioactivity remained in $18:3(n - 9)$. More than 38% of the remaining radioactivity was found in $22:5(n - 3)$ and $22:6(n - 3)$ which are produced by desaturation and elongation.

Elongation by two carbons occurs in microsomes and mitochondria. The latter require acetyl-CoA, NADH, and NADPH for the elongation of saturated and monounsaturated acyl-CoA (Bourre et al., 1978; Mead et al., 1977). The products of elongation are utilized in the mitochondria, not in myelin (Murad and Kishimoto, 1978). Microsomal elongation differs by requiring NADPH and malonyl-CoA (Bourre et al., 1978). Highest activities are found during active myelination (Murad and Kishimoto, 1978; Brophy and Vance, 1975). The rate-limiting step for microsomal elongation is the condensation reaction with malonyl-CoA (Bernert et al., 1979). Elongation enzymes are quite specific (Fig. 5.3). The two best substrates are those that are elongated *in vivo*, whereas the other three are desaturated prior to elongation. In addition, $18:1(n - 9)$ and $18:3(n - 3)$ are effective inhibitors of the elongation of $18:3(n - 6)$, but $18:1(n - 7)$ and $18:2(n - 6)$, the immediate precursor of the substrate, are poor inhibitors (Cook, 1981). In spite of the difference in inhibition of elongation by $18:3(n - 3)$ and $18:2(n - 6)$, neither are good substrates for elongation (Cook, 1982). The elongation of $18:3(n - 6)$ required ATP but was inhibited by CoA. The free acid was a better substrate than the CoA derivative. This suggests that the intermediate for elongation might be an acyladenylate compound (Cook, 1982).

Desaturation of saturated fatty acids is predominately by the 9-desaturase with 16:0 and 18:0 as substrates (Carreau et al., 1979; Cook, 1979). The monoenoic fatty acids with longer chains are formed by elongation of 18:1 (Bourre et al., 1976). Desaturation can be rapid and extensive. When C6 glioma cells were incubated for 6 h with labeled 18:0, 46% of the label in the phospholipids was in 18:1 (Cook et al., 1982).

Polyunsaturated fatty acids in the brain are made from linoleic acid, $18:2(n - 6)$, and linolenic acid, $18:3(n - 3)$, by appropriate combinations

FIGURE 5.2 Distribution of radioactivity in various fatty acids after administration of a single-labeled fatty acid. *Left:* [1-^{14}C]palmitic acid incubated with C6 glioma cells for 6 h in a serum-free medium. Distribution in phospholipids. Results from Cook et al. (1982). *Center:* [1-^{14}C]stearic acid injected subcutaneously into 15-day-old mice. Distribution in neuronal lipids at 20 h after injection. Results from Morand et al. (1979). *Right:* [1-^{14}C]linolenate injected intracerebrally into 21-day-old rats. Distribution in oligodendroglial phospholipids at 12 h after injection. Results from Cohen and Bernsohn (1978).

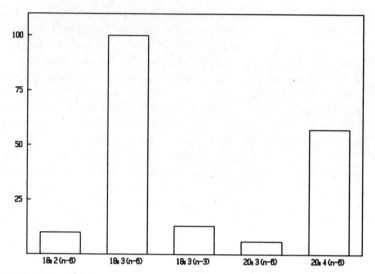

FIGURE 5.3 The relative rate of incorporation of labeled malonyl-CoA into elongation products. Incubations included 100 μ*M* fatty acid as indicated suspended with Triton WR 1339, 50 μM [2-^{14}C]malonyl-CoA, cofactors, and rat brain microsomes (Cook et al., 1982).

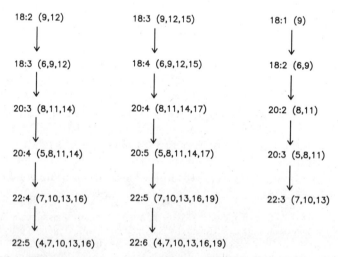

FIGURE 5.4 The sequence of reactions in formation of polyunsaturated fatty acids (Naughton, 1981). The desaturation steps occur at the 6, 5, and 4 positions alternating with elongation reactions. Other reactions such as the elongation of 18:2(n − 6) to 20:2(n − 6) also take place to a small extent.

184

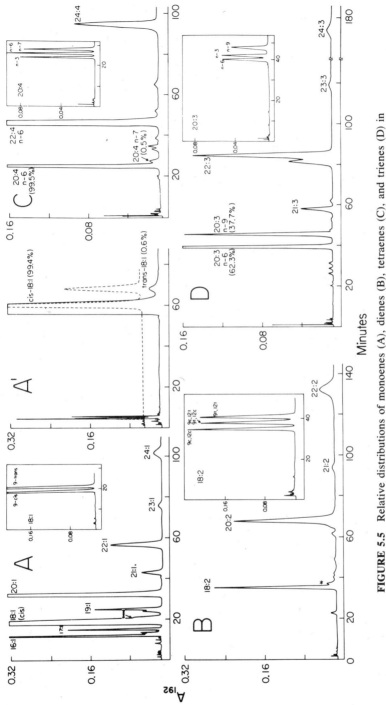

FIGURE 5.5 Relative distributions of monoenes (A), dienes (B), tetraenes (C), and trienes (D) in fatty acid methyl esters derived from glycerophospholipids of bovine brain. Numbers in parentheses indicate isomer proportions on an area basis. The chromatogram A′ is a separation of the 18:1 collected from A. (Reproduced from Aveldano et al., 1983. By permission of *J. Lipid Res.*)

of desaturation and elongation (Fig. 5.4). Quite low amounts of the essential fatty acids, linoleic and linolenic, are found in the brain suggesting that transport might be rate limiting. The major polyunsaturated fatty acids in brain are $22:6(n - 3)$, $20:4(n - 6)$, $22:4(n - 6)$, and $22:5(n - 6)$. Other tetraenoic fatty acids include $24:4(n - 6)$ and a very small amount of $20:4(n - 7)$ (Fig. 5.5). Among the low proportions of dienoic and trienoic fatty acids are $22:3$ (two isomers), $20:3(n - 6)$, $20:3(n - 9)$, $22:2$, and $20:2$. The $20:3(n - 9)$ is formed from oleic acid (Fig. 5.4). Large amounts of this fatty acid are an indicator of essential fatty acid deficiency.

5.5   RELEASE OF FREE FATTY ACIDS

5.5.1   Pathological Response

The content of free fatty acids and prostaglandins (Section 5.6.2) rises markedly as part of the pathophysiological response to injury (Bazán and Rodriguez de Turco, 1980; N.G. Bazán et al., 1982). The enzymes involved in the hydrolysis of phospholipids to give free fatty acids are reviewed in Chapter 2. The increase in free fatty acids in rat brain as a function of time after decapitation was first described by Bazán and Joel (1968) in an abstract. Electroconvulsive shock also elevates free fatty acid levels in rat brain (Bazán, 1970; Bazán, 1971a; Bazán et al., 1980). Transient increases in free fatty acid levels as found during electroconvulsive shock permit reacylation of the fatty acids with lack of permanent injury and thus is compatible with survival. Increases in free fatty acids are also found during and after drug-induced seizures (Marion and Wolfe, 1978, Rodriguez de Turco et al., 1983). For bicuculline-induced status epilepticus, free arachidonic acid is increased 2-fold during the first generalized tonic-clonic convulsion and 13- to 17-fold at 5–6 min after bicuculline injection (Rodriguez de Turco, et al., 1983). A prolonged elevation of free fatty acids associated with ischemia leads to edema and permanent brain damage (Bazán and Rodriguez de Turco, 1980). The rapid production of free fatty acids during ischemia is found in rodent (Aveldano and Bazán, 1975a) and monkey (Bazán, 1971b) brains. It is faster in gray matter than in white matter. The rate and extent of free fatty acid release differs regionally (Fig. 5.6) (N.G. Bazán et al., 1982). Newborn rat brains (Rodriguez de Turco et al., 1977) and the brain of the toad, a poikilotherm (Aveldano and Bazán, 1975a), release free fatty acids very slowly when subjected to ischemia or anoxia. Bovine retina releases substantial amounts of free fatty acids into culture medium, particularly when serum

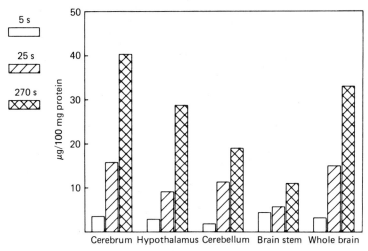

FIGURE 5.6   Concentrations of arachidonic acid in regions of rat brain at 5 (open bars), 25 (striped bars), and 270 (hatched bars) s of ischemia. (Data from N.G. Bazán et al., 1982.)

albumin is present in the medium to bind the fatty acids (Aveldano and Bazán, 1974).

When young rats were subjected to bilateral ligation of the common carotid arteries, a procedure that greatly reduces but does not prevent cerebral blood flow, free fatty acid concentrations were also markedly elevated at 2, 4, and 6 h (Kuwashima et al., 1978). Only trace amounts of free 20:4, 22:4, and 22:6 were found in forebrains of normal rats. At 2 h of ischemia the concentrations were 50, 4.4, and 9.2, and at 4 h they were 84, 10.5, and 28 μg/g tissue, respectively. A substantial proportion of these fatty acids were released from myelin and mitochondria.

Elevated levels of free fatty acids are associated with decreased mitochondrial function and uncoupling of oxidative phosphorylation (Wojtczak, 1976). *In vitro*, these effects are blocked by fatty acid–free serum albumin (Ansevin, 1980) and can be reproduced by adding unsaturated free fatty acids to brain mitochondria (Kuwashima et al., 1976). Mitochondria isolated from rat brains subjected to severe incomplete ischemia, as described in the paragraph above, were markedly impaired in ability to make ATP and reduce oxygen at 2 and 4 h of ischemia (Kuwashima et al., 1978). Mitochondria isolated from guinea pig cerebral cortex had increased levels of free fatty acids (32%) and decreased concentrations of ethanolamine glycerophospholipids (22%) within 30 s of decapitation ischemia (Majewska et al., 1977, 1978). The infusion of octanoic acid or other short-chain fatty acids into rabbits elevates intracranial pressure with eventual coma (Trauner and Adams, 1982) and has been proposed as a model for Reye's syndrome. The release of free fatty acids is decreased somewhat by barbiturates such as pentobarbital (Shiu and Nemoto, 1981; Tang and Sun, 1982).

Very low levels of oxygen are required for triggering the accumulation of free arachidonic acid (Gardiner et al., 1981). In rats subjected to severe hypoxia and displaying high-amplitude slow waves with periods of severe depression, the free arachidonic acid level was elevated from 5 in the control to 23 nmol/g tissue. At the same time there was a small decrease in energy charge due to a large fall in phosphocreatine concentration but no change in cAMP concentration. A more severe hypoxia with an almost flat electroencephalogram in 2–4 min was associated with a free arachidonic acid level of 170 nmol/g tissue, a profound decrease in energy, and an elevation of cAMP. The accumulation of free fatty acid in hypoxia occurs only when energy homeostasis is disrupted.

During hypoglycemia brain tissue may hydrolyze possible endogenous substrates, including carbohydrates, proteins, RNA, and phospholipids. In several studies prolonged and/or severe hypoglycemia has caused a loss of 5–15% of the phospholipid content of the brain (Hinzen et al., 1970). In experiments with rats by Agardh et al. (1981), after 5 min of hypoglycemic coma the brain phospholipids were reduced by 8% and free fatty acids were elevated sixfold. Continuation of hypoglycemia beyond 5 min did not further change the phospholipid and free fatty acid contents. The total fatty acid content of the rat cortex decreased by 11.7 μmol/g tissue while the free fatty acid content increased by 0.63 μmol/g tissue. The difference is much greater than could be accounted for by beta oxidation; thus most of the released free fatty acids were likely transported from the cortex into the blood. The apparent loss of free fatty acid in micromoles per gram of tissue included 2.0, 16:0; 2.5, 18:0; 4.7, 18:1; 0.9, 20:4; and 0.7, 22:6.

The effects of complete and severe incomplete ischemia and recirculation on adult rat brain frontoparietal cortex fatty acids and phospholipids were examined by Rehncrona et al. (1982). Injury to brain tissue is greater during severe incomplete ischemia than during complete ischemia. The former was achieved by clamping both common carotid arteries and lowering the mean arterial blood pressure to 50 mm Hg for 30 min. This resulted in a blood pH of 6.97 at 5 min of recirculation, which gradually increased with a near normal value of 7.32 at 90 min of recirculation. Free fatty acid levels were 158 ± 8 nmol ± S.E.M/g tissue in control rats. Complete and incomplete ischemia caused similar elevations, 4-fold at 5 min and 10-fold at 30 min. During recirculation after 30 min complete ischemia, free fatty acid levels declined from 1800 to 1640 at 5 min, 480 at 30 min, and 120 nmol/g tissue at 90 min, a drop to a normal value. After 30 min incomplete ischemia free fatty acid levels declined markedly, from 1580 to 1030 at 5 min, then more slowly to 610 at 30 min and 210 nmol/g tissue at 90 min. The patterns of change for individual fatty acids were similar in the two types of ischemia with a marked increase in relative content of arachidonic acid from 10 to 30% during ischemia. During the same time period no significant decreases were found in total or individual esterified fatty acids. The increase in free fatty acids was nearly 1.5% of the control level of esterified fatty acids. The lowest levels (statistically not significant) of esterified fatty acids were found at 30 min recirculation with a decrease of 6.5% after complete ischemia and 5.7% after incomplete ischemia. During recirculation most of the released fatty acids must be transported into the blood. At 30 min of recirculation following incomplete ischemia, decreases in phospholipid levels were 6% for ethanolamine glycerophospholipids, 9% for inositol plus serine glycerophospholipids, and 5% for choline glycerophospholipids. Only the decrease in inositol plus serine glycerophospholipids was statistically significant. These results do not explain why the outcome is worse after severe incomplete ischemia than after complete ischemia.

Similar experiments were done by Yoshida et al. (1982) except that severe incomplete ischemia was produced in rats by cauterizing the vertebral arteries before ligating the common carotid arteries. The levels of arachidonic and docosahexaenoic acids decreased faster during recirculation than the levels of palmitic and stearic acids (Fig. 5.7).

During recirculation of gerbils peroxide levels were elevated (Yoshida et al., 1980), indicating free radical peroxidation may also contribute to the damage after ischemia. This is supported by the finding that alpha-tocopherol and reduced ubiquinone levels in rat cerebrum are significantly lower during recirculation after severe ischemia (Yoshida et al., 1982). Peroxidation of polyunsaturated fatty acids may have important deleterious effects on the microcirculation and thus impede recovery after injury by incomplete ischemia or trauma (Demopoulos and Flamm, 1980).

5.5.2 Regulation of Free Fatty Acid Release

Gullis and Rowe published a number of papers on phospholipase A_2 activities in brain and regulation of free fatty acid release by noradrenaline and cAMP. Rowe (1977) could not reproduce these results. Gullis has retracted all of his data in this area (Rowe, 1977; Gullis and Hamprecht, 1977). However, it is still quite likely that cAMP and/or catecholamines may be involved in the regulation of fatty acid release. Activities of plasmalogenase (Horrocks et al., 1978) and phospholipases A_1 and A_2 (Edgar

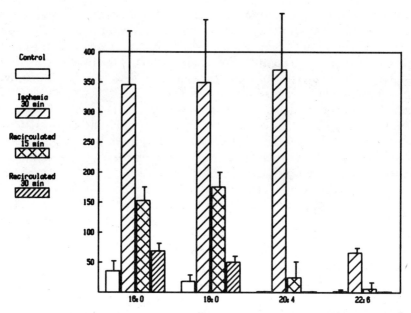

FIGURE 5.7   The concentrations of free fatty acids (nmol/g tissue) in rat cerebrum during and after severe ischemia (Yoshida et al., 1982). The open bars are the control values, the wide-striped bars represent 30 min of ischemia, the hatched bars represent 30 min ischemia plus 15 min recirculation, and the narrow-striped bars represent 30 min ischemia plus 30 min recirculation.

et al., 1982) with ethanolamine glycerophospholipids as substrates are elevated twofold after ischemia produced by bilateral ligation of the common carotid arteries of gerbils. The phospholipase A_1 and A_2 activities are elevated within 1 min. All of these phospholipases were assayed in extracts of acetone-dried powders so it is likely that the changes in activity were produced by changes in covalent bonds or in very strongly bound cofactors. The increases in phospholipase A_1 and A_2 activities coincide with or are preceded by increases in cAMP concentration, which regulates protein kinases and phosphorylation of proteins. A cascade regulation of phospholipase A_2 activity by cAMP in brain was proposed by Bazán (1976) but has not yet been tested experimentally. The evidence in favor of this hypothesis has been summarized (N.G. Bazán et al., 1982; Edgar et al., 1982; Majewska et al., 1978). Catecholamines may also stimulate free fatty acid release (Aveldano de Caldironi and Bazán, 1979).

Regulation through lipomodulin is also a possiblility (Blackwell et al., 1980; Hirata, 1981). Lipomodulin inhibits phospholipases when bound but does not bind when it is phosphorylated. Thus, the elevated cAMP may cause phosphorylation of lipomodulin, which then dissociates from the phospholipase, which is then no longer inhibited. The anti-inflammatory activity of glucocorticoids may be explained by their induction of lipomodulin synthesis. The existence of lipomodulin in brain has not been reported.

The entry of Ca^{2+} into a cell may also activate phospholipases. Intracellular Ca^{2+} may be released whenever the energy charge is low, thus causing an increased free fatty acid level (Agardh et al., 1981). The entry of Ca^{2+} is also associated with increased diacylglycerol levels (Aveldano de Caldironi and Bazán, 1975b; N.G. Bazán et al., 1982; Bazán and Rodriguez de Turco, 1980) and the latter are good substrates for an active lipase. An activation of fatty acid release by Ca^{2+} was also noted with synaptosomes (Majewska et al., 1981).

Edema and lipid peroxidation can be produced by free radicals in cortical slices with the greatest degree of lipid peroxidation in myelin, mitochondria, and synaptosomes (Chan et al., 1982). The phospholipid content was decreased and the contents of free oleic, arachidonic, and docosahexaenoic acids were markedly increased in synaptosomes incubated with a free radical-inducing system. The level of free unsaturated fatty acids was increased fourfold. Chan et al. (1982) suggested that free-radical and lipid peroxides may activate phospholipases, particularly phospholipase A_2, to release free arachidonic and other fatty acids, thus inhibiting Na^+, K^+-ATPase and inducing edema.

These hypotheses should be tested with purified phospholipases when they become available.

5.6 UTILIZATION OF FATTY ACIDS

5.6.1 Acylation

After an intracerebral injection of labeled fatty acid or precursor, there is a rapid labeling of choline and other glycerophospholipids (Koeppen et al., 1980). *De novo* synthesis of glycerophospholipids involves the formation of phosphatidate from dihydroxyacetone phosphate or from *sn*-glycerol-3-phosphate. The specific activity of *sn*-glycerol-3-phosphate acyltransferase increases at the onset of myelination (Carey, 1975a). The initial step for acylation of fatty acid is the formation of acyl-CoA by long-chain fatty acid–CoA ligase (EC 6.2.1.3). This microsomal enzyme has a relatively low activity in brain, less than 10% of the rate in liver (Murphy and Spence, 1980). The order of ligase activity in brain with fatty acids is $18:2 > 18:1 > 16:0 > 22:1$ (Murphy and Spence, 1982). The ligase activity can be reversed by long-chain fatty acyl-CoA hydrolase (EC 3.1.2.2) (Brophy and Vance, 1976). Both the ligase and hydrolase activities increase during early development but are lower in activity in adult brain (Carey, 1975b; Cantrill and Carey, 1975; Smith and Sun, 1981).

Triacylglycerols are trace components of brain but attain a relatively high specific radioactivity within a short time after brain tissue is presented with labeled fatty acids (Horrocks and Harder, 1983). Fatty acids formed from glucose are mostly found in glycerophospholipids whereas added fatty acids are mostly incorporated into triacylglycerols in rabbit cerebral cortex slices (Carey, 1975b). A high specific radioactivity of triacylglycerols is also observed after intracerebral injection of a labeled fatty acid (Cook, 1978; Sun and Yau, 1976). This has led to the suggestions that fatty acid metabolism in brain is regulated by incorporation into and release from triacylglycerols (Carey, 1975b; Sun and Yau, 1976; Cook, 1981) and that triacylglycerols are a reservoir functioning between free fatty acids and glycerophospholipids (Dwyer and Bernsohn, 1979; Mizobuchi et al., 1982). Recent experiments by Cook et al. (1982) with cultured neural tumor cells suggest that exogenous unsaturated fatty acids may be incorporated into endogenous triacylglycerol and later released for incorporation into glycerophospholipids. Release from triacylglycerols is due to triacylglycerol lipase (EC 3.1.1.3) (Vyvoda and Rowe, 1973; Cabot and Gatt, 1978; Arnaud et al., 1981; Mizobuchi et al., 1981). The fatty acid and the diacylglycerol can then be incorporated into glycerophospholipids.

5.6.2 Prostaglandin Formation

Prostaglandins are formed and released after stimulation of neural tissues (Wolfe, 1982). The normally very small pool of free arachidonate (section 5.1.2) is augmented by stimulation. Larger amounts of free arachidonate are associated with larger contents of prostaglandins (Bosisio et al., 1976). Prostaglandins $F_{2\alpha}$, E_2, D_2, I_2, and thromboxane B_2 as well as the lipoxygenase product, 12-hydroxyeicosatetraenoic acid, have been found in brain (Galli et al., 1980; Wolfe, 1982). Damage to the brain generally greatly increases the synthesis of one or more of these compounds which may contribute greatly to pathophysiological reactions (Wolfe, 1982).

Cerebral ischemia causes a massive release of arachidonic acid (Section 5.5.1). When gerbils are subjected to complete ischemia by bilateral common carotid occlusion, only small increases in prostaglandin levels are found in the brain because insufficient oxygen is present (Gaudet and Levine, 1979; Spagnuolo et al., 1980). During reperfusion after brief ischemia, very large quantities of arachidonic acid metabolites accumulated

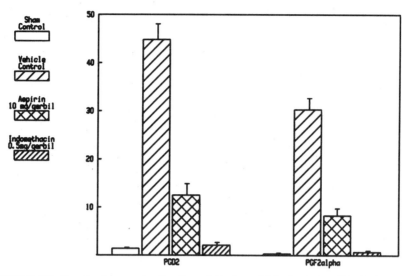

FIGURE 5.8 Levels of prostaglandins D_2 and $F_{2\alpha}$ in gerbil brains (ng $\pm$ SEM/g tissue) of sham-operated controls (open bars) and after 5 min of occlusion and 5 min reperfusion with effects of pretreatment with vehicle (wide-striped bars), aspirin (10 mg) (hatched bars), and indomethacin (0.5 mg) (narrow-striped bars) by intraperitoneal injection 30 min before surgery (Gaudet et al., 1980).

with a peak of 5 min, the earliest time for assays. The highest concentrations were found for $PGF_{2\alpha}$ and PGD_2 (Fig. 5.8). Unilateral common carotid occlusion produces cerebral ischemia in about 40% of gerbils with an incomplete loss of oxygen but with behavioral signs of ischemia (Gaudet and Levine, 1980). In these brains PGD_2 and $PGF_{2\alpha}$ concentrations were markedly elevated at 15 min and 2 h after occlusion. The elevation was greater in the nonoccluded than in the occluded hemispheres. Treatment with indomethacin prevented the elevation of these prostaglandins. Decapitation ischemia increases the levels of $PGF_{2\alpha}$ and TxB_2 substantially (Fig. 5.9).

During convulsions the level of $PGF_{2\alpha}$ increases to very high levels. Pentamethylenetetrazol-induced convulsions increased this prostaglandin from 1.2 in control tissue to 9.9 at 15 s and 183 ng/g tissue at 75 s (Marion and Wolfe, 1978). For durations of clonic convulsions of over 50 s, a significant correlation was found for duration and concentration of $PGF_{2\alpha}$ (Seregi et al., 1981). Since indomethacin blocks production of this prostaglandin without affecting the seizure threshold, the $PGF_{2\alpha}$ is not directly related to convulsions.

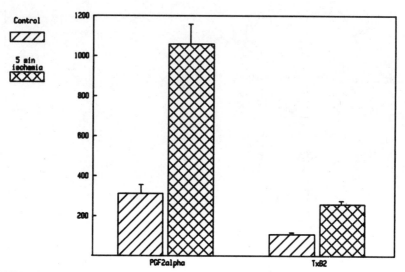

FIGURE 5.9   Levels of PGF$_{2\alpha}$ and TxB$_2$ (pg $\pm$ SEM/mg protein) in gerbil brain cortex in controls (microwave irradiation, striped bars) and after 5 min decapitation ischemia (hatched bars) (Spagnuolo et al., 1980). These control values are considerably higher than those shown in Figure 5.8.

Metabolites of arachidonic acid damage cerebral arterioles (Kontos et al., 1980). A prolonged constriction of basilar arteries and damage to the endothelia was produced with 15-hydroperoxy arachidonic acid (Sasaki et al., 1981). Free-radical and lipoxygenase metabolites of polyunsaturated fatty acids may play an important part in the reduction of blood flow to tissues of the central nervous system after trauma, ischemia, or other injury (Demopoulos et al., 1980).

5.7   SUMMARY

Fatty acids from brain glycerophospholipids are of increasing interest, particularly the arachidonate and other polyunsaturated fatty acids that can be converted by cyclooxygenase and lipoxygenase enzymes to compounds with much biological activity. The polyunsaturated fatty acids can also be peroxidized by free-radical reactions. All fatty acids in glycerophospholipids are continually turned over and exchanged with free fatty acids in the blood. During many pathological conditions, the release of free fatty acids greatly exceeds the capacity of the brain for reacylation or excretion into the blood. This release is so rapid that special techniques must be used to ascertain the basal level *in vivo*.

Fatty acids are generally not oxidized in the brain, although ketone bodies may replace a portion of the glucose required by the brain. The ketone bodies are also very good precursors for fatty acid synthesis. This is particularly important for suckling animals during brain development when fatty acid synthesis is quite active and the demand for fatty acids for growth is very large. All of the required enzymes for elongation and desaturation are present in the brain for the formation of arachidonic, adrenic, and docosahexaenoic acids from essential fatty acid precursors and for the synthesis of very long chain fatty acids for sphingolipids. All of the essential fatty acid precursors and a substantial portion of the other fatty acids in the brain are obtained by transport from the blood.

ACKNOWLEDGMENT

The writing of this review was supported in part by NIH Research Grants NS-08291 and NS-10165.

REFERENCES

Agardh, C-D., Chapman, A.G., Nilsson, B., and Siesjö, B.K., *J. Neurochem., 36,* 490–500 (1981).

Ansevin, C.F., *Neurology, 30,* 160–166 (1980).

Arnaud, J., Nobili, O., and Boyer, J., *Biochim. Biophys. Acta, 663,* 401–407 (1981).

Aveldano, M.I., and Bazán, N.G., *FEBS Lett., 40,* 53–56 (1974).

Aveldano, M.I., and Bazán, N.G., *Brain Res., 100,* 99–110 (1975).

Aveldano, M.I., VanRollins, M., and Horrocks, L.A., *J. Lipid Res., 24,* 83–93 (1983).

Aveldano de Caldironi, M.I., and Bazán, N.G., *J. Neurochem., 25,* 919–920 (1975).

Aveldano de Caldironi, M.I., and Bazán, N.G., *Neurochem. Res. 4,* 213–221 (1979).

Bazán, H.E.P., Careaga, M.M., Sprecher, H., and Bazán, N.G., *Biochim. Biophys. Acta, 712,* 123–128 (1982).

Bazán, N.G., Jr., *Biochim. Biophys. Acta, 218,* 1–10 (1970).

Bazán, N.G., *J. Neurochem., 18,* 1379–1385 (1971a).

Bazán, N.G., Jr., *Lipids, 6,* 211–212 (1971b).

Bazán, N.G., *Adv. Exp. Med. Biol., 72,* 317–335 (1976).

Bazán, N.G., and Bazán, H.E.P., in N. Marks and R. Rodnight, Eds., *Research Methods in Neurochemistry,* Vol. 3, Plenum Press, New York, 1975, pp. 309–324.

Bazán, N.G., Jr., Bazán, H.E.P., Kennedy, W.G., and Joel, C.D., *J. Neurochem., 18,* 1387–1393 (1971).

Bazán, N.G., Jr., and Cellik, S., *Anal. Biochem., 45,* 309–314 (1972).

Bazán, N.G., Jr. and Joel, C.D., *Federation Proc., 27,* 751 (1968).

Bazán, N.G., and Joel, C.D., *J. Lipid Res., 11,* 42–47 (1970).

Bazán, N.G., and Rodriguez de Turco, E.B., *Adv. Neurol., 28,* 197–205 (1980).

Bazán, N.G., Aveldano de Caldironi, M.I., Cascone de Suarez, G.D., and Rodriguez de Turco, E.B., in L. Batistin, G. Hashim, and A. Lajtha, Eds., *Neurochemical and Clinical Neurology,* Alan R. Liss, New York, 1980, pp. 167–169.

Bazán, N.G., Aveldano de Caldironi, M.I., and Rodriguez de Turco, E.B., *Prog. Lipid Res., 20,* 523–529 (1982).

Bazán, N.G., Rodriguez de Turco, E.B., and Morelli de Liberti, S.A., *Neurochem. Res., 7,* 839–843 (1982).

Bernert, J.T., Jr., Bourre, J.M., Baumann, N.A., and Sprecher, H., *J. Neurochem., 32,* 85–90 (1979).

Blackwell, G.J., Carnuccio, R., DiRosa, M., Flower, R.J., Parente, L., and Persico, P., *Nature, 287,* 147–149 (1980).

Bosisio, E., Galli, C., Galli, G., Nicosia, S., Spagnuolo, C., and Tosi, L., *Prostaglandins, 11,* 773–781 (1976).

Bourre, J.M., in N. Baumann, Ed., *Neurological Mutations Affecting Myelination,* Inserm Symposium, Elsevier/North-Holland Biomedical Press, Amsterdam, 1980, pp. 187–206.

Bourre, J.M., *Reprod. Nutr. Develop., 22,* 179–191 (1982).

Bourre, J.M., Daudu, O., and Baumann, N., *Biochim. Biophys. Acta, 424,* 1–7 (1976).

Bourre, J.M., Pollet, S., Paturneau-Jouas, M., and Baumann, N., *Adv. Exp. Med. Biol., 83,* 103–109 (1977).

Bourre, J.M., Pollet, S., Paturneau-Jouas, M., and Baumann, N., *Adv. Exp. Med. Biol., 101,* 17–26 (1978).

Brophy, P.J., and Vance, D.E., *Biochem. J., 152,* 495–501 (1975).

Brophy, P.J., and Vance, D.E., *Biochem. J., 160,* 247–251 (1976).

Cabot, M.C., and Gatt, S., *Biochim. Biophys. Acta, 530,* 508–512 (1978).

Cantrill, R.C., and Carey, E.M., *Biochim. Biophys. Acta, 380,* 165–175 (1975).

Carey, E.M., *Biochim. Biophys. Acta, 398,* 231–243 (1975a).

Carey, E.M., *J. Neurochem., 24,* 237–244 (1975b).

Carreau, J.P., Daudu, O., Mazliak, P., and Bourre, J.M., *J. Neurochem., 32,* 659–660 (1979).

Cenedella, R.J., Galli, C., and Paoletti, R., *Lipids, 10,* 290–293 (1975).

Chan, P.H., Yurko, M., and Fishman, R.A., *J. Neurochem., 38,* 525–531 (1982).

Cohen, S.R., and Bernsohn, J., *J. Neurochem., 30,* 661–669 (1978).

Cook, H.W., *Biochim. Biophys. Acta, 531,* 245–256 (1978).

Cook, H.W., *Lipids, 14,* 763–767 (1979).

Cook, H.W., *Neurochem. Res., 6,* 1217–1229 (1981a).

Cook, H.W., *Lipids, 16,* 920–926 (1981b).

Cook, H.W., *Arch. Biochem. Biophys. 214,* 695–704 (1982).

Cook, H.W., Clarke, J.T.R., and Spence, M.W., *J. Lipid Res., 23,* 1292–1300 (1982).

Cremer, J.E., Teal, H.M., and Cunningham, V.J., *J. Neurochem., 39,* 674–677 (1982).

D'Adamo, A.F., Jr., Gidez, L.I., and Yatsu, F.M., *Exp. Brain Res., 5,* 267–273 (1968).

D'Adamo, A.F., Smith, J.C., and Frigyesi, G., *J. Neurochem., 24,* 597–600 (1975).

DeMedio, G.E., Goracci, G., Horrocks, L.A., Lazarewicz, J.W., Mazzari, S., Porcellati, G., Strosznajder, J., and Trovarelli, G., *Ital. J. Biochem., 29,* 412–432 (1980).

Demopoulos, H.B., Flamm, E.S., Pietronigro, D.D., and Seligman, M.L., *Acta Physiol. Scand. Suppl., 492*, 91–118 (1980).

Dhopeshwarkar, G.A., and Mead, J.F., *Adv. Lipid Res., 11*, 109–142 (1973).

Dhopeshwarkar, G.A., and Subramanian, C., *Lipids, 14*, 47–51 (1979).

Dhopeshwarkar, G.A., Subramanian, C., McConnell, D.H., and Mead, J.F., Biochim. Biophys. Acta, 255, 572–579 (1972).

Dhopeshwarkar, G.A., Subramanian, C., and Mead, J.F., *Biochim. Biophys. Acta, 248*, 41–47 (1971).

Dwyer, B.E., and Bernsohn, J., *Biochim. Biophys. Acta, 575*, 309–317 (1979).

Edgar, A.D., Strosznajder, J., and Horrocks, L.A., *J. Neurochem., 39*, 1111–1116 (1982).

Galli, C., Spagnuolo, C., and Petroni, A., in B. Samuelsson, P.W. Ramwell, and R. Paoletti, Eds., *Advances in Prostaglandin and Thromboxane Research*, Raven Press, New York, 1980, pp. 1235–1239.

Gardiner, M., Nilsson, B., Rehncrona, S., and Siesjö, B.K., *J. Neurochem, 36*, 1500–1505 (1981).

Gaudet, R.J., and Levine, L., *Biochem. Biophys. Res. Commun., 86*, 893–901 (1979).

Gaudet, R.J., and Levine, L., *Stroke, 6*, 648–652 (1980).

Gaudet, R.J., Alam, I., and Levine, L., *J. Neurochem., 35*, 653–658 (1980).

Gullis, R., and Hamprecht, B., *Nature, 265*, 764 (1977).

Hinzen, D.H., Becker, P., and Müller, U., *Pflüegers Arch., 321*, 1–14 (1970).

Hirata, F., *J. Biol. Chem., 256*, 7730–7733 (1981).

Horrocks, L.A., and Harder, H.W., in A. Lajtha, Ed., *Handbook of Neurochemistry*, 2nd ed., Vol. 3, Plenum Press, New York, 1983, pp. 1–16.

Horrocks, L.A., Spanner, S., Mozzi, R., Fu, S.C., D'Amato, R.A., and Krakowka, S., *Adv. Exp. Med. Biol., 100*, 423–438 (1978).

Kawamura, N., and Kishimoto, Y., *J. Neurochem., 36*, 1786–1791 (1981).

Kimes, A.S., Sweeney, D., London, E.D., and Rapoport, S.I., *Brain Res., 274*, 291–301 (1983).

Koeppen, A.H., Mitzen, E.J., and Papandrea, J.D., *J. Neurochem., 34*, 261–268 (1980).

Kontos, H.A., Wei, E.P., Povlishock, J.T., Dietrich, W.D., Magiera, C.J., and Ellis, E.F., *Science, 209*, 1242–1245 (1980).

Koper, J.W., Cardozo, M.L., and Van Golde, L.M.G., *Biochim. Biophys. Acta, 666*, 411–417 (1981).

Kuwashima, J., Fujitani, B., Nakamura, K., Kadokawa, T., Yoshida, K., and Shimizu, M., *Brain Res., 110*, 547–557 (1976).

Kuwashima, J., Nakamura, K., Fujitani, B., Kadokawa, T., Yoshida, K., and Shimizu, M., *Jap. J. Pharmacol., 28*, 277–287 (1978).

Lunt, G.G., and Rowe, C.E., *Biochim. Biophys. Acta, 152*, 681–93 (1968).

Majewska, M.D., Lazarewicz, J.W., and Strosznajder, J., *Bull. Acad. Pol. Sci., Ser. Sci. Biol., 25*, 125–131 (1977).

Majewska, M.D., Manning, R., and Sun, G.Y., *Neurochem. Res., 6*, 567–576 (1981).

Majewska, M.D., Strosznajder, J., and Lazarewicz, J., *Brain Res., 158*, 423–434 (1978).

Marion, J., and Wolfe, L.S., *Prostaglandins, 16*, 99–110 (1978).

McGee, R., Jr., *Biochim. Biophys. Acta, 663*, 314–328 (1981).

Mead, J.F., Dhopeshwarkar, G.A., and Gan Elpano, M., *Adv. Exp. Med. Biol.*, *83*, 313–328 (1977).

Mizobuchi, M., Morisaki, N., Matsuoka, N., Saito, Y., and Kumagai, A., *J. Neurochem.*, *38*, 1365–1371 (1982).

Mizobuchi, M., Shirai, K., Matsuoka, N., Saito, Y., and Kumagai, A., *J. Neurochem.*, *36*, 301–303 (1981).

Morand, O., Baumann, N., and Bourre, J.M., *Neurosci. Lett.*, *13*, 177–181 (1979).

Morisaki, N., Saito, Y., and Kumagai, A., *Atherosclerosis*, *42*, 221–227 (1982).

Murad, S., and Kishimoto, Y., *Arch. Biochem. Biophys.*, *185*, 300–306 (1978).

Murphy, M.G., and Spence, M.W., *J. Neurochem.*, *34*, 367–73 (1980).

Murphy, M.G., and Spence, M.W., *J. Neurochem.*, *38*, 675–679 (1982).

Naughton, J.M., *Int. J. Biochem.*, *13*, 21–32 (1981).

Pardridge, W.M., and Mietus, L.J., *J. Neurochem.*, *34* 463–466 (1980).

Patel, M.S., and Owen, O.E., *J. Neurochem.*, *28*, 109–114 (1977).

Patel, M.S., and Tonkonow, B.L., *J. Neurochem.*, *23*, 309–313 (1974).

Patel, T.B., and Clark, J.B., *Biochem. J.*, *184*, 539–546 (1979).

Patel, T.B., and Clark, J.B., *Biochem. J.*, *188*, 163–168 (1980).

Pleasure, D., Lichtman, C., Eastman, S., Lieb, M., Abramsky, O., and Silberberg, D., *J. Neurochem.*, *32*, 1447–1450 (1979).

Rehncrona, S., Westerberg, E., Akesson, B., and Siesjö, B.K., *J. Neurochem.*, *38*, 84–93 (1982).

Robinson, A.M., and Williamson, D.H., *Physiol. Rev.*, *60*, 143–187 (1980).

Rodriguez de Turco, E.B., Cascone, G.D., Pediconi, M.F., and Bazán, N.G., *Adv. Exp. Med. Biol.*, *83*, 389–396 (1977).

Rodriguez de Turco, E.B., Morelli de Liberti, S., and Bazán, N.G., *J. Neurochem.*, *40*, 252–259 (1983).

Rowe, C.E., *Biochem. J.*, *164*, 287–288 (1977).

Sasaki, T., Wakai, S., Asano, T., Watanabe, T., Kirino, T., and Sano, K., *J. Neurosurg.*, *54*, 357–365 (1981).

Seregi, A., Folly, G., Antal, M., Serfozo, P., and Schaefer, A., *Prostaglandins*, *21*, 217–226 (1981).

Shiu, G.K., and Nemoto, E.M., *J. Neurochem.*, *37*, 1448–1456 (1981).

Smith, R.E., and Sun, G.Y., *Develop. Neurosci.*, *4*, 337–344 (1981).

Spagnuolo, C., Sautebin, L., Galli, G., Ralagni, G., Galli, C., Mazzari, S., and Finesso, M., *Prostaglandins*, *18*, 53–61 (1980).

Sun, G.Y., and Horrocks, L.A., *J. Lipid Res.*, *14*, 206–214 (1973).

Sun, G.Y., and Yau, T.M., *J. Neurochem.*, *27*, 87–92 (1976).

Tang, W., and Sun, G.Y., *Neurochem. Int.*, *4*, 269–273 (1982).

Trauner, D.A., and Adams, H., *J. Neurol. Neurosurg, Psychiat.*, *45*, 428–430 (1982).

Uda, M., Shiojima, K., Shigematsu, H., Singh, I., and Kishimoto, Y., *Arch. Biochem. Biophys.*, *216*, 186–195 (1982).

Volpe, J.J., and Kishimoto, Y., *J. Neurochem.*, *19*, 737–753 (1972).

Volpe, J.J., Lyles, T.O., Roncari, D.A.K., and Vagelos, P.R., *J. Biol. Chem.*, *248*, 2502–2513 (1973).

Volpe, J.J., and Marasa, J.C., *Biochim. Biophys. Acta, 431*, 195–205 (1976a).

Volpe, J.J., and Marasa, J.C., *J. Neurochem., 27*, 841–845 (1976b).

Volpe, J.J., and Marasa, J.C., *Brain Res., 129*, 91–106 (1977).

Vyvoda, O.S., and Rowe, C.E., *Biochem. J., 132*, 233–248 (1973).

Webber, R.J., and Edmond, J., *J. Biol. Chem., 252*, 5222–5226 (1977).

Webber, R.J., and Edmond, J., *J. Biol. Chem., 254*, 3912–3920 (1979).

Wegener, G., *Naturwissenschaften, 70*, 43–45 (1983).

Wojtczak, L., *J. Bioenerg. Biomembr., 8*, 293–311 (1976).

Wolfe, L.S., *J. Neurochem., 38*, 1–14 (1982).

Yao, J.K., Dyck, R.J., VanLoon, J.A., and Moyer, T.P., *J. Neurochem., 36*, 1211–1218 (1981).

Yeh, Y.Y., *Federation Proc., 40*, 1588 (1981).

Yoshida, S., Abe, K., Busto, R., Watson, B.D., Kogure, K., and Ginsberg, M.D., *Brain Res., 245*, 307–316 (1982).

Yoshida, S., Inoh, S., Asano, T., Sano, K., Kubota, M., Shimazaki, H., and Ueta, N., *J. Neurosurg., 53*, 323–331 (1980).

six

PHOSPHOLIPIDS IN CULTURED CELLS OF NEURAL ORIGIN

EPHRAIM YAVIN

Department of Neurobiology
The Weizmann Institute of Science
Rehovot, Israel

CONTENTS

6.1   INTRODUCTION: LIPIDS AND THE NEURAL CELL
       SURFACE   202

6.2   METHODS FOR NERVOUS TISSUE CULTURE   204

       6.2.1   Organotypic Explants, 204
       6.2.2   Dissociated Cell Cultures, 207
       6.2.3   Clonal Neuronal and Glial Cell Lines, 210

6.3   CHEMICALY DEFINED MEDIA, LIPID CONSTITUENTS,
       AND NEURAL CELL GROWTH   212

6.4   COMPOSITION AND METABOLISM OF PHOSPHOLIPIDS   214

       6.4.1   Acyl, Alkyl, and Alk-1-Enyl Bond Composition of
                Phospholipids, 216
       6.4.2   Polar Head Group Composition and Metabolism in
                Isolated Neuronal and Glial Preparations, 221
       6.4.3   Metabolic Regulation of Polar Head Groups in
                Developing Cerebral Cell Cultures, 222
       6.4.4   N-Base Analogs As Probes For Studying Phospholipid
                Metabolism, 227

6.5   PHOSPHOLIPIDS AND NEURAL CELL GROWTH AND
       FUNCTION   228

       6.5.1   Stimulation of Phospholipid Turnover Following
                Ligand–Cell Interaction, 229
       6.5.2   Effects of Fatty Acids and Alteration of Phospholipid
                Composition on Neural Cell Phenotype, 230

6.6   SUMMARY   233

       REFERENCES   234

6.1   INTRODUCTION: LIPIDS AND THE NEURAL CELL SURFACE

The nervous tissue is a highly specialized and very complex network
composed of several morphologically distinct and functionally diverse cell

populations. The unique properties of neural cells and the regulatory mechanisms by which they assemble and operate in concert depend ultimately on molecular determinants associated with the plasma membrane. These determinants consist of specific ion channels, receptor complexes, catalytic, regulatory, and recognition proteins, and different carrier transport systems which segregate physically in the lipid bilayer into a mosaic of well-defined microscopic and functional domains. For example, the plasma membrane of the neuron is characterized by an abundance of synaptic contacts that transmit, receive, and process signals and provide the basis for neuronal circuitry. The spatial stability of the synapse must rely on the close interaction of its molecular constituents, that is, ion channels, receptors, and catalytic proteins. Another aspect of plasma membrane molecular mosaicism and functional segregation is the reciprocal interaction of two cell types of different origin, that is, neurons and glia, to form the myelin membrane. This highly specialized membrane–membrane interaction which presumably involves distinct recognition sites enables the oligodendrocyte in the central nervous system (CNS) and the Schwann cell in the peripheral nervous system (PNS) to form the myelin membrane ensheathment on specific sections of the neuronal plasma membrane. Formation of synapses and myelination of axons are each well-timed and spatially ordered developmental processes. From the ontogenic point of view both cellular events are manifested in molecular terms by the acquisition of new determinants, redistribution and perhaps modulation of preexisting ones, and disappearance of nonessential ones.

Lipid constituents are indisputably involved in these changes, as amply reviewed in several chapters of this book. The importance of lipids as structural constituents of nervous system membranes is reflected by the fact that of the total solids in the mature brain, more than 50% consist of lipids. Some of these, for example, plasmalogens, phosphoinositides, sphingolipids, and glycolipids, accumulate during active periods of myelination. The significance of these compositional changes on membrane fluidity and the consequent effect on neuronal events such as propagation of action potentials, synaptic transmission, or receptor expression is poorly understood. The meaning of metabolic turnover of the phospholipid constituents in the mature brain, an organ in which most cells do not divide, is also not yet clear. The dynamic state of phospholipids in the developing and mature brain must be the result of complex mechanisms in which substrates, metabolic intermediates, and enzymatic pathways are regulated in concert to maintain cells in a constant metabolic flux to match their physiological needs.

The focus of this chapter is to illustrate to neurochemists the potential as well as the pitfalls of nerve cell cultures as a tool for further understanding the role of lipids during the aforementioned metabolic and developmental processes of the nervous system.

6.2   METHODS FOR NERVOUS TISSUE CULTURE

Tissue and cell culture of the nervous system is a most valuable addition to the tools now available in neurobiology to explore regulatory mechanisms of development and membrane associated activities. Many phenomena that characterize the nervous system, such as nerve cell recognition, ontogenesis of the neurotransmitter apparatus and specific receptors, as well as formation of myelin, can be mimicked in culture in a fairly well defined environment isolated from the complex influences of the whole organism.

The various facets of tissue and cell culture of the nervous system are elaborate and have been reviewed extensively in many chapters and books. In this section an account is given of both the advantages and disadvantages of the principal culture techniques. More detailed experimental information is available in several excellent reviews and books (Herschman, 1973; Federoff and Hertz, 1977; Giacobini 1980; Mandel et al., 1976; Nelson and Lieberman, 1981; Murray, 1971; Sato, 1973). The choice of a particular tissue culture system for studying nervous tissue depends on the scope of the research and the methodological tools for investigation. The principal techniques are (1) use of tissue fragments or slices which, when appropriately manipulated, maintain an organotypic structure for relatively long periods; (2) use of dispersed cells maintained in monolayer or as aggregates in suspension for limited time periods; and (3) continuous cell lines derived from tumors of nervous tissue origin. Typical phase contrast micrographs illustrating each of these preparations are shown in Figure 6.1.

6.2.1   Organotypic Explants

The earliest successful attempt to maintain nervous tissue *in vitro* for extended periods was accomplished by Ross Harrison (1907) at the beginning of the ninteenth century. Harrison's observations on growth of axonal fibers from pieces of the tadpole neural tube bathed in frog lymphatic fluid in culture were also the first major contribution of tissue culture to neurobiology; they supported Ramon y Cajal's theory of cellular rather than syncytial organization of the nervous system. In subsequent

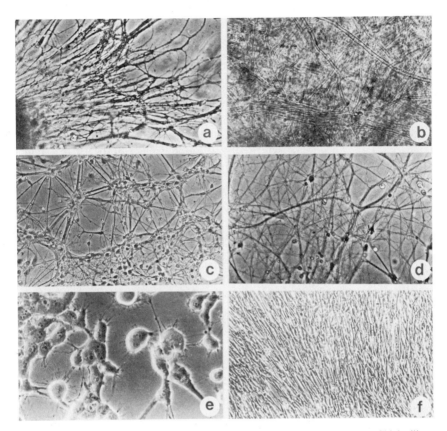

FIGURE 6.1 Phase contrast micrographs of various neural cells in culture. (*a*) Chick ciliary ganglia explant, 5 days *in vitro*. (×215, courtesy of Dr. A. Shahar.) (*b*) Myelin tracts in newborn rat cerebellum explant after 25 days in culture (×656, courtesy of Dr. A. Shahar.) (*c*) Dissociated rat cerebral neurons in serum-free medium after 3 weeks (×165). (*d*) Fiber network of the same preparation (×340). (*e*) Neuroblastoma N1E115 cells (×830). (*f*) C6 rat astrocytoma cells (×165).

years investigators have been concerned with improving conditions for this type of culture by studying growth requirements and by advancing the techniques for microscopic visualization of the various preparations. Today nearly every identifiable CNS and PNS region from most vertebrate species has been at one time adapted to culture (for a review see Murray and Kopech, 1953).

The explant technique has been exploited most widely to investigate the morphological, ultrastructural, and bioelectric properties of the cells using light, electronmicroscopy, and electrophysiological techniques with less emphasis on biochemical approaches. The three-dimensional organization of the cells in the explant and the histotypic preservation of the cells and their connections made it suitable for examining myelinogenesis, one of the most characteristic properties marking intercellular cooperativity in the nervous system. Explants derived from spinal ganglia, spinal cord, and cerebellum actively myelinate *in vitro* (for review, see Murray, 1971) and histochemical and ultrastructural approaches have been used to observe the influence of growth factors, hormones, and pharmacological agents on the integrity of the myelin membrane. Other studies using myelinating explants have examined biochemical processes related to the normal and pathologic brain. Amino acids and some of their intermediates implicated in congenital disorders, such as phenylketonuria and maple syrup urine disease, have been investigated for their possible role in demyelination (Silberberg, 1967, 1969). It was found that indole acids induced toxicity and progressive myelin degeneration at relatively low concentrations (Silberberg, 1967). It was also found that addition of α-ketoisocaproate at levels found in maple syrup patient sera prevented myelination in cerebellar explants (Silberberg, 1969).

Cultured explants have been used to investigate the involvement of the immune system in certain demyelinating disorders (Bornstein, 1963). Antisera raised in animals injected with antigenic preparations from the CNS and PNS were tested for their ability to interfere with myelin formation. Similar to the experimental allergic encephalomyelitis (EAE) syndrome sera from EAE rabbits had marked cytopathic effects on the glial and myelin sheaths of the CNS (Raine and Bornstein, 1961) but not PNS (Raine and Bornstein, 1970) cultures. Similarly, sera from experimental allergic nephritis (EAN) raised in rabbits immunized with PNS preparations demyelinated peripheral nerves in culture (Raine and Bornstein, 1979). Sera from multiple sclerosis patients were shown to contain a myelinotoxic activity which has been associated with an immunoglobulin fraction (Dowling et al., 1968). Thus, the ability to cause demyelination and induce remyelination is a great advantage of the explant system for studying inborn and immune disorders of the nervous system.

Formation of functional synaptic connections has been another line of study pursued in organotypic CNS cultures and was recently reviewed (Crain, 1978). In spite of some concern that the timing and pattern specificity of synapses formed *in vitro* may not reflect the *in vivo* situation (Giacobini, 1980), preparations of dorsal root ganglia innervating explants of spinal cord and medulla may have great potential for studying highly ordered and structured neurogenesis (Crain, 1980). The explant technique can provide a model to study some aspects of synapse plasticity and regeneration in culture but cannot explore in detail the developmental potential of the individual neuron isolated from its immediate cellular environment to express its synaptic capability (Patterson, 1980). For identification of the molecules involved in synaptic connectivity, dissociated cells and synaptically competent, established cell lines may prove more useful; an evaluation of these will be given below.

While morphological, ultrastructural, and electrophysiological correlates can be studied in the explant at the level of the single cell, biochemical analysis is hampered by insufficient amounts of tissue for reliable estimates. The most serious drawback of the explant technique from the metabolic standpoint is that because of poor circulation, parts of it gain only a limited access to nutrients and gases. This may create regions of active metabolism which are confined to the periphery of the explant where outgrowth occurs and tissue thickness is minimal compared to such metabolically deficient regions in the core of the explant. Another problem relates to cell heterogeneity within the explant when the metabolic fate of compounds studied in glia versus neurons is not similar.

6.2.2 Dissociated Cell Cultures

Culture of mechanically or enzymatically dissociated vertebrate neural cells has received increasing attention in the past decade. In using such dispersed cells, neurobiologists have gained access to the individual cell for studies of its sociobehavior; although initially severed of its contacts, the single cell in culture reestablishes functional connections that can be manipulated.

6.2.2.1 Dissociated Cells Grown as Monolayers

Primary cultures of dissociated cells in Maximow slide assemblies, Rose chambers, and petri dishes have been investigated by light and electron microscopy. The preparations of choice consisted either of sympathetic and dorsal root ganglia obtained from the PNS or spinal cord and cerebellum from the CNS. Synaptogenesis and myelin formation in long-term CNS and PNS cultures were reported (Bornstein and Model, 1972; Shahar et al., 1975; Kim, 1972). Myelin structures seen earlier in culture, after 8–10 days, were attributed to the presence of polylysine-coated dishes, which enhance neuritic extension and promote appropriate glia–neuron interaction (Yavin and Yavin, 1977). In other experiments triiodothyronine stimulated incorporation of radiolabeled precursors into sulfatides and cerebrosides of 11–14-day-old cultures of dissociated mouse cerebrum (Bhat et al., 1979), suggesting that manipulation of culture conditions can enhance or prevent expression of a neural function. Recently Sarlieve and co-workers (1983) have shown the presence of myelinlike structures in dissociated fetal mouse cells by discontinuous gradient centrifugation. They confirmed essentially similar observations reported by Berg and Schachner (1982) in mouse cerebellar cultures and by Yavin and Yavin (1977) in rat cerebral cells.

The excitability properties of dissociated CNS neurons in culture was recently reviewed (Nelson et al., 1981). Bioelectric activity has been recorded in dissociated cells from the chick spinal cord and fetal mouse cerebellar cultures. In the latter preparations the electrophysiological maturation was indicated by synaptic coupling between neurons, repetitive action potentials by direct electrical stimulation, and both spontaneous and evoked excitatory and inhibitory postsynaptic potentials. These experiments illustrate that disruption of tissue integrity obstructs neither the electrical coupling of neuronal circuits nor the ability of single cells to fire on stimulus (Nelson et al., 1981).

Developmental aspects of dissociated neural tissue in monolayer cultures have been also studied by biochemical techniques. Unlike morphological, ultrastructural, and electrophysiological approaches which are basically devised to observe single cells, biochemical methods address cell populations. This immediately raises some problems related to reproducibility of culture conditions. Variables such as age of the animal from which tissue is obtained, cell density, feeding regimen, and serum uniformity are all important factors that need to be standardized to maintain a stable population of cells throughout the experimental period. Unstable cell populations result from overgrowth of relatively nonproliferating neurons by more rapidly dividing neuroglia and fibroblast cells. Measurements of biochemical parameters should therefore be accompanied by an assessment of cell proliferation using methods such as [^{3}H]thymidine uptake to measure DNA synthesis or labeled mitotically active cells. It is also desirable to estimate the changes in the percent of neuronal and glial cells by using specific molecular markers, which are becoming more and more available (Raff et al., 1979).

Primary cultures of dissociated cells have been useful mainly to illuminate the similarities or disparities to *in situ* studies. This is perhaps best illustrated in studies involving the ontogenesis of the cholinergic apparatus, that is, the enzymes synthesizing and catabolizing acetylcholine, the receptors for binding the neurotransmitter and the carrier transport system for free choline (for review see Richelson, 1976). In all these studies a surprising degree of parallelism between *in vitro* and *in culture* development was demonstrated. Similarities also have been shown for the synthesis and degradation of catecholamines in dissociated sympathetic neurons (Mains and Patterson, 1973) for different enzymes of neurotransmitter metabolism. Conversely, dissimilarities have also been encountered in some systems, as critically reviewed by Giacobini (1980). These include (1) abnormal onset and levels of neurotransmitter-associated enzymes and altered neurotransmitter receptor pharmacology, (2) functionally deficient (i.e, lack of transmitter) and nonspecificty of synapses, and (3) distorted cell–cell connectivity and cell regression to a primitive nondifferentiated state.

6.2.2.2   Dissociated Cells as Aggregates in Suspension

A major criticism of monolayer cultures is the potential for random and uncoordinated cell–cell interaction because of the lack of three-dimensional contacts and the interaction with physiologically nonrelevant surfaces such as plastic, synthetic polymers, or collagen. To overcome these limitations, a number of laboratories (Seeds, 1973) have utilized dissociated cells maintained as aggregates in suspension, a method pioneered by Moscona (1965). The initial events and the factors required for histotypic assembly of dispersed cells derived from homologous or heterologous brain regions are best studied using this method. Dissociated cells from fetal mouse isocortex reaggregate in such cultures to form histotypic structures similar to the pyramidal cell assembly in the Ammon horn. Using this technique, DeLong and Sidman (1970) postulated that the neurological defect in the Reeler mouse is associated with a misalignment and misorientation of the migratory neurons. Suspension cultures also have been utilized to study myelinogenesis at ultrastructural and biochemical levels (Matthieu et al., 1980). Although the myelin was scarce and immature by biochemical criteria, its onset paralleled *in vivo* development.

6.2.2.3   Homotypic Cultures

The culture systems previously described are all composed of heterogenous populations of cells. However, for genetic and biochemical analysis it is generally agreed that homotypic populations are more desirable. Three major techniques for preparation of such homogeneous cell populations are currently available: free-hand dissection, bulk isolation, and differential growth selection. Of these three the latter technique thus far provides the hope for viable cell populations that can be studied over long periods in culture. Attempts to obtain relatively homogeneous populations of cells from normal tissue fall into one of two categories: The first involves the gross separation of cells into neurons, neuroglia, and nonneuronal cells, while the second is concerned with isolation of subsets of neurons and neuroglia according to highly specific cell surface molecular determinants. Work in the first category was pioneered in Varon's laboratory. Using differential cell adhesiveness, Varon and Raiborn (1969) and later McCarthy and Partlow (1976) obtained enriched neuronal-like preparations that survived several days in culture. In other systems investigators employed derivatized or polymer-coated surfaces (for review see Varon and Manthorpe, 1980) and even lipids (Margolis et al., 1978). Enriched neuronal cultures were obtained by using poly-L-lysine-coated petri dishes (Yavin and Yavin 1974). Poly-L-lysine promotes indiscriminate attachment and spreading of many cell types; by doing so, it minimizes the undesired selectivity caused by low plating efficiency, thus increasing the relative proportion of viable neurons attached to the dish. By selecting donor animals of the appropriate age prior to the *in vivo* glial growth spurt, a further enrichment of neuronal over glial cells can be obtained. Other conventional methods used to enrich the proportion of neuronal cells in a heterotypic culture involve the use of antimitotic drugs (Godfrey et al., 1975) which inhibit glial and fibroblast proliferation.

Separation of neurons and neuroglia cells by affinity probes such as α-bungarotoxin (Dvorak et al., 1978) or use of other probes such as sugar-binding lectins, toxins, or neurohormones cross-linked to appropriate matrices can provide additional means for isolation of cells (Varon and Manthorpe, 1980). The introduction of monospecific antibodies generated by the hybridoma technique provides the basis for a second and perhaps more powerful group of ligands in which the antigenic diversity of cell determinants can be utilized for cell separation. The advantage of the hybridoma technique is that there is no need to isolate and characterize particular cell-specific antigens as a prerequisite for the antibody preparation. During the next decade the research in this area will expand enormously as new clones are bound to provide specific probes not only for sorting out cell populations but also for investigating the role and developmental regulation of the corresponding antigens.

6.2.3 Clonal Neuronal and Glial Cell Lines

Dissociated cells or explants do not remain stable indefinitely. As already noted, the different proliferative capacities of the various populations of cells leads to an undesirable cell selection, and, in most cases, neuronal cells are lost first. Since neuroglia exhibit a limited capacity for growth and can survive several passages, they have been used to study glial cell properties in culture. These properties have been recently discussed in a book edited by Schoffeniels et al. (1978). A major obstacle for biochemical investigation of explants and dissociated cell cultures remains the nonhomogeneous nature of the cells and the limited amount of material available for analytical purposes.

To overcome these problems, work has been directed to establish genetically homogeneous cultures of neurons or glial cells that proliferate indefinitely and differentiate synchronously under defined experimental conditions. Such ideal cultures not only should provide desired quantities of cells but also should exhibit the potential for analyses of genetic regulation, homotypic and heterotypic cell–cell interaction, and effects of epigenetic factors on neural cell behavior. Studies in this direction have led to the establishment of cell lines derived from tumor tissue. A cell line was adapted for culture using neuroblastoma tumor C1300. The morphological, biochemical, and electrophysiological properties of this cell line have since been extensively investigated (for a detailed literature survey see Kimhi, 1981). These studies demonstrate that neuroblastoma cells express in culture many of the properties found in normal differentiated neurons. With the introduction of somatic cell hybridization techniques analysis of the regulation of gene expression in neurogenesis became possible (Minna et al., 1972). Currently a number of hybrid cells with different properties have been isolated (Hamprecht 1977). Another cell line, PC12-pheochromocytoma, isolated by Greene and Tishler (1976) from rat adrenal medulla, has been extensively used for studying nerve growth factor effects on differentiation. An additional source of neural cell lines has been obtained from nitrosourea-induced rat tumors (Schubert et al., 1974).

Clonal cell lines of glial origin were established about the same time as the neuroblastoma. The most widely used, the C6 cell line, was established by Benda et al. (1968). Numerous clones have been isolated since and their properties investigated (for further reference see Pffeifer et al., 1978). The morphological, ultrastructural, and physiological characterization of glial cells and their subsets has been difficult as no exclusive marker could be associated with one particular population of cells. However, a number of biochemical markers exhibit some "selective" association with glial cells; these include the S100 protein, 2′,3′-cyclic nucleotide 3′-phosphohydrolase, glycerophosphate dehydrogenase, glial fibrillary acidic protein, myelin basic proteins, carbonic anhydrase, and several surface-specific antigens. Despite this problem of partial specificity, significant contributions have been made to our understanding of the role of glial cells in the nervous system through the use of established cell lines. Some of these aspects include studies on adrenergic receptors, the role of glial-secreted or glial-responding growth factors, synthesis and degradation of S100 protein, the role in uptake and storage of neurotransmitters, and Na$^+$/K$^+$ transport mechanisms (for further references see Schoffeniels et al., 1978; Pffeifer et al., 1978).

6.3   CHEMICALY DEFINED MEDIA, LIPID CONSTITUENTS, AND NEURAL CELL GROWTH

In addition to physiological salts, nutrients and vitamins of a defined nature (Waymouth, 1954), culture media usually contain serum or occasionally other biological fluids as necessary additives. Serum presents a serious disadvantage for the rigorous preservation of standard culture conditions because of its great variability and the unidentified nature of many of its constituents.

Attempts to isolate and identify the various growth-promoting agents of serum parallel the history of tissue culture. As noted by Barnes and Sato in a recent review (1980), such attempts have been hampered by the abundance of unknown constituents (Brooks, 1975), many of which have no well-defined biological function and no established assays. Using another approach, Sato and co-workers have succeeded in replacing serum with defined hormones, growth factors, and various nutritional agents to sustain survival and growth of several established cell lines (Hayashi and Sato, 1976; Bottenstein and Sato, 1979). From studies such as these it would appear that further formulations may be necessary to sustain highly differentiated or to induce dedifferentiated cells in serum-free medium.

Since serum is a rich source of lipids, its removal may affect cellular properties and lipid metabolism. Thus, delipidated serum or its complete removal from C6 rat glioma cell medium resulted in a two- to threefold increase in associated lipogenic enzyme activities (Volpe and Marasa, 1975). Evidence was obtained that a combination of linoleic and linolenic acids could restore cell division of serum-deprived nonproliferating C6 rat astrocytoma and N18 mouse neuroblastoma cells (Yavin et al., 1975b). Removal of lipids from the nutrient medium had a significant effect on myelination of organotypic mouse spinal cord cultures (Kim and Pleasure, 1978). The levels of myelin basic protein and the activity of 2',3'-cyclic nucleotide phosphohydrolase, both markers for myelin, were reduced. The authors concluded that lipid deprivation was not compensated for by enhanced cellular synthesis. Another possibility is that "delipidation" had removed other lipid-soluble cofactors necessary to stimulate synthesis.

The concentration and composition of lipids isolated from calf or horse serum is not similar and is age dependent within species as recently shown by Spector et al. (1981). It has been shown also that the concentration of phospholipids in fetal bovine serum is almost threefold lower than that found in newborn bovine serum. Differences are also encountered in the composition of fatty acids; fetal bovine serum is rich in arachidonic acid but low in linoleic acid in comparison to other sera of mammalian sources. Horse serum on the other hand is rich in linoleic acid and has no detectable amounts of $22:6(n - 3)$ docosahexaenoic acid (Spector et al., 1981). In most established cell lines the specific profile of cellular lipid fatty acids resembles the profile found in the serum (Geyer et al., 1962). This phenomenon may have a physiological significance with respect to the ability or inability of cells to express their phenotypic functions. The increasing use of serum-free media poses some intriguing questions with regard to essential fatty acid (EFA) requirements in mammalian cells. Linoleic acid is added to most, but not all (Barnes and Sato, 1979), defined media and in at least one case it is required to sustain growth of SV40-transformed 3T3 cells (Rockwell et al., 1980). On the other hand, many established cell lines do not require EFA for growth (Evans et al., 1964). Dissociated cerebral cells from mouse embryo grown in serum-defined medium were found deficient in essential fatty acids, as reflected by an increase of $20:3(n - 9)$ content (Bourre et al., 1983). Addition of EFA or arachidonic and docosahexaenoic acids to the growth medium stimulated proliferation of glial elements and restored the profile of fatty acid in comparison to postnatal brain. It should be noted, however, that most of these cell lines have not been examined for functional correlates which as a consequence of EFA deficiency may have been altered. For instance, enhanced contractility of heart cells would have been affected in the absence of EFA (Gerschenson et al., 1967). Also noted is the fact that addition of EFA has an improved effect on mitochondrial function and impulse propagation in electrically excitable cells (Saum et al., 1981). These observations suggest that EFA may be involved in the specific functions of differentiated cells as well as being important in growth regulation (Holley et al., 1974).

Recently, serum-free medium in conjunction with several hormones and growth factors has been successfully used with cultures of primary neural cells. Embryonic chick sensory ganglia cultures in the absence of serum and in the presence of several supplements were investigated (Bottenstein et al., 1980). The neurons survived for less than a week under these conditions. Honegger et al. (1979) maintained dissociated fetal brain cells under serum-free conditions in suspension cultures in the presence of insulin, hydrocortisone, triiodothyronine, transferin, and trace elements. Myelinogenesis and synaptogenesis were apparent in these cultures, although the onset of these functions was somewhat delayed. The activities of several neurotransmitter-associated enzymes were also similar or slightly lower compared to aggregates grown in 15% fetal calf serum. Some of the Bottenstein–Sato supplements (1979) have been successfully used by Messer et al. (1981) to grow dissociated cerebellar cultures.

Survival of dissociated cerebral neurons in monolayer cultures in the near absence of serum was reported (Yavin and Yavin, 1980). Morphological and biochemical maturation acquired by these cells in the absence of added supplements (Zurgil and Zisapel, 1981) was explained by the presence of growth factors released from nonsurviving cells at early times after dissociation (Yavin and Yavin, 1980). Recently, addition of a number of growth factors, which included insulin, somatostatin, transferin, hydrocortisone, and a tripeptide, greatly curtailed cell death and enabled long-term growth of neuronal-enriched cell cultures (Yavin et al., 1982). Dissociated dorsal root ganglia cells can also survive for about 2 weeks in serum-free medium in the presence of insulin and without any other supplements (Snyder and Kim, 1980). More work is needed to define the exact hormonal and nutritional requirements as well as the influence of factors released from the neural tissue itself in order to prepare the ideal growth "cocktail."

6.4   COMPOSITION AND METABOLISM OF PHOSPHOLIPIDS

Phospholipids are ubiquitous components of eukaryotic cells. Therefore, no phospholipid species has been exclusively associated with a particular cell type or a subcellular membrane structure. Despite that, evidence exists for enrichment of phospholipid species in certain membranes. In addition, partial asymmetric distribution of phospholipids between the inner and outer faces of the membrane have been described, yet nothing is known concerning the origin, maintenance, and role of this asymmetry (Rothman and Lenarz, 1977).

Typical analyses of phospholipid composition extracted from tissue or cells in culture are routinely conducted with respect to the fatty acid profile or tabulated according to the polar head groups. For example, comparison of the composition of the cellular phospholipids of neuronal and glial cells as illustrated in Table 6.1 may erroneously lead to the interpretation that subsets of cells of the nervous tissue are similar and may resemble cells from other tissues. This is a misleading conclusion as it is based on the assumption that the existing methods of classification can account for the molecular heterogeneity and metabolic complexity of cellular phospholipids. In fact, when compiled according to the polar head groups as well as according to the acyl, alkyl, and alk-1-enyl bonds, chain length, and degree of unsaturation, the molecular composition of phos-

Table 6.1 Phospholipid Composition in Several Cell Lines and Bulk Isolated Neural Cells[a]

	Cell Line	CPG	EPG	PEPG	SPG	IPG	SP	Reference
				(% distribution)				
Neuronal	N1E115	51.6	10.4	12.4	5.2	9.6	6.0	Yavin, 1977a
	M1	54.1	12.6	15.2	4.2	10.7	3.2	Robert et al., 1978
	N2A	57.1	12.8	12.8	15.4	10.7	2.0	Charalampous, 1979
Glial	Hamster astrocyte	50.4	9.2	11.5	2.4	4.8	11.1	Eichberg et al., 1976
	C6 astrocytoma	50.2	6.3	10.7	0	5.1	17.5[c]	Eichberg et al., 1976
		52.2	18.0	10.5	4.5	3.8	8.1	Robert et al., 1976
	NN astroblast	47.4	15.7	10.0	6.9	7.2	8.6	Robert et al., 1976
	RN6	47.5	19.2	14.8	3.6	2.2	12.6	Binaglia et al., 1976
Neuron × glia hybrid	NG108-15	58.6	9.9	9.4	4.5	6.8	4.4	Yavin and Zutra, 1979
		64.1	16.1	16.1	3.7	10.0	3.8	McGee, 1981
Bulk isolated	Neurons (rat)	56.8	26.0[b]		5.6	7.0	4.6	Norton and Poduslo, 1971
	Astrocytes (rat)	52.7	29.2[b]		7.6	5.1	5.4	Norton and Poduslo, 1971
	Oligodendrocytes	47.3	22.5[b]		7.6	6.6	10.0	Poduslo and Norton, 1972

[a] CPG—Phosphatidylcholine; EPG—Phosphatidylethanolamine; PEPG—Ethanolamine plasmalogen; SPG—Phosphatidylserine; IPG—Phosphatidylinositol; SP—Sphingomyelin.
[b] Including PEPG.
[c] Including alkyl ether phospholipid.

pholipids gives rise to a great number of permutations. Until such an analytical evaluation of the structural heterogeneity of these compounds becomes available, the metabolic machinery that controls their assembly and disassembly and the relationship to function will remain unsolved. For example, fast and slow metabolic pools, partial degradation and resynthesis, and other kinetic data obtained by isotopic means are indicative of this extensive heterogeneity. Furthermore, the possible association of such diverse phospholipid species with specific membrane microdomains may be the clue in understanding the role of these constituents in a number of vital processes such as chemical and electrical excitability, neurotransmitter–receptor interaction, fusion of synaptic vesicles, and electrical insulation.

6.4.1 Acyl, Alkyl, and Alk-1-Enyl Bond Composition of Phospholipids

The hydrophobic residue of the common phosphoglyceride consists of a long-chain hydrocarbon linked via an *O*-acyl, *O*-alkyl, or *O*-alk-1-enyl bond to the hydroxyl group of the glycerophosphoric acid moiety. These hydrophobic residues are derivatives of fatty acids, alcohols, and aldehydes of varying chain length and degree of unsaturation, and each imparts some specific lipid properties to the phospholipid molecule in its interaction with neighboring lipids or membrane proteins. Analysis of these phospholipid constituents and their variability should provide some clues for unraveling the potential biological significance of phospholipid molecular species encountered in biological membranes. In studying the phospholipid hydrocarbon chain composition of cultured cells, it becomes apparent that neural cells maintained in organotypic "arrays" or as homotypic/heterotypic clusters or even as established cell lines are subject to biochemical variability, some of which was already discussed in Section 6.1. This variability stems from environmental conditions that can enhance or delay biochemical development and maturation as well as aging and cell death, thus creating uncontrolled cell selection pressures. These culture variables necessitate a careful examination of the structural lipid components, particularly with respect to fatty acid residues.

In one of the first studies employing dissociated fetal rat cerebral cells, it was found that the fatty acid composition of phosphatidylcholine and phosphatidylethanolamine lipid species resembled that of the developing nervous system (Yavin and Menkes, 1974a). Palmitic and oleic acids were the predominant fatty acids in the lecithin species, while stearic and oleic acid dominated the ethanolamine phospholipid species. The polyunsaturated fatty acid content of the latter glycerophospholipid was fivefold greater than that of the lecithin and reached a value of about 27% of the total acyl group content.

The fatty acid composition of whole-lipid extracts isolated from newborn rat cerebral explants has been recently studied (Giesing and Zilliken, 1980). Nearly 40% of the fatty acids consisted of two and more double bonds, which may reflect the fact that these cell preparations were non-myelinating organotypic cultures. Unlike the adult brain, cerebral cortex explants from the newborn rat (Giesing and Zilliken, 1980) as well as fetal cerebral cells (Yavin and Menkes, 1973) contained notable quantities of triacylglycerols. The high levels of triacylglycerols in the developing brain tissue under culture conditions has been correlated with the metabolic state of the cells, which may accumulate excess fatty acids in the form of triacylglycerols from the serum-supplemented medium.

The composition of fatty acids in neuronal- and glial-enriched cell cultures from mouse and rat cerebrum was compared to that of SV40-transformed neuronal- and glial-like cell lines (Montaudon et al., 1981). A significant reduction in the relative percent of eicosaenoic and docosaenoic polyunsaturated fatty acids (PUFA) in the transformed as opposed to normal cells was found. The lower levels of PUFA were attributed to cell transformation rather than to epigenetic environmental factors. A significant reduction (over 50%) of the lipid phosphorus content expressed per milligram of protein in the transformed compared to nontransformed cultures was reported (Montaudon et al., 1981). Slight changes in fatty acid labeling of Schwann cell–enriched cultures from Trembler mouse mutant compared to normal cells were also reported (Bourre et al., 1981).

Apart from fatty acids, the composition of O-alkyl and O-alkenyl species was investigated in several cell lines of neuronal and glial origin. Hamster astroblast NN cells and C6, a rat astrocytoma, were found by Robert et al. (1976) to contain more than 80 mol % of diacyl bonds with less than 15% of O-alk-1-enyl bonds. Nearly 40% of the ethanolamine phosphoglyceride fraction in both cell lines was identified as vinylether-containing plasmalogen. When the fatty acid profile of the NN and C6 cellular phospholipids was studied, it was found similar to that of viral-transformed neural cells which contain a remarkably low content of docosapentaenoic (22:5) and docosahexaenoic (22:6) fatty acids of the $n - 3$ linolenic acid family. Similar observations made in N18 (Yavin et al., 1975a) and M1 (Robert et al., 1978a) murine neuroblastoma, human retinoblastoma (Hyman and Spector, 1981), and PC12 rat pheochromocytoma (Williams and McGee, 1982) appear to document a common trend characteristic of most neural cell lines propagated indefinitely in culture. In general, lack of PUFA in transformed or established neural cell lines is somewhat disappointing in view of the abundance of PUFA normally found in the nervous system (Svennerholm, 1968; Clausen, 1969).

6.4.1.1 Uptake and Metabolism of Fatty Acids

The development of techniques for routine cultivation of neural cells provided a new approach for studying metabolism of lipid constituents with long half lives. In one of the first studies using frontal lobe explants, Menkes (1971, 1972) demonstrated that labeled palmitic and stearic acids were incorporated into neutral lipids, glycolipids, and phospholipids, either unchanged or after desaturation, chain elongation, or both. The ability of brain explants to incorporate and metabolize fatty acids was age dependent, that is, it was less effective in explants taken from the adult brain (Menkes, 1971).

An interesting approach for studying lipid metabolism in explants has been reported by Giesing and Zilliken (1980). These investigators determined lipid fatty acid composition in individual explants of homologous brain tissue explanted in the same culture dish several days apart. Innervation of the more mature by the more recent explanted cerebral cortex fragments caused a significant stimulation of eicosatetraenoic [arachidonic, $20:4(n-6)$] and docosahexaenoic $22:6(n-3)$ acid synthesis. The authors accredit this phenomenon to the neuritic bridges established between the explants. Although this approach may be of potential use, lack of compartmentation between explants does not rule out other possibilities, such as secretion of cellular substances that stimulate phospholipid biosynthesis.

The rate of uptake of a series of radioactively labeled saturated and unsaturated fatty acids was measured in dissociated mixed cerebral cell cultures (Yavin and Menkes, 1974a, 1974b). Uptake was greatest for stearic acid and decreased progressively with decreasing chain length. Cellular phospholipids and triacylglycerols were labeled preferentially from all fatty acid precursors. Changes in the labeling pattern of phospholipid fatty acids demonstrated a precursor–product relationship for lauric $(12:0)$, myristic $(14:0)$, palmitic $(16:0)$, and stearic $(18:0)$ fatty acids (Yavin and Menkes, 1974b). Dissociated cerebral cells can readily incorporate essential fatty acids such as linoleate and linolenate and possess all the necessary enzymes to synthesize long-chain polyunsaturated fatty acids (Yavin and Menkes, 1974a). Labeled linoleic and linolenic acids were readily converted into their higher homologs. When the kinetics of incorporation of [^{14}C]linolenate was studied, it was found that during the initial phases of incubation label entered preferentially into free fatty acids, triacylglycerols, and lecithin in the cell. Incorporation into ethanolamine phosphoglycerides increased slowly with time in a biphasic manner and paralleled desaturation and chain elongation of the linolenic acid. By lowering the incubation temperature, it was shown that the conversion of linolenic acid into its higher homologs proceeds by at least two distinct, temperature-sensitive steps. The rate-limiting step appeared to be the conversion of eicosapentaenoic to docosapentaenoic fatty acid. As a result of lowering the temperature, the polyunsaturated fatty acid profile of ethanolamine phosphoglycerides was greatly impaired. The capacity to elongate and desaturate linolenic acid was lost in long-term cultures (Yavin et al., 1975a), in a manner that paralleled the loss of neuronal cells (unpublished observations).

The recognition that both genetic and epigenetic factors may contribute to the observed PUFA pattern alterations in established cell lines prompted studies on elongation and desaturation patterns of essential fatty acids. In one approach essential fatty acids or their higher homologs were administered directly to the culture medium in an attempt to modulate the phospholipid fatty acid composition. In a second approach radioactively labeled precursors were used to study rates of uptake and precursor–product relationships of the various metabolic intermediates or to search for abnormal metabolic pathways.

Labeled linoleic and linolenic acids added to neuroblastoma C1300 clone N18 were taken up at nearly equal rates (Yavin et al., 1975a). Linoleic acid was preferentially incorporated into phosphatidylcholine whereas linolenic acid entered mainly into phosphatidylethanolamine. Eicosapolyenoic fatty acids were preferentially taken up into ethanolamine plasmalogen, which generally agrees with reported values from tissue analysis (Clausen, 1969). Fatty acid precursors were initially elongated and subsequently desaturated to provide the expected profile of long-chain polyunsaturated fatty acid intermediates. However, there was no radioactivity present in the docosahexaenoic fatty acids, which suggested that the Δ-4-desaturase is not functional in these cells (Yavin et al., 1975a). This has also been documented in lines of glial and neuronal origin (Robert et al., 1977, 1978a); when grown in fetal calf serum made deficient in essential fatty acids, the fatty acid profile of the phospholipids in these cells was low in polyunsaturated fatty acids. On the other hand, addition of linoleic and linolenic or their corresponding higher homologs (eicosatetraenoic and docosahexaenoic acids) to the growth medium resulted in the appearance of all these substances as acyl components of cellular phospholipids. Linolenic acid was less effectively taken up than linoleic acid in all these cell lines (Robert et al., 1977, 1978a). The Δ-4-desaturase activity was missing in all cell lines, suggesting an abnormality perhaps related to culture conditions. The lack of significant amounts of docosahexaenoic acid in the nerve cells is rather puzzling. Although this fatty acid cannot be synthesized by the cells, it can be taken up from the extracellular medium. Indeed most tissue culture sera contain 4–5% of docosahexaenoic acid (Spector et al., 1981). The possibility that this fatty acid has no essential role in nervous system function is unlikely in view of its high concentration in synaptosomes (Breckenridge et al., 1972). Alternatively, it may be that the failure to concentrate or synthesize docosahexaenoic acid represents a regression of cellular differentiation that affects some yet unknown phenotypic functions.

It is interesting to note that not all neural cell lines have lost their capability to synthesize docosahexaenoic fatty acid. Hyman and Spector (1981) recently reported that Y79 retinoblastoma cells contained a Δ-4-desaturase activity which converted linoleic acid to docosapentaenoic $22:5(n - 6)$ and linolenic acid to docosahexaenoic fatty acids. Retinoblastoma cells elongated and desaturated linolenic acid added to the culture medium so as to increase by nearly 70% the content of docosahexaenoic acid in phospholipids as compared to untreated cultures, particularly in phosphatidylethanolamine species. On the other hand, cultured skin fibroblasts did not possess such an effective elongation–desaturation system (Hyman and Spector, 1981). Supplements of docosahexaenoic fatty acid were taken up by retinoblastoma and by fibroblast cells into cellular phospholipids. It is not known whether phosphatidylethanolamine and phosphatidylserine species in both types of cells were the main acceptors, as has been demonstrated in a C1300 neuroblastoma clone (Robert et al., 1978a). Such a relationship between the polar head group and degree of fatty acid unsaturation has been indicated by the concomitant addition of N-methyl containing ethanolamine bases and eicosapentaenoic $20:5$ $(n - 3)$ acid (Yavin and Robert, 1979).

Elongation and desaturation of essential fatty acids have been studied in detail in two other clones of neuronal origin. The neuroblastoma–glioma hybrid clone NG108-15 had a low content of arachidonic acid (about 6%) when grown in the regular medium supplemented with 5% fetal bovine serum (McGee, 1981). Upon addition of 0.125 μM linoleate, a twofold increase in arachidonic acid and docosatetraenoic acid $22:4$ ($n - 6$) was observed. After addition of arachidonate, more than 40% of the total cellular fatty acids was present as PUFA and nearly half of this was docosatetraenoic acid, the elongation product of arachidonic acid (McGee, 1981). This remarkable elongation activity has been previously demonstrated in another cell line of neural origin (Robert et al., 1978a) and also more recently in a PC12 pheochromocytoma cell line (Williams and McGee, 1982). Unlike neuroblastoma or the hybrid cells, PC12 cells contain a relatively high percentage (13–16%) of arachidonic acid (Williams and McGee, 1982), which is not surprising since the horse serum in which these cells grow is enriched with linoleic acid (Spector et al., 1981). Addition of arachidonate to the growth medium increases cellular arachidonate and docosatetraenoate 22:4 in a time- and concentration-dependent fashion. These authors did not report whether either the hybrid or the pheochromocytoma cell line had a Δ-4-desaturase deficiency.

6.4.1.2. *Prospects for Metabolic Studies of Fatty Acids*

Further research in the area of fatty acid metabolism in neural tissue is foreseen in two main domains: (1) the establishment of homogeneous neuron or glial cell populations to study synthesis, catabolism, and fatty acid exchange, particularly of the long-chain polyunsaturated type, into specific phosphoglycerides and (2) the investigation of whether transformation, aging, or other epigenetic factors affect enzymatic activities (such as lack of Δ-4-desaturase) and alter plasma membrane fatty acid composition and its functions.

6.4.2. Polar Head Group Composition and Metabolism in Isolated Neuronal and Glial Preparations

Important information on the dynamic state of phospholipids in cells of nervous tissue origin has been gained through studies using bulk isolated neuronal- and glial-enriched cell preparations (Porcellati and Goracci, 1976). Uptake and utilization of labeled precursors such as glycerol, inorganic phosphorus, fatty acids, and nitrogen-containing bases have clearly established the cytidine nucleotide pathway as the major route to formation of new phosphoglycerides. Other reactions such as base exchange also have been demonstrated (Goracci et al., 1973). Studies using bulk isolated neurons and glial cells seem to indicate that neuronal phospholipids have a faster turnover rate than glial phospholipids (Binaglia et al., 1973). Bulk isolated neurons, astrocytes, and oligodendrocytes from the CNS consist in principle of similar phospholipid species compared to established cell lines of neuronal or glial origin (summarized in Table 6.1). As indicated by this comparative table, the classification of phospholipids according to the polar head group reveals differences in the relative proportion of some minor phospholipid (i.e., phosphatidylinositol) species. Also, in at least two cases (Yavin, 1977a; Robert et al., 1978b) murine neuroblastoma cell lines seem to have a higher proportion of ethanolamine plasmalogen. In accord with studies using nonneural cells, some of these differences may reflect an environmental aspect of cell growth in culture, such as contact inhibition (Diringer and Koch, 1973), proliferating capacity (Bergeron et al., 1970), or nutrient availability (Wood and Falch, 1973; Diringer and Koch, 1974).

Significant differences in the composition of phospholipids in whole brain have been attributed to developmental changes (for review see Rouser et al., 1972). Some parallelism has been found in developing fetal rat brain in culture (Yavin and Menkes, 1974a; Giesing and Zilliken, 1980). After 2 days in culture, when cells are at the initial stage of fiber outgrowth, the levels of phosphatidylcholine, ethanolamine plasmalogen, and phosphatidylethanolamine are 79.0, 15.8, and 32 nmol lipid phosphorus/ mg protein, respectively (Yavin, 1976a). After 3 weeks, following the formation of an extensive network of fibers, mixed cerebral cultures consist of many synapses and are abundant in myelin figures (Yavin and Yavin, 1977). At this time the levels of phosphatidylcholine, ethanolamine plasmalogen, and phosphatidylethanolamine attain a maximum value of 120, 51.4, and 61.5 nmol/mg protein, respectively (Yavin, 1976a). This major increase in cellular phospholipids, which is accompanied by significant changes in the relative proportion of ethanolamine plasmalogen, parallels changes observed in the developing CNS (Ansell, 1973, and also this text).

Changes in composition and content of polar head groups appear to be associated with the cell cycle (Diringer and Friis, 1977; Hoffman et al., 1980). A twofold decrease in membrane microviscosity during the transition from mitosis to G1 phase was found by DeLaat et al., (1977) in neuroblastoma cells. Changes in phospholipid composition due to growth of neuroblastoma cells in suspension or in monolayer cultures was also reported (Charalampous, 1979). According to this study, monolayer cultures contained significantly higher concentrations of phospholipids per cell and also more phosphatidylcholine than cells grown in spinner cultures.

6.4.3. Metabolic Regulation of Polar Head Groups in Developing Cerebral Cell Cultures

Although recent methods have improved cellular viability, particularly of glial cells (Pleasure et al., 1981), bulk isolated neurons and glial preparations cannot be kept alive for periods longer than several hours. Cells in culture, on the other hand, are more suitable for long-term metabolic studies. Despite the fact that enriched neuronal and glial cell cultures did not exist until recently, important information on phospholipid metabolism has been gained through studies with such mixed neuron–glia cultures. In one of the early studies incorporation of labeled choline and CDP-choline into phospholipids of a myelin fraction isolated from brain explants after 2–4 weeks in culture was reported by Chida and Shimizu (1973). The majority of radioactivity from both radiolabeled compounds was found in lecithin, with lesser amounts present in sphingomyelin. It was not clear whether the CDP-nucleotide was incorporated intact or whether it was degraded prior to uptake by the cells.

The uptake and utilization of serine, ethanolamine, and choline for phospholipid biosynthesis in cultured dissociated cells from rat embryo cerebral hemispheres have been studied in some detail (Yavin and Kanfer, 1975a; Yavin, 1976b; Yavin and Ziegler, 1977). Unlike serine, which is a nonessential amino acid and therefore can be generated from intracellular sources, supplies of ethanolamine and choline for phospholipid synthesis are presumably derived from extraneural sources. A highly efficient uptake for ethanolamine and choline with apparent K_m of 8 and 16 μM, respectively, was reported (Yavin and Kanfer, 1975a). Choline uptake did not follow simple Michaelis Menten saturation kinetics; a second low-affinity uptake component of 0.96 mM was also found (Yavin, 1976b). Similar high- and low-affinity uptake components have been established in other cells of neural origin, although other mechanisms for choline uptake have been proposed (Massarelli et al., 1979). The reciprocal pattern of inhibition of choline and ethanolamine by a number of analogs such as 2-chloroethylamine and hemicholinium-3 suggested the existence of separate active transport systems for these compounds. It was also noted that the specificity of the high-affinity choline uptake component depends on the number of N-methyl groups present; dimethylaminoethanol and monomethylaminoethanol were both competitive inhibitors (K_i = 6 and 60 μM, respectively) of the high- but not the low-affinity choline uptake component (Yavin, 1980).

Based on these studies, it was concluded that cerebral cells, and presumably the intact brain, possess a very efficient mechanism for incorporating choline and ethanolamine from the extracellular compartment, even if these metabolites are present at very low concentrations.

The metabolic fate of nitrogen-containing bases after they become incorporated within the cells has also been investigated. When analyzing the distribution of radioactivity in water-soluble choline and ethanolamine intermediates following short-term pulses, it became apparent that at low precursor concentration most of the label was found in phosphocholine and phosphoethanolamine. Furthermore, kinetic analyses demonstrated that the phosphorylated bases accumulated within the cells prior to the appearance of label in phospholipids in a time-dependent manner, consistent with a precursor–product relationship. On reducing the incubation temperature from 37°C to 22°C, phospholipid synthesis was almost completely abolished, whereas phosphorylation itself was barely affected.

These observations suggested that phosphorylation, which is independent of transport, is perhaps the major mechanism for maintaining adequate intracellular levels of free choline and ethanolamine for phospholipid biosynthesis (Yavin and Kanfer, 1975, Yavin, 1976b).

An interesting finding that bears directly on the question of the interrelation between the high-affinity choline transport system and acetylcholine and phosphocholine synthesis emerged from these studies (Yavin, 1976b). At low choline concentrations most of the [^{14}C]choline label was present in the phosphocholine fraction with little or no label in acetylcholine. In contrast, at high choline concentrations a large proportion of radioactivity was incorporated into acetylcholine. The difference in the extent of formation of these choline-containing compounds as a function of choline concentration was interpreted as an indication for the existence of two independent enzymatic activities, choline phosphokinase and choline acetyltransferase, each with a different affinity for the choline substrate. This observation may be of potential significance for understanding choline reutilization mechanisms at the synaptic endings (Kessler and Marchbanks, 1979).

A general increase in the phospholipid content of cerebral cells during growth *in vitro* was previously noted (Yavin, 1976a). In particular, the levels of 1-alkenyl, 2-acyl, and 1,2-diacyl containing ethanolamine phosphoglycerides were greatly elevated. Kinetic data obtained using labeled ethanolamine indicated that the CDP-nucleotide pathway is the major route by which brain cells synthesize these phospholipids. The rates of labeling of ethanolamine plasmalogen and phosphatidylethanolamine from labeled phosphoethanolamine were practically identical. However, a relatively greater increase in plasmalogen labeling was observed whenever free ethanolamine was present in the incubation medium. Using a double-label pulse technique, it was postulated that in addition to the *de novo* synthesis via the CDP-nucleotide pathway an independent pattern of plasmalogen synthesis existed (Yavin and Kanfer, 1975b). Support for this observation was obtained indirectly from a study of the role of serine as a possible source for the ethanolamine moiety of phosphatidylethanolamine (Yavin and Ziegler, 1977). Free serine is incorporated in cerebral cells via an energy-independent Ca^{2+}-stimulated base-exchange pathway as well as by an energy-related pathway as implied by studies using oligomycin and the Ca^{2+} ionophore A23187. The energy-independent base exchange has been acknowledged as the major pathway for phosphatidylserine formation in mammalian cells. That phosphatidylserine can be also decarboxylated has also been known for years, yet its contribution as a significant source for phosphatidylethanolamine had not until recently been quantitatively evaluated. Using radioactively labeled serine as a

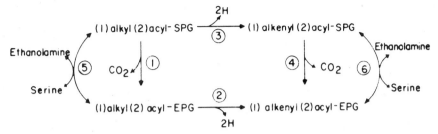

FIGURE 6.2   Metabolic interconversion scheme of ether bond-containing serine (SPG) and ethanolamine (EPG) phosphoglycerides by means of decarboxylation (1,4) desaturation (2,3) and nonhomologous base exchanges (5,6). For further details see Yavin and Ziegler (1977).

marker and a simplified mathematical model to fit the data, it was found that a considerable portion of phosphatidylethanolamine may arise via phosphatidylserine decarboxylation. Based on this mathematical compartmentation model, analysis of the flux from 1-alkyl,2-acyl serine phosphoglyceride via 1-alkyl,2-acyl ethanolamine phosphoglyceride (by decarboxylation) into ethanolamine plasmalogen (by dehydrogenation) was estimated in spite of the fact that in the latter reaction, the precursor–product crossover point could not be experimentally determined. Figure 6.2 outlines a metabolic scheme proposed to account for the possible interconversions of the ether bond-containing serine and ethanolamine phosphoglycerides.

In this scheme serine displacement by free ethanolamine to form 1-alkyl,2-acyl ethanolamine phospholipids and ultimately ethanolamine plasmalogen appears compatible with previous observations on free ethanolamine–stimulated plasmalogen synthesis (Yavin and Kanfer, 1975b). Thus serine, a common amino acid, can fulfill the cellular needs for ethanolamine for maintaining ethanolamine phospholipid levels when other potential sources are restricted.

A different approach for studying plasmalogen biosynthesis was undertaken by Witter and Debuch (1982). These workers used 1-alkyl glycerophosphoryl ethanolamine (GPE) to investigate the ability of mixed astrocyte/oligodendrocyte primary cultures to incorporate and metabolize this ether lipid precursor. Nearly one-third of the labeled substrate was incorporated by the cells within a period of 3 h. A very effective acylation at the 2-position took place, resulting in net accumulation of 1-alkyl,2-acyl GPE. Only very small amounts of labeled plasmalogen, the immediate product of the alkyl-acyl phospholipid, was detected after 3 h incubation even when the level of the substrate was highly elevated. Although the authors attribute their inability to demonstrate desaturation to the relatively short periods of incubation, the possibility exists that the substrate is taken up by the cells in a form not metabolically available for the desaturase activity.

A metabolic pathway previously considered to be of minor significance in the biosynthesis of phosphatidylcholine in the brain, namely a two-step methylation of phosphatidylethanolamine with S-adenosylmethionine as methyl donor, has attracted great interest as a possible mechanism for transduction of biological signals via phospholipid modification (Hirata and Axelrod, 1980). Although the functional significance of this pathway has been questioned (Vance and Kruijff, 1980), its presence in cultures of rat cerebral neurons (Yavin and Yavin, 1980) and chick neuronal and glial cells (Dainous et al., 1982) has been reported. The rapid incorporation of the nitrogenous bases monomethyl- and dimethylaminoethanol into cellular phospholipids offered an opportunity to study the synthesis of the various phospholipid intermediates containing either none, one, or two N-methyl groups by following the incorporation of the labeled methionine. Addition of methyl-labeled methionine to culture medium at tracer levels or at millimolar concentration enabled measurements of the rates of phospholipid methylation from phosphatidylethanolamine, phosphatidylmonomethyl-, and phosphatidyldimethylaminoethanol precursors (Yavin, 1984). At tracer doses the rates of methylation from the above respective phospholipids were 0.45, 1.17, and 1.70 pmol/h/µg DNA. At 1 mM methionine, synthesis of phosphatidylcholine proceeds from [^{14}C]phosphatidylethanolamine or [^{14}C]phosphatidyldimethylaminoethanol at initial rates of 8 and 17 pmol/h/µg DNA, respectively (Yavin, 1985). While the latter phospholipid analog can be generated from its monomethyl precursor, methylation of phosphatidylethanolamine does not result in the accumulation of phosphatidyldimethylaminoethanol, suggesting two segregated and metabolically distinct pathways. The methylation pathway contributes a significant portion of choline from endogenous sources, most likely through conversion of phosphatidyl serine.

A kinetic model (depicted in Fig. 6.3) to estimate the rates of synthesis and degradation of the various N-methylethanolamine lipid intermediates using N-base analogs and [^{3}H-methyl]methionine is currently under investigation.

Lipid transmethylation in cultured cells of neural origin has been recently studied in C6 astrocytoma (Strittmater et al., 1979) and PC12 pheochromocytoma (Maeda et al, 1981) cell lines. Compared to four other lines of nonneural origin, membrane preparations from a pheochromocytoma PC12h subclone displayed the lowest capability to methylate phosphatidylethanolamine (Maeda et al., 1981).

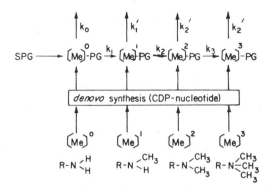

FIGURE 6.3   Model for phosphatidylcholine synthesis via the cytidine nucleotide and transmethylation pathways in cerebral cell cultures. Me^0–Me^3 represent the various degrees of methylation of ethanolamine; PG, phosphoglyceride; SPG, phosphatidylserine.

6.4.4.   *N*-Base Analogs as Probes for Studying Phospholipid Metabolism

Inorganic ^{32}P-labeled phosphate (^{32}P$_i$) has been widely used for studying the dynamic aspects of phospholipid metabolism in cell cultures (Howard and Howard, 1974). Eichberg et al. (1976) used cultured astrocytes and noticed a rapid labeling of phosphatidylcholine, choline plasmalogen, phosphatidylinositol, and phosphatidic acid by ^{32}P$_i$ in comparison to the strikingly lower levels of labeling of ethanolamine phosphoglycerides. The specific radioactivity of choline plasmalogen was the highest among all phospholipid species at an early cell passage but became reduced significantly at a late cell passage.

Base analogs such as monomethyl- and dimethylethanolamine have been used in neuroblastoma cells to estimate the rates of phospholipid synthesis via the CDP-nucleotide pathway (Yavin, 1977a,b). Following nitrogen-base analog addition, the newly synthesized phospholipids accumulated rapidly in cells at a rate of 90 and 120 pmol/µg DNA/h for monomethyl and dimethyl derivatives, respectively, and displaced the preexisting phospholipids (Yavin, 1977a). This process could be reversed by adding ethanolamine or choline precursors. The biochemical basis for these substitutions has been ascribed to the competition between the nitrogen-base precursors at the level of anabolic processes. By measuring the changes in pool sizes of the various *N*-methyl containing phospholipid derivatives, the apparent rates of synthesis, degradation, and reutilization of polar head groups in whole cells could be estimated. For example, the apparent doubling time for phosphatidylcholine synthesis in intact cells was 11 h (Yavin, 1977b). Unlike isotopic studies these initial velocity measurements did not involve the constraint of stable and labile pools since the lipid analog was totally absent in cells at the beginning of the experiment. These studies also suggested that internal recycling of the polar head group may be a vital process for maintaining cellular phospholipids under steady-state conditions.

The assessment of rates of assembly and degradation of membrane lipid components is a most fundamental question of membrane biogenesis. Using formaldehyde-induced plasma membrane vesicles that maintain the "right side out" lipid asymmetry, the apparent rates at which dimethylethanolamine phosphoglycerides were synthesized and subsequently translocated from the interior to the exterior cell surface was investigated (Yavin and Zutra, 1979). It was found that the appearance of new ^{32}P-labeled phospholipid analog molecules in whole cells was almost identical with that observed in isolated plasma membrane vesicles, suggesting a rapid transport of the phospholipid from its site of synthesis to the cell surface. This was accompanied by a progressive depletion of phosphatidylcholine, the major vesicle phospholipid. Treatment of plasma membrane–derived vesicles isolated during the course of phosphatidyldimethylethanolamine accumulation with phospholipase A2 revealed evidence for a two-component system that translocates the newly synthesized lipid from the inner to the outer sites of the membrane.

6.5   PHOSPHOLIPIDS AND NEURAL CELL GROWTH AND FUNCTION

Much of the information on the physicochemical properties and organization of lipid assemblies has been gained through studies with artificial membranes of well-defined chemical composition. Unlike artificial membranes, the phospholipids in biological membranes display marked intramolecular variability of their polar head groups and polar hydrocarbon residues. Therefore, extrapolation from model systems to native membranes can only be qualitative in nature. The intramolecular variety of the phospholipid species and the asymmetry that characterizes phospholipid organization in biological membranes (Rothman and Lenarz, 1977) poses some intriguing questions concerning the relationship between the structural variability of this large group of compounds and its role in membrane-associated cellular functions. In other words, to what extent does any particular interaction between membrane constituents and specific phospholipids determine the magnitude of a cellular response?

6.5.1 Stimulation of Phospholipid Turnover Following Ligand–Cell Interaction

A wealth of experimental evidence exists to indicate that membrane-associated cellular functions such as expression of enzymatic activities, receptor and antigenic recognition sites, transport processes, and electrical properties are intimately related to specific phospholipids. In particular, the phenomenon of increased phosphatidylinositol turnover in response to a variety of hormonal and drug stimuli via Ca^{2+}-requiring processes has received increasing attention (Michell, 1975). Stimulation of phospholipid labeling in short-term organ cultures of the pineal gland has been studied by Eichberg et al. (1973). Norepinephrine and other phenylethylamine derivatives as well as the adrenergic blocker propranolol enhanced the incorporation of $^{32}P_i$ into phosphatidylinositol and phosphatidylglycerol. Work from the same laboratory failed to demonstrate a similar effect using norepinephrine and carbamylcholine on mouse N1E neuroblastoma and C2 rat glioma cell lines (Eichberg et al., 1975). Since norepinephrine has been shown to stimulate cAMP production, the authors concluded that phosphatidylinositol-enhanced turnover and adenylate cyclase activation are independent events. Ligand-induced specific labeling of phosphatidylinositol (PI) and phosphatidic acid (PA) has been reported in several systems and was recently reviewed (Michell et al., 1981; Michell, 1975). The PI response is activated by receptor-mediated stimuli, in particular those involved in cGMP production and increased calcium uptake (Michell et al., 1981). One such agent is gonadotrophin-releasing hormone (GnRH) which, after 1 and 10 min incubation, induces a two- and threefold increase of PI and PA labeling in cultured pituitary cells, respectively (Naor et al., 1985). Incidently, these cells incorporate 45% of the total ^{32}P label into PI and less than 35% into phosphatidylcholine after incubation of short duration with the isotope. Since neither prostaglandins nor cyclic nucleotides are believed to be second messengers in the GnRH interaction with pituitary cells, it is suggested that the PI response and calcium and phospholipid turnover may act as alternative mechanisms for peptide action.

Stimulation of phosphatidylethanolamine transmethylation following ligand–cell surface interaction is another aspect of phospholipid involvement in signal transduction (Hirata and Axelrod, 1980). Addition of adrenergic receptor agonists such as isoprenaline, epinephrine, and norepinephrine as well as benzodiazepine significantly enhanced ^3H{methyl}methionine methylation of phosphatidylcholine in C6 rat astrocytoma cells (Strittmater et al., 1979). Whether transmethylation is an essential step for signal transduction or is merely a result of physiologi-

cally nonrelevant perturbation of the membrane lipids still awaits an une-
quivocal demonstration. This exciting area of research concerning the
role of phospholipids in mediating information through the bilayer will
certainly expand in the future as more neural receptors are isolated and
characterized.

6.5.2   Effects of Fatty Acids and Alteration of Phospholipid Composition on Neural Cell Phenotype

Mammalian cells are able, in principle, to control and modulate via the
cellular metabolic machinery the composition and distribution of phospholipids. This has prompted many investigations aimed at perturbing the
regular pattern of cellular phospholipids for detection of subtle changes
in cellular activities. Such alterations of phospholipid composition can be
easily accomplished in culture by supplementing the medium with the
appropriate precursor, that is, fatty acids (Wisnieski et al., 1973; Horwitz
et al., 1974) or nitrogen containing bases (Ferguson et al., 1975; Schroeder
et al., 1976). Unlike most isotope studies in which incorporation of labeled
precursors is carried out for relatively short time periods (i.e., minutes
or hours), the modification of the phospholipid profile requires a longer
duration, usually several days. Modification of acyl chain groups and
altered cellular activities in cultured cells (of nonneural origin) has been
recently reviewed (Spector et al., 1981). Evidently, neural cell lines have
been used only to a limited extent for such studies. Lack of polyunsaturated fatty acids in neuroblastoma cells, in contrast to the large quantities found in the nervous system, is one such example that should generate interest as to whether such a deficiency in any way affects the
phenotypic expression of the cells. Studies in this direction are already
underway. The effect of fatty acid supplements on high-affinity transport
of L-glutamate and taurine in M1 neuroblastoma cells has been investigated (Balcar et al., 1980).. Addition of linoleic or linolenic acid at concentrations of 30–40 μM under conditions in which the higher homologs,
docosapolyenoic acids, are formed resulted in a fourfold increase in the
apparent V_{max} for L-glutamate transport but not for taurine transport. The
K_m value for L-glutamate was also significantly altered. Using a similar
approach, alterations in the V_{max} and K_m of the ectoenzymes 5'-nucleo-
tidase and Mg^{2+}-ATPase in M1 cells following linoleic, linolenic, or docosahexaenoic acid addition have been reported (Robert et al., 1980).
Supplements of the latter fatty acid caused changes in the apparent V_{max}
and K_m for Mg^{2+}-ATPase and resulted in a nearly 30% reduction of enzymatic activity. Neither of these studies provided direct evidence for a
particular phospholipid that may be involved in these modulations. Ho-

negger and Matthieu (1980) have shown that addition of linoleic acid to reaggregating fetal rat brain cells grown in chemical-defined medium resulted in an increase of myelin-related enzymes. In accord with the general concepts discussed above, these alterations could either affect the composition of neighboring phospholipids surrounding the protein or cause a macroscopic change in membrane fluidity, which in turn could indirectly influence membrane protein disposition (Shinitzky and Henkart, 1979).

Recently Saum et al. (1981) and Williams and McGee (1982) have documented some identifiable functional alterations of neural cell lines following phospholipid fatty acid substitutions. Unsaturated fatty acids added to NG108-C15 hybrid cells grown in the regular serum-supplemented medium caused marked changes in the profile of cellular polyunsaturated fatty acids (McGee, 1981). A marked increase of approximately 60% in the amount of phosphatidylethanolamine present was also observed, thus suggesting, as has already been pointed out (Yavin and Robert, 1979), a possible metabolic relationship between the degree of unsaturation and the polar head group composition. Apart from these metabolic alterations, the effects of arachidonic acid supplements on the electrical excitability of these hybrid cells was investigated (Saum et al., 1981). While the resting membrane potential and its resistance did not seem to be affected, a 40% decrease in the maximum rate of rise of action potential (dv/dt) was detected. It is not yet clearly established whether these changes relate to a macroscopic fluidization of the membrane due to the fatty acid substitution or to subtle changes in some specific phospholipid species associated with the activity of the Na^+ channel. This effect is remarkable in the sense that it provides diverse probes for analyzing structure–function relationships at the physiological level. Of similar interest is the depolarization-induced neurotransmitter release phenomenon studied in PC12 rat pheochromocytoma cells after fatty acid substitutions (Williams and McGee, 1982). Carbamylcholine-stimulated or veratridine-activated Na^+ channel–mediated exocytosis was diminished in PC12 cells enriched with unsaturated fatty acids. In contrast, none of the fatty acid supplements had any effect on the K^+-stimulated exocytic release of norepinephrine. This suggested to these authors that the K^+-dependent Ca^{2+} channel depolarization and the subsequent Ca^{2+}-dependent exocytosis process were unaffected by the fatty acid changes. However, the extent to which these bulk phospholipid alterations have a direct impact on the nicotinic receptor complex or the Na^+ channel component remains to be established. Short-term exposure of Neuro 2A neuroblastoma cells to oleic and linoleic acid, but not stearic acid, under conditions that presumably do not lead to extensive phospholipid modification, caused a significant membrane potential depolarization (from

−51 to −36 mV) followed by a slow repolarization (Boonstra et al., 1982). The effects of unsaturated fatty acids on cellular cation permeability suggested by these experiments requires further rigorous testing to rule out transient perturbations related to transport of fatty acids through the plasma membrane.

Marked changes in the morphological appearance of neuroblastoma cells in serum-deprived growth media have been noted; the rapid extension of slender processes was one of the first characteristic properties that marks morphological differentiation of neuroblastoma cells (Seeds et al., 1970). This observation has been extended by Monard et al. (1977) who showed that approximately 60% of NB2A neuroblastoma cells extend neurites when grown in a delipidated serum-containing medium. Addition of oleic acid and to a lesser extent linolenic acid complexed with albumin appeared to prevent this spontaneous process, suggesting the involvement of lipid or lypophilic substances in suppressing the expression of a neuronal property. Thus, the studies of Boonstra et al. (1982) and Monard et al. (1977) may provide the basis for investigating the possibility that membrane depolarization and morphological differentiation are two mutually related phenotypic events both triggered by fatty acids.

Concommitant addition of eicosapentanoic acid and dimethylaminoethanol base supplements had a marked effect on growth parameters of N1E115 neuroblastoma cells (Yavin and Robert, 1979). After 72 h in serum-free medium and in the presence of these supplements, cell doubling time was markedly reduced and extension of many processes was observed. Polar head group substitution of phospholipids by N-methyl ethanolamine bases caused a marked decrease in the adhesiveness of M1 neuroblastoma cells to the surface of the dish (Robert et al., 1978). On the other hand, cell–cell adhesion in B103 neural cells was not affected by changes in fatty acid composition induced by addition of elaidic (18:1-*trans*) or oleic (18:1-*cis*) fatty acids (Moya et al., 1979). It would be interesting to investigate the influence of substituted polyunsaturated fatty acids under these conditions.

Lipid-induced morphological differentiation accompanied by changes in the content of microtubules and microfilaments in NG41A3 neuroblastoma cells treated with phosphatidylcholine/phosphatidylserine-containing liposomes has been demonstrated (Chen et al., 1976). Whether the effect of the phospholipid vesicles is due to adsorption or fusion with the plasma membrane or to internalization is still unclear; the studies point out, however, that a close relationship exists between lipid constituents and cytoskeletal elements. More recently Sandra et al. (1981), using a variety of phospholipid vesicles, also demonstrated a rapid stimulation of neuritic outgrowth in N3P2 neuroblastoma cells. Oleic acid and palmitic acid, 10 μg/ml each, added in the absence of serum, were also neurite outgrowth promoters. The latter finding is somewhat in contrast to the inhibitory activity of fatty acids described by Monard et al. (1977), although the experimental conditions and the cell lines were rather different. This discrepancy emphasizes the need for more direct evidence to correlate these lipid effects to morphological differentiation through alterations in membrane properties (i.e., fluidity and permeability), to changes in lipid metabolism, or to the restructuring of the cytoskeletal elements.

6.6   SUMMARY

Tissue culture of the nervous system has now become an indispensable *in vitro* tool for investigating a wide variety of cellular and molecular events that constitute the phenotypic behavior of the neural cell surface. In spite of some drawbacks and reservations, which have been amply discussed in the preceeding sections, neural cells isolated and cultured *in vitro* constitute a valid model for studying the molecular basis of homotypic and heterotypic cell–cell interactions. The detailed molecular aspects of these interactions, which ultimately lead to the functional assembly of the nervous system, are far from being clear.

The library of neuronal, glial, and hybrid cell lines presently available has contributed much information in delineating a number of genetically controlled, biochemical, and electrophysiological properties of nerve cells. Similarly primary mixed neuronal/glial or enriched neuronal or glial cultures have added a great deal to our understanding of the concepts and basic requirements for the formation of myelin and synaptic contacts.

Studies on phospholipids in neural tissue in culture have expanded remarkably since they were last reviewed in the mid-seventies (Mandel et al., 1976; Ansell, 1973), largely due to the development of better and more reproducible methods for cell culture as well as because of improved semicroanalytical techniques. Although the principal metabolic pathways of phospholipid biosynthesis have been discerned, the dynamic aspects of their metabolic regulation in the living cell still remain obscure. One of the most puzzling aspects of this metabolic regulation is the rapid modulation of lipid constituents in response to a variety of physiological stimuli. The generation of free arachidonic acid from phospholipids such as PI to provide precursors for prostaglandins, prostacyclin, thromboxane, and leukotrienes takes place as a consequence of cell surface receptors stimulation. It is hoped that by using the previously discussed tissue culture approaches, experiments can be designed to resolve the sequelae of these metabolic events.

The effects of phospholipid turnover on the magnitude or effectiveness of physiological processes such as neuroreceptor expression, active transport, electrical insulation, and excitability or synaptic vesicle fusion are also not yet understood. Nerve cell cultures offer the possibility of studying the implications of these specific surface phenomena on phospholipid regulation. Some aspects of this regulation, such as the intramolecular arrangement of phospholipids with respect to degree of unsaturation, acyl and alkenyl ether bonds, and polar head group content, have been discussed. The profound morphological and functional changes induced by phospholipids or free fatty acid supplements is yet another feature of the potential exploitation of a well-defined and easily altered environment such as that achieved from studies using serum-free media. Systematic manipulation of the chemical composition and the physical environment of the nerve cells should also provide clues toward understanding the aforementioned physiological functions such as receptor expression and ion channel activity. Neural cell cultures that grow in defined medium also offer the opportunity to study the direct role that lipids may have as signal transducers.

In spite of the optimism stated in the preceeding paragraphs, it should be stressed that the valuable information obtained from culture systems represents the reductionist view; the artificial environment and relative simplicity must be reinforced with data obtained from *in vivo* studies. Thus, any pertinent question that can be studied *in vitro* in defined systems should remain within the framework of a physiologically relevant phenomenon.

ACKNOWLEDGMENTS

I wish to express my appreciation to Dr. S. Rybak for her excellent editorial work and invaluable comments, to Dr. J. Robert for library help and comments, and to Drs. Debuch, McGee, and Spector for preprints and reprints.

REFERENCES

Ansell, G.B., in G.B. Ansell, J.N. Hawthorne, and R.M.C. Dawson, Eds., *Form and Function of Phospholipids*, Elsevier, Amsterdam, 1973, pp. 377–422.

Balcar, V.J., Borg, J., Robert, J., and Mandel, P., *J. Neurochem., 34,* 1678–1681 (1980).

Barnes, D., and Sato, G., *Nature, 281,* 388–389 (1979).

Barnes, D., and Sato, G., *Cell, 22,* 649–655 (1980).

Benda, P., Lightbody, J., Sato, G., Levine, L., and Sweet, W., *Science, 161*, 370–371 (1968).

Berg, G., and Schachner, M., *Neurosci. Lett., 28*, 75–80 (1982).

Bergeron, J.J.M., Warmsley, A.M.H., and Pasternak, C.A., *Biochem. J., 419*, 489–492 (1970).

Bhat, N.R., Sarlieve, L.L., Subba Rao, G., and Pieringer, R.A., *J. Biol. Chem., 254*, 9342–9344 (1979).

Binaglia, L., Goracci, G., Porcellati, G., Roberti, R., and Woelk, H., *J. Neurochem., 21*, 1067–1082 (1973).

Binaglia, L., Karageosian, K., and Stoffel, W., in G. Porcellati, L. Amaducci, and C. Galli, Eds., *Advances in Experimental Medicine and Biology*, Vol. 72, Plenum Press, New York, 1976, pp. 131–137.

Boonstra, J., Nelemans, S.Ad., Bierman, A., van Zoelen, E.J.J., van der Saag, P.T., and deLaat, S.W., *Biochim. Biophys. Acta, 692*, 321–329 (1982).

Bornstein, M.B., *NCI Monograph, 11*, 197–214 (1963).

Bornstein, M.B., and Appel, S.H., *J. Neuropathol. Exp. Neurol., 20*, 141–157 (1961).

Bornstein, M.B., and Model, P.G., *Brain Res., 37*, 287–293 (1972).

Bottenstein, J.E., and Sato, G., *Proc. Natl. Acad. Sci. USA, 76*, 514–517 (1979).

Bottenstein, J.E., Skaper, S.D., Varon, S.S., and Sato, G.H., *Exp. Cell Res., 125*, 183–190 (1980).

Bourre, J.M., Faivre, A., Dumont, O., Nouvelot, A., Loudes, C., Puymirat, J., and Tixier-Vidal, A., *J. Neurochem., 41*, 1234–1242 (1983).

Bourre, J.M., Morand, O., Dumont, O., Boutry, J.M., and Hauw, J.J., *J. Neurochem., 37*, 272–275 (1981).

Breckenridge, W.C., Gombos, G., and Morgan, I.G., *Biochim. Biophys. Acta, 266*, 695–707 (1972).

Brooks, R.F., in A. C. Allison, Ed., *Structure and Function of Plasma Proteins*, Plenum Press, New York, 1975, pp. 1–112.

Charalampous, F.C., *Biochim. Biophys. Acta, 556*, 38–51 (1979).

Chen, J.S., DelFa, A., Di Luzio, A., and Calissano, P., *Nature, 263*, 604–606 (1976).

Chida, N., and Shimizu, Y., *Tohoku J. Exp. Med., 111*, 41–49 (1973).

Clausen, J., in A. Lajhta, Ed., *Handbook of Neurochemistry*, Vol. 1, Plenum Press, New York, 1969, pp. 273–300.

Crain, S.M., in S. Federoff and L. Hertz, Eds., *Cell Tissue and Organ Culture in Neurobiology*, Academic Press, New York, 1978, pp. 147–190.

Crain, S.M., in R.K. Hunt, Ed., *Current Topics in Developmental Biology*, Vol. 16, Academic Press, New York, 1980, pp. 87–115.

Dainous, F., Freysz, L., Mozzi, R., Dreyfus, H., Louis, J.C., Porcellati, G., and Massarelli, R., *FEBS Lett., 146*, 221–223 (1982).

DeLaat, S.W., van der Saag, P.T., and Shinitzky, M., *Proc. Natl. Acad. Sci. USA, 74*, 4458–4461 (1977).

DeLong, G.R., and Sigman, R.L., *Develop. Biol., 22*, 584–600 (1970).

Diringer, H., and Friis, R.R., *Cancer Res., 37*, 2979–2984 (1977).

Diringer, H., and Koch, M.A., *Biochem. Biophys. Res. Commun., 51*, 967–971 (1973).

Diringer, H., and Koch, M.A., *Z. Physiol. Chem., 355*, 93–97 (1974).

Dowling, P.C., Kim, S.U., Murray, M.R., and Cook, S.D., *J. Immunol., 101,* 1101–1104 (1968).

Dvorak, D.J., Gipps, E., and Kidson, C., *Nature, 271,* 564–566 (1978).

Eichberg, J., Shein, H.M., and Hauser, G., *J. Neurochem., 24,* 67–70 (1975).

Eichberg, J., Shein, H.M., and Hauser, G., *J. Neurochem., 27,* 679–685 (1976).

Eichberg, J., Shein, H.M., Schwartz, M., and Hauser, G., *J. Biol. Chem. 248,* 3615–3622 (1973).

Evans, V.J., Bryant, J.C., Kerr, H.A., and Schilling, E.L., *Exp. Cell Res., 36,* 439–474 (1964).

Federoff, S., and Hertz, L., Eds., *Cell, Tissue and Organ Culture in Neurobiology,* Academic Press, New York, 1977, p. 693.

Ferguson, K.A., Glaser, M., Bayer, W.H., and Vagelos, P.R., *Biochemistry, 14,* 146–151 (1975).

Giesing, M., and Zilliken, F., *Neurochem. Res., 5,* 257–270 (1980).

Gerschenson, L.E., Harary, I., and Mead, J.F., *Biochim. Biophys. Acta, 131,* 50–58 (1967).

Geyer, R.P., Bennett, A., and Rohr, A., *J. Lipid Res., 3,* 80–83 (1962).

Giacobini, E., in E. Giacobini, A. Vernadakis, and Shahar, A. Eds., *Tissue Culture in Neurobiology,* Raven Press, New York, 1980, pp. 187–204.

Giacobini, E., Vernadakis, A., and Shahar, A., Eds., *Tissue Culture in Neurobiology,* Raven Press, New York, 1980, p. 512.

Godfrey, E.W., Nelson, P.G., Schrier, B.K., Breuer, A.C., and Ransom, B.R., *Brain Res., 90,* 1–21 (1975).

Goracci, G., Blomstrand, Ch., Arienti, G., Hamberger, A., and Porcellati, G., *J. Neurochem. 20,* 1167–1180 (1973).

Green, L.A., and Tischler, A.S., *Proc. Natl. Acad. Sci. USA, 73,* 2424–2428 (1976).

Hamprecht, B., *Int. Rev. Cytol., 49,* 99–170 (1977).

Harrison, R.G., *Proc. Soc. Exp. Med. Biol., 4,* 140–143 (1907).

Hayashi, I., and Sato, G.H., *Nature (London), 259,* 132–134 (1976).

Herschman, H.R., in D.J. Schneider, R.H. Angeletti, R.A. Bradshaw, A. Grasso, and B.W. Moore, Eds., *Proteins of the Nervous System,* Raven Press, New York, 1973, pp. 95–115.

Hirata, F., and Axelrod, J., *Science, 209,* 1082–1090 (1980).

Hoffmann, R., Erzberger, P., Frank, W., and Ristow, H.J., *Biochim. Biophys. Acta, 618,* 282–292 (1980).

Holley, R.W., Baldwin, J.H., and Kiernan, J.A., *Proc. Natl. Acad. Sci. USA, 71,* 3976–3978 (1974).

Honegger, P., and Mattieu, J.M., in N. Baumann, Ed., *Neurological Mutations Affecting Myelination* INSERM Symp. *14* Elsevier North Holland, Amsterdam, 1980, pp. 481–488.

Honegger, P., Lenoir, D., and Favrod, P., *Nature, 282,* 305–307 (1979).

Horwitz, A.F., Hatten, M.E., and Burger, M.M., *Proc. Natl. Acad. Sci. USA, 71,* 3115–3119 (1974).

Howard, B.V., and Howard, W.J., *Adv. Lipid Res., 12,* 51–95 (1974).

Hyman, B.T., and Spector, A.A., *J. Neurochem., 37,* 60–69 (1981).

Kessler, P.D., and Marchbanks, R.M., *Nature, 279,* 542–544 (1979).

Kim, S.U., *Exp. Cell Res., 73,* 528–530 (1972).

Kim, S.U., and Pleasure, D., *Brain Res., 157,* 206–211 (1978).

Kimhi, Y., in P.G. Nelson and M. Lieberman, Eds., *Excitable Cells in Tissue Culture,* Plenum Press, New York, 1981, pp. 173–245.

Maeda, M., Tanaka, Y., and Akamatsu, Y., *Biochim. Biophys. Acta, 663,* 578–582. (1981).

Mains, R.E., and Patterson, P.H., *J. Cell Biol., 59,* 361–366 (1973).

Mandel, P., and Ciesielski-Treska, J., and Sensenbrenner, M., in W. Gispen, Ed., *Molecular and Functional Neurobiology,* Elsevier, Amsterdam, 1976, pp. 112–157.

Margolis, L.B., Dyathlovitskaya, E.V., and Bergelson, L.D., *Exp. Cell. Res. 111,* 454–457 (1978).

Massarelli, R., Wong, T.Y., Froissart, C., and Robert, J., in S. Tucek, Ed., *Progress in Brain Research,* Vol. 49, Elsevier, Amsterdam, 1979, pp. 89–96.

Matthieu, J.-M., Honegger, P., Favrod, P., Poduslo, J.F., Constantino-Ceccarini, E., and Krstic, R., in E. Giacobini, A. Vernadakis, and A. Shahar, Eds., *Tissue Culture in Neurobiology,* Raven Press, New York, 1980, p. 441–459.

McCarthy, K.D., and Partlow, L.M., *Brain Res., 114,* 391–414 (1976).

McGee, R., *Biochim. Biophys. Acta, 663,* 314–328 (1981).

Menkes, H., *J. Neurochem., 18,* 1433–1443 (1971).

Menkes, H., *Lipids, 7,* 135–141 (1972).

Messer, A., Mazurkiewicz, J.E., and Maskin, P., *Cell. and Mol. Neurobiol., 1,* 99–114 (1981).

Michell, R.H., *Biochim. Biophys. Acta, 415,* 81–157 (1975).

Michell, R.H., Kirk, C.J., Jones, L.M., Downes, C.P., and Creba, J.A., *Phil. Trans. Roy. Soc. Lond. B, 296,* 123–137 (1981).

Minna, J., Glazer, D., and Nirenberg, M., *Nature New Biol., 235,* 225–231 (1972).

Monard, D., Rentsch, M., Schurch-Rathgeb, Y., and Linsday, R.M., *Proc. Natl. Acad. Sci. USA, 74,* 3893–3897 (1977).

Montaudon, D., Louis, J.-C., and Robert, J., *Lipids, 16,* 293–297 (1981).

Moscona, A.A., and Wilmer, B.M., Ed., *Cells and Tissues in Culture,* Academic Press, New York, 1965, pp. 489–529.

Moya, F., Silbert, D.F., and Glaser, L., *Biochim. Biophys. Acta, 550,* 485–499 (1979).

Murray, M., and Kopech, G., *A Bibliography of the Research in Tissue Culture 1884–1950,* Academic Press, New York, 1953, p. 1741.

Murray, M.R., in A.A. Lajtha, Ed., *Handbook of Neurochemistry,* Vol. 5, *Metabolic Turnover in the Nervous System,* Part A, Plenum Press, New York, 1971, pp. 373–438.

Naor, Z., Molcho, J., Zakut, H., and Yavin, E. (Submitted for publication).

Nelson, P.G., and Lieberman, M., Eds., *Excitable Cells in Tissue Culture,* Plenum Press, New York, 1981, p. 422.

Nelson, P.G., Neale, E.A., and MacDonald, R.L., in P.G. Nelson and M. Lieberman, Eds., *Excitable Cells in Tissue Culture,* Plenum Press, New York, 1981.

Norton, W.T., and Poduslo, S.E., *J. Lipid Res., 12,* 84–90 (1971).

Patterson, P.H., in J. Taxi, Ed., *Ontogenesis and Functional Mechanisms of Peripheral Synapses,* Elsevier North Holland, Amsterdam, 1980, pp. 3–13.

Pfeifer, S.E., Betschart, B., Cook, J., Mancini, P., and Morris, R., in S. Federoff and L. Hertz, Eds., *Cell Tissue and Organ Culture in Neurobiology,* Academic Press, New York, 1978, pp. 287–346.

Pleasure, D., Hardy, M., Johnson, G., Lisak, R., and Silberberg, D., *J. Neurochem.*, *37*, 452–460 (1981).

Poduslo, S.E., and Norton, W.T., *J. Neurochem.*, *19*, 727–736 (1972).

Poduslo, S.E., Miller, J., and McKhann, G.M., *J. Biol. Chem.*, *253*, 1592–1597 (1978).

Porcellati, G., and Goracci, G., in R. Paoletti, G. Porcellati, and G. Jacini, Eds., *Lipids*, Vol. 1, Raven Press, New York, 1976, pp. 203–214.

Raff, M.C., Fields, K.L., Hakomori, S.-I., Mirski, R., Pruss, R.M., and Winter, J., *Brain Res.*, *174*, 273–308 (1979).

Raine, C.S., and Bornstein, M.B., *J. Neuropathol. Exp. Neurol.*, *29*, 177–191 (1970).

Raine, C.S., and Bornstein, M.B., *Lab. Invest.*, *40*, 423–432 (1979).

Richelson, E., in A.M. Goldberg and I. Hanin, Eds., *Biology of Cholinergic Function*, Raven Press, New York, 1976, pp. 451–483.

Robert, J., Mandel, P., and Rebel, G., *J. Neurochem.*, *26*, 771–777 (1976).

Robert, J., Montaudon, D., and Rebel, G., *Ann. Nutr. Alim.*, *34*, 423–436 (1980).

Robert, J., Rebel, G., and Mandel, P., *Biochimie*, *59*, 417–423 (1977).

Robert, J., Rebel, G., and Mandel, P., *J. Neurochem.*, *30*, 543–548 (1978a).

Robert, J., Rebel, G., Mandel, P., and Yavin, E., *Life Sci.*, *22*, 211–216 (1978b).

Rockwell, G.A., McClure, D., and Sato, G.H., *J. Cell Physiol.*, *103*, 323–331 (1980).

Rothman, J.E., and Lenarz, J., *Science*, *195*, 743–753 (1977).

Rouser, G., Kritchevsky, G., Yamamoto, A., and Baxter, C.F., in R. Paoletti and D. Kritchevsky, Eds., *Advances in Lipid Research*, Vol. 10, Academic Press, New York, 1972, pp. 261–360.

Sandra, A., Paltzer, W.B., and Thomas, M.J., *Expt. Cell Res.*, *132*, 473–477 (1981).

Sarlieve, L.L., Fabre, M., Rebel, G., Susz, J., Vincendon, G., and Matthieu, J.M., in H. Peeters, Ed. *Protides of the Biological Fluids* Vol., 30 Pergamon Press, Oxford, 1983, pp. 107–110.

Sato, G.H., Ed., *Tissue Culture of the Nervous System*, Plenum Press, New York, 1973.

Saum, W.R., McGee, R., and Love, G., *Cell. and Mol. Neurobiol.*, *1*, 319–324 (1981).

Schoffeniels, E., Franck, G., Hertz, L., and Tower, D.B., Eds., *Dynamic Properties of Glial Cells*, Pergamon Press, Oxford, 1978, p. 466.

Schroeder, F., Perlmutter, J.F., Glaser, M., and Vagelos, P.R., *J. Biol. Chem.*, *251*, 5015–5026 (1976).

Schubert, D., Heinemann, S., Carlisle, W., Tarikas, H., Kimes, B., Patrick, J., Streinbach, J.H., Culp, W., and Brandt, B.L., *Nature (London)*, 249, 224–229 (1974).

Seeds, N.W., in G.H. Sato, Ed., *Tissue Culture of the Nervous System*, Plenum Press, New York, 1973, pp. 35–53.

Seeds, N.W., Gilman, A.G., Amano, T., and Nirenberg, M., *Proc. Natl. Acad. Sci. USA*, *66*, 160–168 (1970).

Shahar, A., Grunfeld, Y., Spiegelstein, M.Y., and Monzain, R., *Brain Res.*, *88*, 44–51 (1975).

Shinitzky, M., and Henkart, P., *Int. Rev. Cytol.*, *60*, 121–147 (1979).

Silberberg, D.H., *Arch. Neurol.*, *17*, 524–529 (1967).

Silberberg, D.H., *J. Neurochem.*, *16*, 1141–1146 (1969).

Snyder, E.Y., and Kim, S.U., *Brain Res.*, *196*, 565–571 (1980).

Spector, A.A., Mathur, S.N., Kaduce, T.L., and Hyman, B.T., in *Progress in Lipid Research*, Vol. 19, Pergamon Press, Oxford, 1981, pp. 155–186.

Strittmater, W.J., Hirata, F., Axelrod, J., Mallorga, P., Tallman, J.F., and Henneberry, R.C., *Nature*, 282, 857–860 (1979).

Svennerholm, L., *J. Lipid Res.*, 9, 570–579 (1968).

Vance, D.E., and de Kruijff, B., *Nature*, 288, 277–278 (1980).

Varon, S., and Manthorpe, M., *Advances in Cellular Neurobiology*, Vol. 1, Academic Press, New York, 1980, pp. 405–442.

Varon, S., and Raiborn, C., *Brain Res.*, 12, 180–199 (1969).

Volpe, J.J., and Marasa, J.C., *J. Neurochem.*, 25, 333–340 (1975).

Waymouth, C., *Int. Rev. Cytol.*, 3, 1–68 (1954).

Williams, T.P., and McGee, R., *J. Biol. Chem.*, 257, 3491–3500 (1982).

Wisneiski, B.J., Williams, R.E., and Fox, C.F., *Proc. Natl. Acad. Sci.*, USA, 70, 3669–3673 (1973).

Witter, B., and Debuch, H., *J. Neurochem.*, 38, 1029–1037 (1982).

Wood, R., and Falch, J., *Lipids*, 8, 702–709 (1973).

Yavin, E., in G. Porcellati, L. Amaducci, and C. Galli, Eds., *Advances in Experimental Medicine and Biology*, Vol. 72, Plenum Press, New York, 1976a, pp. 115–122.

Yavin, E., *J. Biol. Chem.*, 251, 1392–1397 (1976b).

Yavin, E., *Biochim. Biophys. Acta*, 489, 278–289 (1977a).

Yavin, E., *Biochim. Biophys. Acta*, 489, 290–297 (1977b).

Yavin, E., *J. Neurochem.*, 34, 178–183 (1980).

Yavin, E., *J. Neurochem.*, in press (1985).

Yavin, E., and Kanfer, J.N., *J. Biol. Chem.*, 250, 2885–2890 (1975a).

Yavin, E., and Kanfer, J.N., *J. Biol. Chem.*, 250, 2891–2895 (1975b).

Yavin, E., and Menkes, J.H., *J. Neurochem.*, 21, 901–912 (1973).

Yavin, E., and Menkes, J.H., *J. Lipid Res.*, 15, 152–157 (1974a).

Yavin, E., and Menkes, H., *Lipids*, 9, 248–253 (1974b).

Yavin, E., and Robert, J., *Trans. Biochem. Soc.*, 7, 341–345 (1979).

Yavin, E., and Yavin, Z., *J. Cell Biol.*, 62, 540–546 (1974).

Yavin, E., and Yavin, Z., in E. Giacobini, A. Vernadakis, and A. Shahar, Eds., *Tissue Culture in Neurobiology*, Raven Press, New York, 1980, pp. 277–289.

Yavin, E., and Ziegler, B.P., *J. Biol. Chem.*, 252, 260–267 (1977).

Yavin, E., and Zutra, A., *Anal. Biochem.*, 80, 430–437 (1977).

Yavin, E., and Zutra, A., *Biochim. Biophys. Acta*, 553, 424–437 (1979).

Yavin, E., Yavin, Z., and Menkes, J.H., *J. Neurochem.*, 24, 71–78 (1975a).

Yavin, E., Yavin, Z., and Menkes, J.H., *Neurobiology*, 5, 214–220 (1975b).

Yavin, Z., and Yavin, E., *Exp. Brain Res.*, 29, 137–147 (1977).

Yavin, Z., and Yavin, E., *Develop. Biol.*, 75, 454–459 (1980).

Yavin, Z., Yavin, E., and Kohn, D., *J. Neurosci. Res.*, 7, 267–278 (1982).

Zurgil, N., and Zisapel, N., *Life Sci.*, 29, 2265–2271 (1981).

THE BIOCHEMICAL BASIS AND FUNCTIONAL SIGNIFICANCE OF ENHANCED PHOSPHATIDATE AND PHOSPHOINOSITIDE TURNOVER

STEPHEN K. FISHER†
BERNARD W. AGRANOFF

Neuroscience Laboratory and Department of Biological Chemistry
The University of Michigan
Ann Arbor, Michigan

† Present address: Department of CNS Research, Medical Research Division of American Cyanamid Co., Lederle Laboratories, Pearl River, NY 10965.

CONTENTS

INTRODUCTION   243

7.1.1   Historical Review, 243

7.1.2   The Phosphatidate–Phosphatidylinositol Cycle, 244

7.1.3   Subcellular Localization of Enzymes Involved in the
        Metabolic Interconversion of Phosphatidate and the
        Phosphoinositides, 247

7.1.4   Neural Preparations Evincing Enhanced Phospholipid
        Turnover, 253

7.2   PHARMACOLOGY OF RECEPTORS THAT ELICIT
      ENHANCED PHOSPHOLIPID TURNOVER   253

7.2.1   Cholinergic Receptors, 258

7.2.2   Adrenergic Receptors, 260

7.2.3   Histaminergic Receptors, 261

7.2.4   Dopaminergic Receptors, 261

7.2.5   Serotonergic Receptors, 262

7.2.6   Nerve Growth Factor, 262

7.2.7   Amino Acid Neurotransmitters, 262

7.2.8   Peptidergic Receptors, 263

7.3   BIOCHEMICAL CHARACTERISTICS AND MECHANISMS   264

7.3.1   General Properties, 264

7.3.2   Stimulated Phospholipid Labeling in Nerve Tissue: A
        Closed Cycle, 264

7.3.3   Is the Hydrolysis of Phosphatidylinositol or of a
        Polyphosphoinositide the Key Initial Response?, 266

7.3.4   Evaluation of Phospholipid Turnover in Brain: Labeling
        and Prelabeling Approaches, 269

7.4   CELLULAR AND SUBCELLULAR LOCALIZATION OF
      ENHANCED PHOSPHOLIPID TURNOVER   271

7.4.1   Neuronal, Glial, or Both?, 271

7.4.2   Subcellular Locus, 272

7.4.3   Is the Site of Enhanced Phospholipid Turnover Pre- or
        Postsynaptic?, 274

7.5   FUNCTIONAL SIGNIFICANCE OF ENHANCED
      PHOSPHOLIPID TURNOVER   277

7.5.1   Does Stimulated Turnover Regulate a Calcium Gate or
Is It the Result of Calcium Mobilization—or
Neither?, 278

7.5.2   Production of Phosphatidate: An Endogenous Calcium
Ionophore?, 281

7.5.3   Generation of Inositol Trisphosphate: An Intracellular
Second Messenger?, 282

7.5.4   Does Inositol Phospholipid Hydrolysis Modulate the
Activities of Enzymes in the Plasma Membrane?, 282

7.5.5   Production of Diacylglycerol: A Link between Lipid
and Protein Phosphorylation?, 283

7.5.6   Does Polyphosphoinositide Turnover Mediate Ion
Fluxes at the Plasma Membrane?, 284

7.5.7   Is Enhanced Phospholipid Labeling Related to
Arachidonate Metabolism?, 285

7.6   SUMMARY   287

REFERENCES   288

7.1   INTRODUCTION

7.1.1   Historical Review

A dynamic role for phospholipids in receptor-mediated cell responses was first proposed some 30 years ago (Hokin and Hokin, 1953, 1955). These early experiments demonstrated that radioactive orthophosphate ($^{32}P_i$) was rapidly incorporated into specific phospholipids of brain and pancreas slices and that the addition of acetylcholine (Ach) resulted in a selective increase in the labeling of an inositol-containing phospholipid, phosphatidylinositol (PI), and of another phospholipid, subsequently identified as phosphatidate (PA; Hokin and Hokin, 1958a). The labeling of other quantitatively major phospholipids such as phosphatidylcholine, phosphatidylserine, phosphatidylethanolamine and sphingomeylin was largely or entirely unaffected. This selective action of Ach on PA and PI labeling suggested a significant biological role for the effect and provided much of the impetus for subsequent investigations. The stimulation of labeling of PI and/or PA from $^{32}P_i$ under the action of a number of agents that stimulate cell surface receptors has been variably referred to as enhanced or stimulated, labeling or turnover, of PI and/or PA or, more generally, as "the phospholipid-labeling effect." It is generally expressed as a simple ratio calculated from the radioactivity obtained in PA or PI following incubation of a tissue preparation in the presence of an agonist divided by that obtained in its absence. The Hokins observed that the stimulatory effect of Ach on PA and PI labeling on the pancreas could be prevented by inclusion of the cholinergic muscarinic antagonist, atropine (Hokin and Hokin, 1953), but not by d-tubocurarine, a cholinergic nicotinic antagonist. While the amount of Ach added to produce stimulated labeling was greater than that required for the demonstration of secretion, the pharmacological studies pointed strongly to a specific muscarinic receptor interaction of both processes. Stimulated labeling could not be detected after detergent, hypoosmotic shock or freeze–thaw pretreatment (L. E. Hokin and M. R. Hokin, 1959). Thus, it was also apparent that demonstration of the receptor-mediated effect on phospholipid labeling required maintenance of the vectorial relationship of the cell membrane with its intracellular and extracellular environment.

In this review emphasis has been placed on those receptor–ligand interactions that result in a selective stimulation of PA and PI turnover in the absence of a significant increase in *de novo* synthesis. This distinguishes the effects produced by neuroeffectors from those that occur on the application of certain drugs (e.g., cationic amphiphilic), which enhance *de novo* synthesis and labeling of most phospholipids. Enhanced phospholipid turnover may be considered a means for the transfer of external information to the cell interior following the activation of distinct classes of receptors (e.g., muscarinic cholinergic, α_1-adrenergic, H_1-histaminergic). It is not observed following activation of those receptors considered to act predominantly through an increased cAMP accumulation (e.g., β-adrenergic, H_2-histaminergic, and 5-HT, (ketanserin-insensitive); Berridge, 1981). The enhanced turnover of PI and PA presently under consideration is distinct from receptor-mediated changes in turnover of other phospholipids, for example, β-adrenergic receptors linked to phosphatidylethanolamine methylation. While an interrelationship between these two processes has been suggested (Dennis, 1982), the link has yet to be established.

7.1.2 The Phosphatidate–Phosphatidylinositol Cycle

As a result of the Hokins studies, PA was established as a minor but measurable cellular membrane component (Hokin and Hokin, 1958a). At that time it also became known that PI was synthesized via a CDP-diacylglycerol intermediate (Agranoff et al., 1958; Paulus and Kennedy, 1960) such that the glycerol phosphate bond of PA was preserved during biosynthesis, in contrast to phosphatidylethanolamine and phosphatidylcholine syntheses, in which cases the lipid phosphate is derived from CDP-ethanolamine and CDP-choline, respectively. It was not until some years later that the formation of CDP-diacylglycerol from PA and CTP was demonstrated (Petzold and Agranoff, 1965, 1967; Carter and Kennedy, 1966), completing the sequence: phosphatidate → CDP-diacylglycerol → phosphatidylinositol (see Fig. 7.1). While incorporation of radioactive glycerol into PA and PI can be measured, this labeling is not increased by receptor activation. The observed labeling effects are thus not attributable to a net increase of synthesis but rather to exchange labeling of the phosphate of preexisting lipid moieties. A clue to how this might be accomplished was provided by the discovery of two additional enzymes. The first is a widely prevalent phospholipase C, PI phosphodiesterase (Dawson, 1959), which cleaves PI to yield diacylglycerol and inositol monophosphate. Recent evidence suggests that this enzyme may be activated by PA, leading to the possibility of a regulatory mechanism (Irvine et al., 1979; Dawson et al., 1980; Hirasawa et al., 1981a). The second enzyme, diacylglycerol (diglyceride) kinase (M. R. Hokin and L. E. Hokin, 1959), phosphorylates preformed diacylglycerol to [^{32}P]PA. A cycle can then be envisioned (Durrell et al., 1969) in which ^{32}P$_i$ is introduced into PA and PI, utilizing 1, 3, 5, and 6 in Figure 7.1, and which consumes 1 mole each of ATP and CTP per mole of cycled diacylglycerol, as follows:

$$\text{Diacylglycerol} + \text{ATP} \rightarrow \text{PA} + \text{ADP}$$
$$\text{PA} + \text{CTP} \rightarrow \text{CDP-diacylglycerol} + \text{PP}_i$$
$$\text{CDP-diacylglycerol} + \text{inositol} \rightarrow \text{PI} + \text{CMP}$$
$$\text{PI} \rightarrow \text{diacylglycerol} + \text{inositol mono-phosphate}$$
$$\text{Inositol monophosphate} \rightarrow \text{inositol} + \text{P}_i$$

$$\text{Net:} \quad \text{ATP} \rightarrow \text{ADP} + \text{P}_i$$
$$\text{CTP} \rightarrow \text{CMP} + \text{PP}_i$$

CDP-diacylglycerol is presumably also labeled but is not detected, since it is ordinarily present in low steady-state amounts (see Section 7.3.1). Diacylglycerol can alternatively be furnished from other sources, for example, from the action of PA phosphatase on PA (see Fig. 7.1). The inositol-containing phospholipids (phosphoinositides) include in addition to PI two further phosphorylated forms termed collectively *polyphos-*

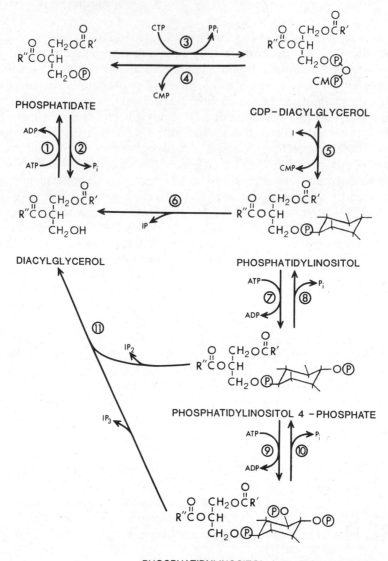

FIGURE 7.1 Enzymatic interconversions of lipids of phosphoinositide metabolism. Names of enzymes used (as well as Enzyme Commission numbers, where available) corresponding to the steps described are: (1) diacylglycerol kinase; (2) PA phosphatase (EC 3.1.3.4); (3) PA:CTP cytidylyltransferase (EC 2.7.7.41); (4) CDP-diacylglycerol pyrophosphatase (EC 3.6.1.26); (5) CDP-diacylglycerol:inositol phosphatidyltransferase (EC 2.7.8.11); (6) PI phosphodiesterase (EC 3.1.4.10); (7) PI kinase (EC 2.7.1.67); (8) PIP phosphatase; (9) PIP kinase (EC 2.7.1.68); (10) PIP$_2$ phosphatase (EC 3.1.3.36); (11) Polyphosphoinositide phosphodiesterase (EC 3.1.4.11). *Myo*-inositol (I) is shown in the chair form and has five equatorial and one axial hydroxyl, vicinal to the phosphodiester linkage (Agranoff, 1979). IP, IP$_2$, and IP$_3$ represent inositol phosphates.

phoinositides: phosphatidylinositol 4-phosphate (PIP) and phosphatidyl-inositol 4,5-bisphosphate (PIP$_2$). The majority of published studies on stimulated phospholipid labeling employ techniques that do not extract the polyphosphoinositides, and if extracted, the thin-layer chromatography (TLC) methods employed usually do not lead to their migration from the origin so that they have often been ignored or mistaken for phosphoprotein or low-molecular-weight contaminants.

The polyphosphoinositides are derived from PI by sequential kinases utilizing ATP (Colodzin and Kennedy, 1965; Kai et al., 1966, 1968). Phosphatases that degrade PIP$_2$ to PIP and thence to PI are also present, and the kinases and phosphatases together constitute an exchange system whereby the phosphomonoester functions of the polyphosphoinositides become rapidly labeled from [^{32}P]ATP. The labeling of the polyphosphoinositides is not stimulated by Ach. Polyphosphoinositides may nevertheless play a role in the origin of the stimulated labeling, since they can be degraded by phosphodiesteratic action to inositol phosphates and diacylglycerol (Keough and Thompson, 1970, 1972; Keough et al., 1972). The significance of polyphosphoinositides has become increasingly recognized as the primary step in initiation of stimulated labeling as is detailed below.

7.1.3 Subcellular Localization of Enzymes Involved in the Metabolic Interconversion of Phosphatidate and the Phosphoinositides

Although when applied to the brain or other neural preparations (e.g., superior cervical ganglion), subcellular fractionation techniques often yield incomplete organelle separation, they suffice to demonstrate that the enzymes of the proposed PA–PI cycle are not all located at the same intracellular locus. These techniques have determined that the synaptic plasma membrane is the primary location for PA phosphatase (Cotman et al., 1971). At least part of cellular diacylglycerol kinase activity is also located in the plasma membrane. Lapetina and Hawthorne (1971) found that 60–70% of the recovered brain enzyme activity was located in particulate fractions and that the enrichment of diacylglycerol kinase in subcellular fractions paralleled that of both 5'-nucleotidase and acetylcholinesterase. A plasma membrane locus for the kinase is in accord with the rapid appearance of labeled PA usually seen following receptor activation in brain as well as in nonneural tissues. The further metabolism of PA occurs in either the mitochondria or endoplasmic reticulum. Petzold and Agranoff (1965, 1967) found that most of the PA-cytidylyltransferase activity in embryonic chick brain was located in a 12,000g pellet while very little activity could be measured in the microsomal fraction. Although this subcellular location did not correspond to the endoplasmic reticulum localization in liver found by Carter and Kennedy (1966), a subsequent fractionation study by Cotman et al. (1971) in rat brain employing both morphological and marker enzyme techniques to assess the purity of subcellular fractions showed that brain PA-cytidylyltransferase was indeed almost exclusively confined to the purified mitochondrial fractions, with little or no activity of this enzyme in the microsomal fraction. It thus appears possible that the enzyme has different subcellular locations in brain and liver. CDP-diacylglycerol is converted to PI via CDP-diacylglycerol: inositol phosphatidyltransferase, located primarily in the endoplasmic reticulum (Benjamins and Agranoff, 1969; Harwood and Hawthorne, 1969; Cotman et al., 1971). This reaction has been demonstrated to be reversible, so that CDP-diacylglycerol may be formed from CMP and PI (Petzold and Agranoff, 1967). CDP-diacylglycerol involved in the synthesis of phosphatidylglycerols is probably localized within a mitochondrial pool, since these lipids are largely confined to mitochondrial membranes. CDP-diacylglycerol may be cleaved via a hydrolase originally found in bacteria (Raetz et al., 1972, 1976) and which has now been identified and partially purified from mammalian brain (Rittenhouse et al., 1981). This enzyme was judged to be lysosomal from its behavior on subcellular fractionation, its cofractionation with lysosomal marker enzymes, and its acidic pH optimum. Completion of the PA-PI cycle is achieved through PI phosphodiesterase (Dawson, 1959), a Ca^{2+}-dependent phospholipase C (Thompson, 1967; Hirasawa et al., 1981b). The presence of high levels of PI phosphodiesterase activity in membrane fractions following osmotic shock suggests that some of the enzyme is membrane bound (Friedel et al., 1969). Moreover, the soluble and particulate forms of the phosphodiesterase have different pH optima and detergent requirements (Michell and Lapetina, 1972; Lapetina and Michell, 1973). However, in an extensive series of experiments Irvine and Dawson (1978) demonstrated that the ratio of soluble-to-bound phosphodiesterase varied with assay conditions employed, including the substrate concentration and form (i.e., membrane-bound or free PI), as well as detergent and Ca^{2+} concentrations. Further, when synaptic plasma membranes were assayed for PI-phosphodiesterase activity in the presence of varying amounts of synaptosomal supernatant, a plot of PI-phosphodiesterase versus lactate dehydrogenase (a soluble fraction marker enzyme) passed through the origin. This provides compelling evidence that most, if not all, of the Ca^{2+}-dependent PI-phosphodiesterase activity in brain is located in the cytoplasmic fraction. There is in addition a Ca^{2+}-independent PI-phosphodiesterase identified in liver lysosomes (Irvine et al., 1977, 1978). The Ca^{2+}-independent enzyme is reportedly detectable in brain lysosomal fractions as well and can be dissociated from the Ca^{2+}-dependent enzyme on a Sephadex G150 column (Irvine et al., 1978). Although the absolute amounts of the two phospholipases differ by more than 100-fold, when the considerably larger cytosolic volume of a cell is compared to that occupied by the lysosomes, the actual activities of the Ca^{2+}-dependent and -independent enzymes in their respective environments *in vivo* may be similar (Irvine et al., 1979). More recently it has been claimed that the lyosomal activity in liver is not PI specific (Matsuzawa and Hostetler, 1980).

PI kinase, which converts PI to PIP, is mainly membrane bound in mammalian brain (Colodzin and Kennedy, 1965; Kai et al., 1966, 1968; Harwood and Hawthorne, 1969). On subcellular fractionation the enzyme cofractionates with 5'-nucleotidase and Na^+, K^+-ATPase, a result that suggests a plasma membrane location. The enzyme has recently been purified from rat brain membranes by Bostwick and Eichberg (1981). In contrast, over 75% of recovered PIP kinase activity is found in the cytosolic compartment and cofractionates with 6-phosphogluconate dehydrogenase (Kai et al., 1968). Furthermore, Harwood and Hawthorne (1969) showed that in subsynaptosomal fractions prepared by osmotic lysis, little PIP kinase activity was associated with plasma or intracellular membranes. There remains the possibility, however, that some PIP kinase may be associated with membrane structures (Jolles et al., 1980). The polyphosphoinositides may be degraded via phosphomonoesterases (phosphatases) and phosphodiesterases. Both PIP and PIP_2 phosphatase (Dawson and Thompson, 1964; Salway et al., 1967; Harwood and Hawthorne, 1969; Nijjar and Hawthorne, 1977) and presumptive PIP and PIP_2 phosphodiesterase activities (Harwood and Hawthorne, 1969; Keough and Thompson, 1972) appêar to be located predominantly in the cytosolic fraction. However, phosphodiesterase activity is also associated with myelin (Deshmukh et al. 1982), and Van Rooijen et al. (1983) have found evidence for membrane-bound phosphodiesterase activity which acts on endogenous PIP and PIP_2 but not PI. Sheltawy et al. (1972) observed that the distribution of PIP_2 phosphatase in brain subcellular fractions was altered when the enzyme was assayed in the presence of "pH 5" factor (Dawson and Thompson, 1964). Under these conditions, the enzyme was found to be associated with membrane structures enriched in 5'-nucleotidase activity, with little or no increase in the relative specific activity of the enzyme in the cytosolic fraction.

Since the various enzymes involved in synthesis and breakdown of the phosphoinositides are located in different subcellular environments, the question arises as to how the phospholipids are transported between different intracellular loci in order to effect a cycle. Although knowledge

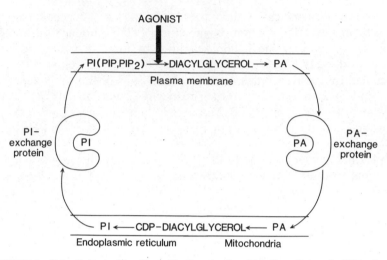

FIGURE 7.2   Subcellular loci implicated in the stimulated labeling of phospholipids. In this diagram the action of the agonist is proposed to initiate a closed labeling cycle with the breakdown of polyphosphoinositides. The formation of diacylglycerol and the formation of PA both occur in the plasma membrane. In nerve tissue PA must be transported to the mitochondria, where it is converted to CDP-diacylglycerol and thence to the endoplasmic reticulum, where PI synthesis occurs. PI is phosphorylated to PIP following return to the plasma membrane via intracellular transport.

concerning this topic is limited, there are indications from other systems that phospholipids may be transferred between subcellular sites by means of exchange proteins (see Chapter 4; Fig. 7.2). While much emphasis has been placed on proteins for transfer of PI and phosphatidylcholine, it is possible that intracellular transfer of other lipids, for example, PA and CDP-diacylglycerol, also occurs via as yet unknown exchange proteins.

A summary of the presumed location of enzymes involved in PA and phosphoinositide interconversions is shown in Table 7.1. Enzymes involved in the degradation of inositol-containing phospholipids are all cytosolic or perhaps loosely associated with the plasma membrane which contains their substrates. It is believed that the inositol lipids are located in the inner plasma membrane leaflet (Michell, 1975), and their polar headgroups, which project into the cytosol, may be envisioned to be accessible to enzymes of phosphomonoesteratic or phosphodiesteratic cleavage. The formation of PA via diacylglycerol kinase also occurs at the plasma membrane site, while the resynthesis of PI involves the endoplasmic reticulum and mitochondria. From this we may predict that isotopic measurement of the breakdown of plasma membrane inositol phospholipids and the appearance of PA to be early events, while the

TABLE 7.1 Subcellular Distribution of Enzymes Involved in Stimulated Phospholipid Turnover

Locus	Enzyme	Reference
Plasma membrane	PA phosphatase	Cotman et al. (1971)
	Diacylglycerol kinase	Lapetina and Hawthorne (1971)
	PI kinase	Kai et al. (1966, 1968); Harwood and Hawthorne (1969)
	PIP phosphodiesterase	Van Rooijen et al. (1983)
	PIP$_2$ phosphodiesterase	Van Rooijen et al. (1983)
Cytosol	Ca^{2+}-Dependent PI phosphodiesterase	Irvine and Dawson (1978)
	PIP phosphodiesterase	Harwood and Hawthorne (1969)
	PIP$_2$ phosphodiesterase	Keough and Thompson (1972)
	PIP phosphatase	Dawson and Thompson (1964); Salway et al. (1967); Harwood and Hawthorne (1969)
	PIP$_2$ phosphatase[a]	Salway et al. (1967); Harwood and Hawthorne (1969)
	PIP kinase	Kai et al. (1968); Harwood and Hawthorne (1969)
Mitochondria	PA-cytidylyltransferase	Petzold and Agranoff (1965, 1967); Cotman et al. (1971)
Endoplasmic reticulum	CDP-diacylglycerol: inositol transferase	Benjamins and Agranoff (1969); Harwood and Hawthorne (1969); Cotman et al. (1971)
Lysosomes	Ca^{2+}-Independent PI phosphodiesterase	Irvine et al. (1978)
	CDP-diacylglycerol hydrolase	Rittenhouse et al. (1981)

[a] See alternative view of Sheltawy et al. (1972).

TABLE 7.2   Neural-related Preparations Demonstrating Enhanced
Phospholipid Turnover

Preparation	Stimulation	References
Central Nervous System		
Whole brain, various regions (*in vivo*)	Neuroeffectors	Friedel and Schanberg (1972, 1975); Friedel et al. (1973, 1974)
Brain slices, various regions	Neuroeffectors	Hokin (1955, 1969, 1979); Abdel-Latif et al. (1974); Hokin-Heaverson (1980); Fisher et al. (1984b)
Brain minces	Neuroeffectors	Reddy and Sastry (1979)
Subcellular fractions (nerve-ending preparations)	Neuroeffectors, electrical depolarization, elevated K^+, A23187	Schacht and Agranoff (1972, 1974); Yagihara and Hawthorne (1972); Bleasdale and Hawthorne(1975); Miller (1977); Griffin and Hawthorne (1978); Yandrasitz and Segal (1979); Fisher and Agranoff (1980, 1981); Fisher et al. (1983a)
Synaptic plasma membranes	Neuroeffectors	Jolles et al. (1980; 1981a,c)
Pineal (gland and dissociated cells)	Neuroeffectors	Eichberg et al. (1973); Hauser et al. (1974); Smith et al. (1979); Nijjar et al. (1980)
Anterior pituitary	Neuroeffectors	Young et al. (1979); Hauser and Parks (1983)
Retina	Light	Anderson and Hollyfield (1981)
Peripheral Nervous System		
Superior sympathetic ganglion	Electrical pulses, neuroeffectors, elevated K^+	Hokin et al. (1960); Larrabee and Leicht (1965); Larrabee (1968); Lapetina et al. (1976); Pickard et al. (1977)

TABLE 7.2 (*continued*)

Preparation	Stimulation	References
Adrenal medulla (slices and dissociated chromaffin cells)	Neuroeffectors	Trifaro (1969a); Mohd.Adnan and Hawthorne (1981); Fisher et al. (1981a); Azila and Hawthorne (1982); Ohsako and Deguchi (1983)
Neuroblastoma	Neuroeffectors	Siman and Klein (1981); Cohen et al. (1983)
Auditory organ (noctuid moth)	Sound	Killian and Schacht (1980)
Electroplax (*Torpedo marmorata*)	Electrical pulses	Bleasdale et al. (1976)

resynthesis of PI might be delayed. As will be discussed in Section 7.3.4, this appears to be the case.

7.1.4   Neural Preparations Evincing Enhanced Phospholipid Turnover

A variety of neural preparations have been shown to demonstrate enhanced phospholipid labeling upon application of an appropriate stimulus (Table 7.2). Preparations from the central nervous system (CNS) include whole brain (*in vivo* studies), brain slices, minces, and subcellular fractions (nerve-ending preparations). Also included as "CNS related" are the pineal and anterior pituitary gland. Although these structures lie outside the blood–brain barrier, they are of central neuroembryological origin and constitute part of the neuroendocrine system. Peripheral nervous system (PNS) related preparations include sympathetic ganglia, adrenal medulla, and electroplax and can be demonstrated to respond to a diverse range of pharmacological and physiological stimuli.

7.2   PHARMACOLOGY OF RECEPTORS THAT ELICIT ENHANCED PHOSPHOLIPID TURNOVER

While there is some evidence that a variety of neuroeffectors can elicit an increased labeling of PA and/or PI from $^{32}P_i$ (Table 7.3), most information relates to the cholinergic and adrenergic systems. The cholinergic

TABLE 7.3 Pharmacological Profile of Phospholipid Turnover in Neural-related Preparations

Receptor	Preparation	Effective Agonists	Effective Antagonists[a]	References
Muscarinic cholinergic	In vivo	Carbamylcholine	Atropine	Friedel and Schanberg (1972); Soukup et al. (1978)
	Brain slices (various regions)	Acetylcholine	Atropine	Hokin and Hokin (1955); Lapetina and Michell (1972); Abdel-Latif et al. (1974); Canessa de Scarnati et al. (1976); Berridge et al. (1982); Brown and Nahorski (1983); Fisher et al. (1984b)
	Brain minces (cerebral cortex)	Acetylcholine	N.T.	Reddy and Sastry (1979)
	Nerve-ending preparations (cerebral cortex or hippocampus)	Acetylcholine, carbamylcholine, muscarine, methacholine, arecoline, bethanechol, oxotremorine, pilocarpine	Atropine, scopolamine, quinuclidinylbenzilate	Schacht and Agranoff (1972, 1974); Yagihara and Hawthorne (1972); Miller (1977); Yandrasitz and Segal (1979); Fisher and Agranoff (1980, 1981); Fisher et al. (1981b, 1983a)

	Agonists	Antagonists	References
Superior cervical ganglion	Carbamylcholine, bethanechol	Atropine, propyl benzilylcholine mustard	Hokin et al. (1960); Lapetina et al. (1976); Pickard et al. (1976); Horwitz et al. (1984)
Pituitary (slices and dissociated cells)	Carbamylcholine, pilocarpine, oxotremorine, acetylcholine	Atropine, scopolamine, quinuclidinylbenzilate	Young et al. (1979); Hauser and Parks (1983)
Adrenal medulla (slices and dissociated cells)	Acetylcholine, carbamylcholine, muscarine, methacholine	Atropine	Trifaro (1969a); Fisher et al. (1981a); Mohd.Adnan and Hawthorne (1981); Ohsako and Deguchi (1982); Swilem et al. (1983)
Neuroblastoma (NG 108–15) (NIE-115)	Carbamylcholine	N.T.	Siman and Klein (1981)
In vivo	Carbamylcholine Norepinephrine	Atropine Phenoxybenzamine, phentolamine	Cohen et al. (1983); Friedel et al. (1973, 1974); Slotkin et al. (1982)
α_1-Adrenergic			
Brain slices (various regions)	Norepinephrine Phenylephrine	N.T. or prazosin	Hokin (1969, 1970); Abdel-Latif et al. (1974); Hokin-Neaverson (1980); Berridge et al. (1982); Brown and Nahorski (1983)

TABLE 7.3 *(continued)*

Receptor	Preparation	Effective Agonists	Effective Antagonists[a]	References
	Brain minces (cerebral cortex)	Norepinephrine	N.T.	Reddy and Sastry (1979)
	Nerve-ending preparations	Norepinephrine	Thymoxamine	Sneddon and Keen (1970)
	Pineal (intact gland and dissociated cells)	Norepinephrine, methylnorepinephrine, phenylephrine, methoxamine	WB-4101, phenoxybenzamine, prazosin, phentolamine	Eichberg et al. (1973); Hauser et al. (1974, 1978); Smith et al. (1979); Nijjar et al. (1980)
H_1-Histaminergic	*In vivo*	Histamine, 2(2-pyridyl)ethylamine	Pyrilamine, tripelennamine	Friedel and Schanberg (1975); Subramanian et al. (1980, 1981)
	Brain slices	Histamine	Mepyramine (pyrilamine)	Daum et al. (1983)
5-Hydroxytryptamine ($5HT_1$?)	Brain slices (various regions)	Serotonin	N.T.	Hokin (1969); Abdel-Latif et al. (1974); Berridge et al. (1982)
	Brain minces	Serotonin	N.T.	Reddy and Sastry (1979)
Dopamine	*In vivo*	Dopamine	N.T.	Friedel et al. (1974)
	Brain slices (various regions)	Dopamine	N.T.	Hokin (1969); Abdel-Latif et al. (1974); Hokin-Neaverson (1980)
	In vivo (snail brain)	Dopamine	N.T.	Althaus et al. (1975)

256

Nerve growth factor (NGF)	Superior cervical ganglion	NGF	Anti-NGF	Lakshamanan (1978a,b; 1979)
	PC 12 cells	NGF	N.T.	Traynor et al. (1982)
Peptides	Synaptic membranes	$ACTH_{1-24}$, β-endorphin	N.T. (analogs of ACTH ineffective)	Jolles et al. (1980; 1981a,c)
	Brain slices	Substance P		Downes (1983); Watson and Downes (1983)
		Neurotensin		Downes (1983); Watson and Downes (1983)
		Vasopressin		Downes (1983)
		CCK-octapeptide		Downes (1983)
	Superior cervical ganglion	Vasopressin		Michell et al. (1985)
	GH_3 pituitary cells	Thyrotropin (TRH)		Martin (1983)
Amino acids	Brain slices	GABA, aspartic acid	(Bicuculline)	Hokin (1969); Friedel et al. (1977); Canessa de Scarnati et al. (1982)

[a] N.T., Not tested.

muscarinic receptor interaction has received the most attention, but as will be seen, even in this system a number of critical issues remain to be resolved.

7.2.1 Cholinergic Receptors

Low concentrations (10^{-5}–10^{-8} M) of classical muscarinic antagonists such as atropine, scopolamine, and quinuclidinylbenzilate (QNB) completely block the Ach- or carbamylcholine-mediated stimulation of PA and PI labeling in neural preparations, while nicotinic antagonists such as d-tubocurarine and hexamethonium are completely ineffective (Hokin and Hokin, 1955; Schacht and Agranoff, 1972; Griffin et al., 1979; Fisher and Agranoff, 1981). In addition, "pure" muscarinic agonists such as muscarine and methacholine are able to elicit the response, while nicotine and 1,1-dimethyl-4-phenylpiperazinium iodide are without effect (Fisher and Agranoff, 1981). We conclude that the muscarinic, not the nicotinic, cholinergic receptor is coupled to enhanced phospholipid turnover. In only one experimental preparation, the superior cervical ganglion, have nicotinic receptors been implicated in stimulated PI labeling (Larrabee and Leicht, 1965). However, results from two other studies employing specific antagonists conflict with this claim and suggest that the cholinergic receptors involved in this system are also muscarinic (Lapetina et al., 1976; Pickard et al., 1977). There are, in fact, few documented examples of tissues containing muscarinic receptors that are not coupled to stimulated phospholipid turnover (e.g., muscarinic receptors in brain microvessels; Zeleznikar et al., 1983). The clear pharmacological distinction between the effector systems of muscarinic and nicotinic receptors is further illustrated by the bovine chromaffin cell, which possesses both types of receptors on its plasma membrane. In this cell it can be shown that only muscarinic receptors are coupled to stimulated PA and PI turnover and cGMP production (Fisher et al., 1981a; Mohd.Adnan and Hawthorne, 1981; Derome et al., 1981; Azila and Hawthorne, 1982; Ohsako and Deguchi, 1983), while nicotinic receptors have no effect on phospholipid labeling but are linked to Ca^{2+} influx and catecholamine release (Kilpatrick et al., 1980; Fisher et al., 1981a; Swilem et al., 1983).

Within the category of muscarinic agonists there are considerable differences in the relative efficacies of individual agonists in eliciting increased PA and PI labeling. This receptor heterogeneity appears to be tissue specific. Thus, in nerve-ending preparations and brain slices bethanechol, oxotremorine, pilocarpine, and arecoline typically elicit a smaller increase in PA and inositol lipid turnover than do muscarine or methacholine, and as such, the four agents may be defined as "partial" rather than "full" agonists (Fisher et al., 1983a, 1984b). In the superior cervical ganglion, however, bethanechol is claimed to be a full agonist with regard to both stimulated PI labeling and the physiological response, that is, ganglionic depolarization (Lapetina et al., 1976; Brown et al., 1980), although more recent evidence indicates a partial agonist status for bethanechol (Horwitz et al., 1984). Relatively high concentrations of muscarinic agonists are required for a maximal effect in nerve-ending preparations and brain slices. The threshold concentration of Ach or carbamylcholine is about 10^{-7} M, while 10^{-3} M or greater concentrations are required for a maximal effect or labeling (Hokin and Hokin, 1955; Hokin et al., 1960; Schacht and Agranoff, 1972, 1974). While the broad range of concentration dependence of this response might appear to militate against a possible physiological role for enhanced phospholipid turnover in synaptic transmission, the agonist concentrations required to evoke the labeling responses are very similar to those required for occupation of all of the receptors (Michell et al., 1976). From this it may be predicted that concentration dependence curves of PA/PI turnover will be displaced to the right (i.e., higher concentration ranges) of the "physiological" response curve, since the latter typically requires the occupation of only a small fraction of the receptors. In the case of nerve endings the nature of the physiological response to the activation of these CNS muscarinic receptors has yet to be identified and thus the hypothesis awaits a more rigorous test. However, Miller (1977) determined the apparent dissociation constants for the Ach-stimulated PA and PI labeling in rat nerve-ending preparations and found them to be in good agreement with published values for the dissociation constant of the Ach-muscarinic receptor complex itself. Similarly, the affinity constants for carbamylcholine, acetylcholine, and muscarine stimulation of PA labeling in guinea pig nerve-ending preparations are in the same range as those obtained by radioligand displacement analysis, performed under the same incubation conditions (Fisher et al., 1983a). The muscarinic receptor in brain, as in other tissues, can be differentiated into "high"- and "low"-affinity states that account for 35 and 65% of the total sites, respectively (Birdsall et al., 1978). This raises the question as to whether both forms of the receptor are coupled to PA turnover. When concentration dependence curves of PA labeling are constructed for carbamylcholine, acetylcholine, and muscarine, more than 88% of the inferred muscarinic receptors are in the low-affinity state (Fisher et al., 1983a). The full agonists such as carbamylcholine also display large differences in their binding affinities for the high- and low-affinity forms of the receptor, whereas for partial agonists such as oxotremorine the difference in affinities is much less. This suggests that the enhancement of PA and PI turnover in brain by muscarinic agonists is related to an agonist-mediated conformational change in the receptor, and that the ability of an agonist to induce this conversion may be predicted by its differential binding to the high- and low-affinity forms of the receptor. Of these two affinity forms, in the CNS it appears that the low-affinity state of the muscarinic receptor is that which is preferentially coupled to stimulated phospholipid labeling.

Still less is known about the concentrations of agonists required for maximal receptor occupancy, enhanced phospholipid labeling, and the relevant physiological responses in the PNS. However, in the adrenal medulla we have observed that maximal stimulation of PA and PI labeling requires a concentration of muscarine (10^{-3} M) that is two orders of magnitude greater than that reported to produce a maximal stimulation of cGMP production (Fisher, Holz, and Agranoff, unpublished results; Derome et al., 1981). Although the information available is very limited, it appears consistent with the existence of a quantitative relationship between occupancy of the muscarinic receptor and an increased turnover of PA and PI. Further details of the behavior of partial agonists and of the relative involvement of high- and low-affinity forms of the muscarinic receptor should greatly facilitate our understanding of both the underlying molecular mechanism of enhanced phospholipid labeling and its physiological consequences.

7.2.2 Adrenergic Receptors

Adrenergic receptors have been implicated in stimulated PI and PA labeling, both from *in vivo* studies (Friedel et al., 1973) and from *in vitro* studies—for example, the addition of norepinephrine to brain slices (Hokin, 1969; Abdel-Latif et al., 1974; Berridge et al., 1982; Brown and Nahorski, 1983), to nerve-ending preparations (Sneddon and Keen, 1970), and to the isolated pineal gland (Eichberg et al., 1973; Hauser et al., 1974) (Table 7.3). All available evidence suggests that α rather than β receptors are involved, and of these, the α_1 subtype response predominates. This assertion is derived primarily from studies on intact pineal glands and on dissociated pinealocytes. In these preparations 10^{-5} M norepinephrine, methylnorepinephrine, phenylephrine, or methoxamine elicits a large increase in PI labeling, which can be blocked by administration of WB-4101, phenoxybenzamine, prazosin, or phentolamine, all of which are classical α-antagonists, but not by sotalol or propranolol, classical β-antagonists (Smith et al., 1979). In addition, three agonists that act preferentially, although not exclusively, on α_2-adrenergic receptors, clonidine, oxymetazoline, and ergometrine produce little or no stimulation of PI labeling. They may act as "partial" agonists in that they can block the stimulation of PI labeling induced by norepinephrine (Smith et al., 1979). This pharmacological profile is then entirely consistent with the activation of α_1-adrenergic receptors in the pineal, a pattern that may well exist in other neural-related preparations.

7.2.3 Histaminergic Receptors

The intracisternal administration of histamine results in increased incorporation of added $^{32}P_i$ into brain phospholipids and specifically into PI (Friedel and Schanberg, 1975; Subramanian et al., 1980, 1981). This effect can be mimicked by the addition of the H_1-agonist 2-(2-pyridyl)ethylamine and is blocked by pyrilamine, an H_1-antagonist. The H_2-agonist 4-methylhistamine is without effect, as is the H_2-antagonist cimetidine. Of particular interest is the observation that the magnitude of stimulated PI labeling detected in response to the administration of histamine correlates well with the appearance of brain H_1-histamine receptors and histaminergic neurotransmission (Subramanian et al., 1981). The observation that addition of histamine to brain slices in the presence of lithium results in the accumulation of inositol monophosphate provides further evidence for an involvement of H_1-histaminergic receptors in stimulated PI turnover (Daum et al., 1983).

7.2.4 Dopaminergic Receptors

The possibility of enhanced PA and PI labeling in response to dopaminergic receptor activation remains questionable. Several earlier studies indicated that dopamine has either a stimulatory (Abdel-Latif et al., 1974; Friedel et al., 1974; Althaus et al., 1975) or a marked inhibitory effect (Hokin, 1970; Hokin-Neaverson, 1980). Evidence purporting to correlate dopaminergic receptor activation and stimulated labeling should be regarded with caution, as exemplified by a study in the pineal gland (Nijjar et al., 1980). In this tissue dopamine addition (like that of norepinephrine) leads to stimulation of PI labeling. However, specific dopaminergic agonists such as apomorphine and piribedil fail to elicit a measurable response, and furthermore, the stimulatory response of dopamine may be blocked by the α-adrenergic antagonists, phenoxybenzamine, and phentolamine. In addition, saturating concentrations of both dopamine and α-adrenergic agonists do not result in a stimulation larger than that elicited by either agent alone, as would have been predicted had both α-adrenergic and dopaminergic receptors been independently involved. The apparent dopamine-mediated stimulation of PI labeling in this preparation can thus be attributed to an activation of the α-adrenergic receptors. Addition of dopamine to nerve-ending preparations from the striatum, a brain region that receives a dense innervation of dopaminergic terminals from the substantia nigra, also fails to elicit a response (Nijjar et al., 1980). Similarly, dopamine addition to superior cervical ganglion is reported not to result in a measurable increase in PI turnover (Michell, 1975).

7.2.5   Serotonergic Receptors

Serotonin addition to brain minces (Reddy and Sastry, 1979) and slices from various brain regions elicits an increased labeling of both PA and PI (Hokin, 1970) and an accumulation of inositol monophosphate in the presence of lithium (Berridge et al., 1982). No antagonist data are yet available, nor is it known whether $5HT_1$ or $5HT_2$ receptors are involved.

7.2.6   Nerve Growth Factor

Lakshmanan has shown that the addition of nerve growth factor (NGF) at very low concentrations (10^{-10}–10^{-7} M 2.5S NGF) to organ cultures of superior cervical ganglia specifically stimulates the incorporation of $^{32}P_i$ into PI (Lakshmanan, 1978a,b, 1979). In addition, NGF has been reported to increase the incorporation of $^{32}P_i$ into PA and PI of pheochromocytoma cells (Traynor et al., 1982). A question has been raised of the possibility of reninlike activity in the NGF preparation that could endogenously generate angiotensin, a known stimulatory agent in hepatocytes (Billah and Michell, 1979; Michell et al., 1981). While this is a possibility, such an explanation must be reconciled with the demonstrated effectiveness of anti-NGF antibodies in blocking the stimulated PI labeling (Lakshamanan, 1978a).

7.2.7   Amino Acid Neurotransmitters

The CNS is atypical of other mammalian tissues in that it maintains relatively high concentrations of free amino acids, some of which may also play a role in neurotransmission, for example, glutamic, aspartic, and 4-aminobutyric acid (GABA). The addition of aspartate or GABA to neural preparations does not result in an increased turnover of PA and PI, and in fact an appreciable inhibition of the basal labeling of all phospholipids occurs (Hokin, 1970; Friedel et al., 1977). In the case of aspartate the effect is not limited to the naturally occurring L-isomer, and the application of this amino acid to liver slices produces a stimulation rather than inhibition of phospholipid labeling (Canessa de Scarnatti et al., 1982).

There is then as yet no firm evidence supporting the coupling of amino acid receptors to stimulated phospholipid labeling.

7.2.8 Peptidergic Receptors

Recent studies have indicated that corticotropin(1-24)tetracosapeptide (ACTH) can exert profound effects on phospholipid turnover (Jolles et al., 1980, 1981a,c). Unlike the studies on stimulated phospholipid labeling studies thus far, these experiments were performed with lysed nerve-ending fractions, and tissues were labeled with added $[^{32}P]ATP$ rather than with $^{32}P_i$. Furthermore, it should be noted that in this case, only PA, PIP, and PIP_2 are labeled, as might be predicted from the location of the enzymes mediating their labeling at the plasma membrane (see Section 7.1.3). PI is presumably unlabeled because its resynthesis occurs in the endoplasmic reticulum, which although present in the lysate is not likely to be accessible. The addition of ACTH stimulates phosphorylation of PIP to PIP_2 and inhibits PA labeling, each effect reaching a maximum within 20–30 s. ACTH stimulation requires the presence of Mg^{2+} ions, is inhibited by Ca^{2+}, and appears to be mediated by an alteration of phosphorylation of lipids rather than of dephosphorylation (Jolles et al., 1981c). Studies with structural analogs of ACTH indicate that the sequence $ACTH_{5-7}$ accounts for the stimulation of PIP_2 labeling, while the sequences $ACTH_{7-10}$ and $ACTH_{10-16}$ account for the inhibition of PA labeling. A stimulatory effect on PIP labeling is also detected when ACTH is shortened from the N-terminus. Results from the addition of β-endorphin are somewhat different. This peptide inhibits the labeling of PA but, unlike ACTH, has no effect on the phosphorylation of PIP (or of PI). Of particular interest is that earlier studies utilizing intact synaptosomes and $^{32}P_i$ as a source of label indicated that ACTH inhibited the labeling of all phospholipid classes (Jolles et al., 1979). While the relatively high concentration of Ca^{2+} used in the studies with intact synaptosomes may have obscured underlying changes in PIP_2 formation, the experiments raise the interesting possibility that broken cell preparations may be used to advantage to unravel the complexities associated with establishing the enzymic steps that mediate the stimulated labeling of PA and PI.

Recent studies have also indicated that the addition of vasopressin, neurotensin, CCK-octapeptide, or substance P to brain slices incubated in the presence of lithium results in an increased accumulation of inositol monophosphate, a product of stimulated lipid turnover (Downes, 1983; Watson and Downes, 1983).

7.3. BIOCHEMICAL CHARACTERISTICS AND MECHANISMS

Of the various neural preparations used, emphasis in this reveiw is placed on the use of isolated nerve endings, that is, "synaptosomal" preparations, which have proven a useful model for biochemical studies on synaptic mechanisms.

7.3.1 General Properties

In the nervous system, as in other tissues, the addition of an appropriate ligand results in a selective increase in the incorporation of added $^{32}P_i$ into PI and/or PA. Labeling of phosphatidylcholine may also be increased slightly (Abdel-Latif et al., 1974). This characteristic pattern of enhancement of labeling is seen in the face of a wide range of differences in the relative proportions of label incorporated into individual phospholipid classes in the absence of a stimulus from one type of preparation to another. For example, there is little or no basal incorporation of $^{32}P_i$ into either phosphatidylcholine or phosphatidylethanolamine in nerve-ending preparations (Schacht and Agranoff, 1972; Yagihara and Hawthorne, 1972), whereas appreciable incorporation of label into these lipids is observed in rat cortical minces or slices (Abdel-Latif et al., 1974; Reddy and Sastry, 1979) and in pineal gland (Eichberg et al., 1973; Hauser et al., 1978). PA and PI are presumed to become labeled via an exchange cycle (see Section 7.1.2), and PIP and PIP_2 are undoubtedly labeled primarily in the 4- and 5-phosphomonoester positions of inositol by the actions of kinases and phosphatases in the presence of $[^{32}P]ATP$. Labeled CDP-diacylglycerol is not normally detected. The liponucleotide is formed slowly, and in the presence of the high concentration of inositol in neural cytoplasm, it is rapidly incorporated into PI via CDP-diacylglycerol: inositol phosphatidyltransferase. In the pineal gland preparation it is possible to deplete the inositol tissue stores, and stimulation by α-adrenergic agents then leads to accumulation of labeled CDP-diacylglycerol (Hauser and Eichberg, 1975). Under these conditions there is also enhanced labeling of the phosphatidylglycerols, a feature uncharacteristic of the labeling pattern of other tissues (Hauser et al., 1978).

7.3.2 Stimulated Phospholipid Labeling in Nerve Tissue: A Closed Cycle

When nerve-ending preparations, brain slices, or minces are incubated with $^{32}P_i$ in a medium that supports oxidative phosphorylation, radioactivity is rapidly incorporated into phosphoinositides and PA. $^{32}P_i$ is converted to $[\gamma - {}^{32}P]ATP$ and enters the labeling cycle via diacylglycerol kinase, which phosphorylates endogenous diacylglycerol to yield labeled PA and PI. PI and PIP kinases sequentially phosphorylate endogenous PI at the 4 and 5 hydroxyl cyclitol positions to form PIP and PIP_2 (Fig. 7.1). On application of an appropriate stimulus, for example, a muscarinic or α_1-adrenergic agonist, electrical pulse, elevated K^+, or the ionophore A23187, there is a selective stimulation of labeling of PA and PI. This could result from (1) either increased *de novo* synthesis or decreased degradation of these lipids, (2) increased amount or specific radioactivity of the precursor $[^{32}P]ATP$ pool, or (3) increased rate of turnover of preexisting phospholipid to increase the availability of diacylglycerol, which is presumed to be rate limiting. The possibility of net increases in PA and PI appears unlikely on the basis of studies in which the stimulated incorporation of other lipid precursor molecules such as labeled glucose and glycerol is compared to that of $^{32}P_i$. In both brain slices and nerve-ending preparations measurable incorporation of these precursors can be detected, yet stimuli that evoke increases in $^{32}P_i$ labeling into PA and PI do not result in a comparable increase (Hokin and Hokin, 1958b; Schacht and Agranoff, 1974; Abdel-Latif et al., 1974; Lapetina and Michell, 1974; Fisher and Agranoff, 1981). The possibility of separate precursor pools for basal and stimulated labeling should, however, also be considered. The situation regarding the incorporation of labeled inositol is less clear. An early study (Hokin and Hokin, 1958b) showed that when Ach was added to brain slices there were comparable increases in the incorporation of both $^{32}P_i$ and $[^3H]$inositol. However, in a subsequent study (Hokin-Neaverson, 1980) there was a smaller percentage increase in labeled inositol incorporation than in $^{32}P_i$ when brain slices were stimulated by the addition of norepinephrine. In nerve-ending preparations the percent stimulation of labeled inositol incorporation is consistently lower than that of $^{32}P_i$ (Schacht and Agranoff, 1974; Yandrasitz and Segal, 1979; Fisher and Agranoff, 1981). This difference suggests either that added inositol does not exchange readily with a precursor pool for stimulated PI synthesis or that much of the basal ^3H incorporated is accounted for by the CDP-diacylglycerol-independent base-exchange pathway (Takenawa et al., 1977) and is hence insensitive to Ach or carbamylcholine addition. Problems associated with the measurement of $[^3H]$inositol incorporation into PI in cell preparations have recently been discussed (Eisenberg and Hasegawa, 1981).

The possibility that increased PA or PI labeling can be explained by an increase in the specific activity of a precursor ATP pool has been studied by a number of groups. Friedel et al. (1974) could detect no increase in specific activity of the *in vivo* nucleotide phosphate pool when dopamine and norepinephrine were administered intracisternally. Similarly, neither neurotransmitter nor 5-hydroxytryptamine changed the radioactivity of the nucleotide phosphate pool when added to slices from various brain regions (Hokin, 1969, 1970). In addition, no increase in the radioactivity associated with the ATP fraction was detected in nerve-ending preparations incubated with Ach, carbamylcholine, or the ionophore A23187 (Yagihara and Hawthorne, 1972; Schacht and Agranoff, 1974; Fisher and Agranoff, 1981). Taken together, these findings exclude the possibility that major changes in the specific activity of the ATP pool are responsible for the labeling pattern. It appears then that the increased labeling of PA and thereby of PI depends on an increased rate of phosphorylation of diacylglycerol. The source of diacylglycerol for the stimulation of phospholipid labeling remains a major question.

7.3.3   Is the Hydrolysis of Phosphatidylinositol or of a Polyphosphoinositide the Key Initial Response?

Until recently, the hypothesis originally put forward by the Hokins that PI hydrolysis is the key initial event in the initiation of enhanced phospholipid turnover was widely accepted, particularly when applied to non-neural tissues such as pancreas, avian salt gland, parotid gland, and platelets. Demonstration of stimulated PI hydrolysis in the nervous system has, however, proved to be elusive. Neither Lapetina and Michell (1974) nor Abdel-Latif et al. (1974) could detect any breakdown of prelabeled PI when Ach was added to brain slices. When nerve endings were prelabeled with either $^{32}P_i$, [^{3}H]glycerol, or [^{3}H]inositol, there was no detectable loss of radioactivity from PI on the addition of muscarinic agonists (Schacht and Agranoff, 1974; Fisher and Agranoff, 1981). Lunt and Pickard (1975), however, observed a 23% decrease in the specific activity of PI following intraventricular injection of carbamylcholine, with the synaptic vesicle fraction of brain demonstrating the largest reduction. Pickard and Hawthorne (1978) also observed PI breakdown in electrically stimulated nerve-ending preparations. However, this latter observation is difficult to interpret in view of the finding that radioactivity is lost from prelabeled PA at the same rate. It appears that there is at present a lack of convincing evidence to suggest that PI hydrolysis is the key initial response in enhanced phospholipid turnover in the nervous systems. An alternate source of diacylglycerol is PA breakdown via PA phosphohydrolase. Some evidence suggesting this possibility was put forward by Yagihara et al. (1973) and Schacht and Agranoff (1974), although similar preparations which can be shown to mediate a muscarinic stimulation of

PA labeling showed no detectable loss of prelabeled PA on the addition of Ach (Fisher and Agranoff, 1981).

A role for polyphosphoinositide breakdown to diacylglycerol in the initiation of stimulated phospholipid labeling now appears possible. These lipids, although constituting less than 2% of the total cellular phospholipid, are relatively enriched in the nervous system (Dawson and Eichberg, 1965), are extremely labile, and typically account for more than 50% of the ^{32}P present in incubated nerve-ending fraction lipids (Schacht and Agranoff, 1972, 1974; Yagihara and Hawthorne, 1972; Fisher and Agranoff, 1981). Moreover, these lipids (unlike PI) are apparently located predominantly in plasma membranes (Michell, 1975) and exist in brain in both a "stable" form associated with the myelin membrane and in a "labile" form that is present in neuronal and glial plasma membranes (Eichberg and Hauser, 1973). Earlier reports did not support a primary role for the polyphosphoinositides in stimulated PA and PI labeling (Hokin, 1965; Palmer and Rossiter, 1965; Schacht and Agranoff, 1972; Yagihara and Hawthorne, 1972), possibly because the changes seen are relatively small. In 1978 Griffin and Hawthorne demonstrated that the introduction of Ca^{2+} into a nerve-ending preparation with the divalent cation ionophore A23187 resulted in the stimulated breakdown of PIP and PIP_2, the release of water-soluble inositol phosphates, and an accelerated appearance of label in PA. Soukup et al. (1978) demonstrated an increased turnover of polyphosphoinositides in brain following intracisternal administration of carbamylcholine which could be blocked by atropine. Results from a nonneural preparation, the iris smooth muscle, had shown that the activation of muscarinic cholinergic and α_1-adrenergic receptors in this tissue results in a breakdown of PIP_2 but not of PI or PIP (Abdel-Latif et al., 1977; Akhtar and Abdel-Latif, 1978, 1980). These various observations raise the possibility that the initial action of pharmacological agents in brain and iris smooth muscle involves the hydrolysis of polyphosphoinositides. A systematic evaluation of the effects of muscarinic agonists and antagonists on the lowering of PIP and PIP_2 labeling in nerve-ending preparations suggested that the reductions, while relatively small (approximately 10%), were indeed mediated through the muscarinic receptor (Fisher and Agranoff, 1981). More convincing evidence was obtained from experiments in which both Ach and A23187 were added (Fisher and Agranoff, 1981). This combination results in a synergistic increase in the labeling of PA and PI, as well as a synergistic decrease in the labeling of PIP and PIP_2, which now become sizable (50–70%). While muscarinic antagonists do not block the effect of the ionophore, they do block the cholinergic potentiation both of increased (PA and PI) and decreased (PIP and PIP_2) labeling, further indicating that the activation of muscarinic receptors in nerve-ending preparations is somehow linked to PIP and PIP_2 turnover (Fisher and Agranoff, 1981). The potentiating effects of the combined ionophore and Ach addition suggest the interaction of different, but impinging, mechanisms. For example, the increase in local Ca^{2+} concentrations produced by ionophore could increase the basal rate of polyphosphoinositide breakdown via action on a specific phosphodiesterase. Receptor activation by ligand, on the other hand, could produce a transmembrane conformational change that increases the number of membrane-bound substrate and enzyme domains participating in the stimulated turnover (Agranoff and Bleasdale, 1978). Experiments in which the polyphosphoinositides are allowed to become labeled to isotopic equilibrium and are then challenged with a muscarinic agonist, ionophore, or the combination also show an accelerated loss of label from both PIP and PIP_2. These results suggest that the hydrolysis of PIP and/or PIP_2, rather than of PI, may trigger events leading to enhanced phospholipid labeling in the nervous system. Very recently this proposition has received direct support from the measurement of stimulated release of inositol bis- and trisphosphate from brain slices following carbachol addition (Berridge et al., 1983).

Additional indirect evidence supporting a role for polyphosphoinositide breakdown in stimulated phospholipid turnover comes from the observation that the response of nerve-ending preparations to both muscarinic agonists and A23187 requires the presence of a minimal Ca^{2+} concentration. Although added Ca^{2+} is not obligatory for the response, addition of the Ca^{2+}-chelating agent EGTA abolishes both the muscarinic stimulation of PA and PI labeling and the loss of radioactivity from prelabeled PIP and PIP_2 (Griffin and Hawthorne, 1978; Griffin et al., 1979; Fisher and Agranoff, 1980, 1981). Experiments with Ca^{2+}-EDTA buffers have indicated that $10^{-7}-10^{-6}$ M free Ca^{2+} is required (Griffin et al., 1979). Using Ca^{2+}-EGTA buffers, we calculated the same concentration requirement for free Ca^{2+} (S. K. Fisher and B. W. Agranoff, unpublished results). Enzymes of both phosphomonesteratic and phosphodiesteratic breakdown of polyphosphoinositides are known to be sensitive to Ca^{2+} depletion, and thus its removal might be expected to inhibit their breakdown (Jolles et al., 1981b). In contrast, the synthesis of PA via diacylglycerol kinase and of PI via CDP-diacylglycerol, at least in nerve-ending preparations, appears to be largely insensitive either to depletion of cellular Ca^{2+} or to its addition in millimolar concentrations (Griffin et al., 1979). Although these experiments clearly point to a requirement for the presence of Ca^{2+} in the overall changes in labeling, they do not establish whether Ca^{2+} mobilization results from receptor–ligand interaction and mediates increased labeling of PA and PI or whether some minimal cytosolic Ca^{2+} concentration is required for expression of a signal that stimulates phospholipid labeling but does not regulate it (see Section 7.5.1).

It now appears that in nonneural systems including parotid gland, hepatocytes, platelets, and blowfly salivary gland, PI breakdown may also be secondary to an initial receptor-linked breakdown of PIP_2 at the plasma membrane (Kirk et al., 1981b; Michell et al, 1981; Vickers et al., 1982; Weiss et al., 1982; Agranoff et al., 1983; Berridge, 1983; Berridge et al., 1983; Poggioli et al., 1983; Rhodes et al., 1983). Thus, polyphosphoinositide breakdown may play a key role not only in brain, in which they are relatively enriched, but in other tissues, where they are trace membrane components (Fisher et al., 1984a).

The closed cycle depicted in Section 7.1.2, then, for a number of tissues including brain, requires phosphorylation of PI to polyphosphoinositide prior to stimulated phosphodiesteratic cleavage:

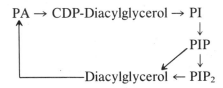

7.3.4 Evaluation of Phospholipid Turnover in Brain: Labeling and Prelabeling Approaches

Stimulated turnover of PA and PI has been traditionally detected by (1) measurement of the incorporation of $^{32}P_i$ into tissue lipids in the presence and absence of ligand, (2) addition of the ligand to prelabeled tissue, in which case-stimulated phospholipid breakdown could occur, or (3) determination of changes in the chemical amounts of lipids upon addition of ligand. Receptor-mediated breakdown of PI, measured either chemically or radiochemically, has been detected in several nonneural preparations, although the magnitudes of these changes differ considerably among tissues, for example, 5–10% of total PI is depleted in the hepatocyte compared to 40–60% in the platelet (Michell et al., 1976; Bell and Majerus, 1979; Billah and Michell, 1979; Cockcroft et al., 1980b; Weiss and Putney, 1981). The concomitant formation of diacylglycerol can also be demonstrated following stimulation of certain tissues, for example, when thrombin is added to platelets (Rittenhouse-Simmons, 1979), or when muscarinic cholinergic agonists are added to pancreas (Banschbach et al., 1981). The increased incorporation of $^{32}P_i$ into PA and PI that occurs on the addition of Ach or norepinephrine to neural-related preparations (nerve endings, brain slices, pineal gland, and adrenal medulla) is not accompanied by measurable alterations in the chemical amounts of phosphoinositides. Prelabeling studies have in fact failed to detect a selective loss of labeled PI following receptor activation in neural systems (Abdel-Latif et al., 1974; Lapetina and Michell, 1974; Schacht and Agranoff, 1974; Fisher and Agranoff, 1981). The failure to detect receptor-mediated PI breakdown in brain might indicate that the pool associated with enhanced turnover is a small fraction of the total tissue PI. It is alternatively possible that the initial event in stimulated phospholipid turnover is not the breakdown of PI, but rather of PIP and PIP_2 (see Section 7.3.3). As a consequence of the absence of measurable chemical or radiochemical breakdown of the phosphoinositides in brain-derived preparations, studies on stimulated lipid turnover in neural preparations have thus largely remained restricted to labeling experiments. Although the use of the labeling approach has been criticized (Michell and Kirk, 1981), the fact remains that an increase in the labeling of PI and often PA as well is observed in those tissues in which PI breakdown can also be demonstrated chemically, indicating the operation of a PA-phosphoinositide cycle, for example, in neutrophils (Cockcroft et al., 1980a,b, 1981), pancreas (Hokin-Neaverson, 1977), hepatocyte (Billah and Michell, 1979), parotid gland (Weiss and Putney, 1981), and ileum (Michell et al., 1976). An exception to this generalization is 5-HT activated breakdown of PI in the blowfly salivary gland, which is not accompanied by increased relabeling of PI or PA. Where investigated, the concentrations of agonists required to elicit increased PI breakdown and labeling are also comparable (Michell et al, 1976; Billah and Michell, 1979; Jones et al., 1979; Kirk et al., 1981a). Furthermore, although increased labeling of PI occurs well after the initial breakdown of an inositol phospholipid, the appearance of label in PA is kinetically indistinguishable from phosphoinositide breakdown (Bell and Majerus, 1979; Lapetina and Cuatrecasas, 1979; Salmon and Honeyman, 1980; Cockcroft et al., 1980b). The problems associated with either the labeling or prelabeling approach may in the future be circumvented by measurement of the release of water-soluble inositol phosphates rather than by changes in the label associated with the individual phospholipids. This has been made feasible by the observation that the inclusion of lithium ions inhibits inositol 1-phosphatase, thus permitting the measurement of inositol monophosphate (Hallcher and Sherman, 1980). When assayed under such conditions, the addition of appropriate agonists to brain slices results in an increased accumulation of inositol monophosphate, reflecting an enhanced inositol phospholipid breakdown (Berridge et al., 1982; Daum et al, 1983; Watson and Downes, 1983; Fisher et al., 1984b). Although the accumulation of inositol monophosphate could result from the phosphodiesteratic cleavage of PI, an alterative possibility involves an initial release of inositol trisphosphate and/or inositol bisphosphate from polyphosphoinositide breakdown and degradation to inositol monophosphate by phosphatases. The latter explanation has recently gained support from the experiments of Berridge (1983) and Downes and Wuseman (1983) in nonneural preparations.

The nature of neural preparations may favor the measurement of those aspects of PA and phosphoinositide metabolism directly related to the initial receptor–ligand interaction at the plasma membrane in the absence of subsequent events in phospholipid turnover at other intracellular loci. Such may not be the case for secretory events, for example, thrombin stimulation of platelets and secretagogue stimulation of pancreas.

7.4. CELLULAR AND SUBCELLULAR LOCALIZATION OF ENHANCED PHOSPHOLIPID TURNOVER

The receptor–ligand interaction takes place at the outer plasma membrane while it is presumed that the inner leaflet is the principal locus of the enzymes and substrates participating in the initiation of stimulated phospholipid labeling. The questions arise of whether other subcellular components play an important role and which neuronal or possibly even glial elements mediate the effect. The answers to these questions bear directly on the elucidation of the physiological significance of the effect.

7.4.1 Neuronal, Glial, or Both?

Despite the fact that the number of glia present in the adult mammalian brain may exceed by several-fold the number of neurons (Cragg, 1968), few studies have attempted to measure the possible contribution made by glia to enhanced phospholipid turnover. Woelk et al. (1974) administered $^{32}P_i$ intracisternally to rats and, following sacrifice 5–60 min later, isolated neuronal- and glial-enriched fractions, which were then assessed for purity by measurement of the activity of the base-exchange enzymes, believed to be exclusively located in neurons (Goracci et al., 1973). The incorporation of $^{32}P_i$ into phospholipids occurred more rapidly in neurons than in the glia, with PI being the most actively labeled lipid in both cell types. Norepinephrine increased the incorporation of $^{32}P_i$ into PI in *both* neurons and glia but had no stimulatory effect on the incorporation of label into sphingomyelin, phosphatidylcholine, or ethanolamine plasmalogens. These results, taken at face value, would indicate a similar capacity of both neurons and glia to respond to norepinephrine. A similar conclusion was reached by Abdel-Latif et al. (1974) from experiments in which neuronal- and glial cell–enriched fractions were obtained from slices of cerebral cortex that had previously been incubated in the presence of $^{32}P_i$. In these experiments Ach, 5-hydroxytryptamine, norepinephrine, and dopamine all increased the incorporation of $^{32}P_i$ into PA and PI in both neurons and glia, although the effect was less marked for glial cells. It is difficult to reconcile these results with more recent evidence pointing to a predominantly neuronal localization of α_1-adrenergic receptors and muscarinic cholinergic receptors in brain. Perhaps the most direct evidence for a neuronal locus of the muscarinic stimulation of phospholipid labeling is the finding that preparations from hippocampus previously lesioned with the excitatory neurotoxin ibotenate result in a loss of stimulated PA and PI labeling (see Section 7.4.3).

7.4.2 Subcellular Locus

While broken cells do not exhibit a receptor-mediated stimulation of PA and PI labeling, two experimental approaches have been taken to determine the subcellular localization of the effect. In the first, the intact neural preparations are either labeled with $^{32}P_i$ in the presence and absence of an agonist or are prelabeled with $^{32}P_i$ followed by the addition of an agonist, usually under "pulse-chase" conditions. Subcellular fractions are then analyzed. The second experimental approach attempts to localize the effect by isolating subcellular fractions that still mediate stimulated labeling. While the use of broken preparations might appear to negate the aforementioned requirement for structural integrity, neural tissues are an exception in this regard, since homogenization of brain results in the formation of nerve-ending particles, which may be considered resealed anucleate neurons.

Studies that have employed the first approach have not given a clear indication of a subcellular locus for enhanced phospholipid turnover. Lapetina and Michell (1972) and Abdel-Latif et al. (1974) observed that following incubation of prelabeled rat cortical slices, increased incorporation of $^{32}P_i$ into PI was observed equally in all subcellular fractions. Similarly, Eichberg et al. (1973) observed that the increased incorporation of $^{32}P_i$ into PI in norepinephrine-stimulated pineal glands was relatively unlocalized. Only in the electrically stimulated superior cervical ganglion was there an indication of a subcellular localization of the response. In these experiments Burt and Larrabee (1973) found the largest increase in PI labeling in bands associated with the nerve endings and mitochondria. Recently Azila and Hawthorne (1982), in an attempt to localize the subcellular site from which prelabeled lipid is lost following the addition of agonists to perfused bovine adrenal medulla, observed a rapid loss of prelabeled PA and PI from all subcellular locations (chromaffin granules, plasma membranes, microsomes, and mitochondria) on addition of carbamylcholine. A central problem with all studies in which labeled tissue is fractionated, and which may seriously limit this approach, is that the initial loss of labeled phospholipid (presumably from the plasma membrane) may be followed by a rapid reequilibration of lipids throughout the cell. In both intact cells and in subcellular fractions, the logistics of intracellular phospholipid transport must be considered (Fig. 7.2).

In regard to the second approach, the Hokins first observed increased turnover of PA in "microsomal" fractions of brain homogenates in response to added Ach (Hokin and Hokin, 1958c). Subsequently, Redman and Hokin (1964) obtained a stimulation of both PA and PI labeling in a "cytoplasmic" (postnuclear) fraction from guinea pig cerebral cortex. On the basis of a $^{32}P_i$ labeling study in the absence of stimulation, Durrell and Sodd (1964) suggested that a "synaptosomal" fraction might mediate the stimulated labeling seen in brain homogenates. Ach stimulation of both PA and PI labeling was indeed localized to a "light" nerve-ending fraction which banded at 1.1 M sucrose (Schacht and Agranoff, 1972). Nuclear, mitochondrial, myelin, and microsomal fractions possessed little ability to incorporate $^{32}P_i$ into PA and PI and did not respond to the addition of Ach. The localization of stimulated PA labeling to a nerve-ending fraction was also reported by Yagihara and Hawthorne (1972), and subsequent studies have also indicated the response to be enriched in nerve-ending fractions (Miller, 1977; Yandrasitz and Segal, 1979; Aly and Abdel-Latif, 1982). Attempts to further localize stimulated labeling in nerve-ending subfractions have been only partially successful. Schacht et al. (1974) labeled nerve-ending fractions with $^{32}P_i$ and, following osmotic lysis, fractionated the tissue on a discontinuous sucrose density gradient. Both PA and PI incremental labeling was greatest in fractions judged to be plasma membrane from morphological and enzyme marker studies. Results obtained by Yagihara et al. (1973) and Bleasdale and Hawthorne (1975) differed in that the increased PA labeling was primarily localized to the synaptic vesicle fraction. The reasons for these inconsistencies are not obvious. The plasma membrane localization of labeled PA is in accord with the known location of diacylglycerol kinase (Section 1.3). On the other hand, since the synaptic vesicle membrane would be expected to fuse with the plasma membrane during exocytosis (Fried and Blaustein, 1973), the composition of these two membranes might be predicted to be similar. As yet, there is no evidence for subsynaptosomal localization of initial inositol phospholipid breakdown in response to agonists.

7.4.3   Is the Site of Enhanced Phospholipid Turnover Pre- or Postsynaptic?

Conceivably, both presynaptic and postsynaptic receptors could be coupled to phospholipid turnover. However, in three experimental preparations, the superior cervical ganglion, the pineal gland, and the hippocampus, in which this question has been addressed, the evidence points to a postsynaptic location for the receptors involved.

The superior cervical ganglion preparation has proven particularly useful in studying this question. Hokin (1965) observed that when cat superior cervical ganglion slices were incubated with [^{3}H]myo-inositol and stimulated by the addition of Ach, much of the increase in the water-insoluble (i.e., lipid-bound) radioactivity was associated with the cell body, as determined autoradiographically. In a subsequent study Hokin (1966) found that removal of the cervical sympathetic trunk, which resulted in the degeneration of presynaptic elements within 2 weeks, failed to appreciably reduce the stimulation of PI labeling in ganglionic slices in response to Ach. The response of the superior cervical ganglion to NGF also appears to be postsynaptic (Lakshmanan, 1978b, 1979). NGF addition to the ganglion resulted in a 151–156% stimulation of labeled inositol incorporation into PI, and this was not diminished by prior central denervation of the superior cervical ganglion. A postsynaptic locus is also indicated for the α_1-adrenergic receptors coupled to PI turnover in the pineal gland. Berg and Klein (1972) showed that norepinephrine stimulation of PI labeling was unaffected by prior superior cervical ganglionectomy. In a later study Smith et al. (1979) detected no reduction of stimulated PI turnover in pineals of rats that had been injected intracerebrally with 6-hydroxydopamine at birth. This treatment should result in the degeneration of presynaptic noradrenergic nerve endings. Pineal dispersions prepared by collagenase and hyaluronidase digestion (and essentially free of presynaptic nerve endings) also responded well to norepinephrine addition. Furthermore, adrenergic agonists with known preferences for postsynaptic receptors, such as phenylephrine and methoxamine, are markedly more effective stimulators of PI turnover than agonists with a preference for presynaptic receptors such as ergometrine and clonidine. These various surgical and pharmacological approaches provide consistent evidence for a postsynaptic location for the norepinephrine-mediated stimulation of phospholipid turnover in the pineal gland.

The suggestion that stimulated PI turnover in these tissues is characteristically postsynaptic is at odds with arguments that have supported a presynaptic locus of the effect in nerve-ending preparations. For example, electron microscopy of nerve-ending fractions used in labeling studies

TABLE 7.4   Alterations in Stimulated PA and PI Labeling and Cholinergic
Parameters following Fornix/Fimbria or Ibotenate Lesions of Hippocampus[a]

Parameter	Fornix/Fimbria Percent Change	Ibotenate Percent Change
Stimulated PA Labeling	N.S.	−45
Stimulated PI Labeling	N.S.	−40
Choline Acetyltransferase	−72	N.S.
Acetylcholinesterase	−56	Not Determined
[³H]QNB	N.S.	−42
Glutamate Decarboxylase	N.S.	−30

[a] Data are based on Fisher et al., 1980, 1981b, N.S., not statistically significant; QNB,
quinuclidinylbenzilate.

indicate a predominance of "synaptosomes," structures that contain mitochondria, synaptic vesicles, and a limited amount of smooth endoplasmic reticulum. The light synaptosomal fraction contained relatively few attached fragments of postsynaptic membrane from the efferent cell body, dendrite, or axon (Schacht et al., 1974). In addition [^{32}P]ATP must be generated from the added $^{32}P_i$ inside the nerve-ending particle and is therefore presumably not accessible to the postsynaptic fragments. From these considerations, and the known existence of presynaptic muscarinic autoreceptors, it seemed reasonable that the muscarinic stimulation of PA and PI turnover in the nerve-ending preparations was presynaptic.

Recent experiments employing nerve-ending fractions prepared from the hippocampus, however, have cast doubt on this interpretation. The hippocampus represents a specialized region of the cerebral cortex and has the considerable experimental advantage that virtually all of its cholinergic input is derived from the septal nuclei and arrives via a single well-defined anatomical tract, the fimbria. This fiber tract may be readily lesioned, either electrolytically or surgically, and the presynaptic cholinergic input to the hippocampus degenerates within a few days. Nerve-ending fractions prepared from guinea pig hippocampus 10 days following lesion showed a marked reduction in the presynaptic marker enzymes cholineacetyltransferase and acetylcholinesterase, but not in either [³H]QNB binding or in the magnitude of stimulation of PA or PI labeling in response to added Ach (Fisher et al., 1980; Table 7.4). These results indicate that the majority of muscarinic receptors present in nerve-ending fractions are not located on cholinergic nerve terminals and that the stimulated turnover of PA and PI is associated with a structure that is postsynaptic to the site of Ach release. More direct support for this assertion came from experiments utilizing the neurotoxin, ibotenic acid. This agent selectively destroys intrinsic cell bodies of the hippocampus, while leaving the presynaptic terminals intact (Schwarcz et al., 1979). Destruction of hippocampal neurons was effected by stereotaxic injection of ibotenate on one side of the hippocampus, the other side serving as a control. Twelve days after injection histological examination revealed that the lesioned side was markedly shrunken in appearance, with an extensive loss of nerve cells from both the hippocampus and dentate gyrus. [³H]QNB autoradiography also revealed a parallel loss of muscarinic receptors from the lesioned side (Fisher et al., 1981). In nerve-ending preparations obtained from the ibotenate-lesioned hippocampus, there was a marked reduction in carbamylcholine-stimulated PA and PI labeling, consistent with the loss of [³H]QNB binding (45–50%). Basal phospholipid labeling (i.e., the incorporation of $^{32}P_i$ into phospholipids in the absence of agonist) based on protein content was not impaired. Nor was there a reduction in cholineacetyltransferase activity, in confirmation of the selective action of the neurotoxin. The results suggest then that the muscarinic receptors mediating the observed stimulation of PA and PI labeling in these nerve-ending preparations are derived from postsynaptic (cholinoceptive) structures. They additionally confirm the neuronal localization of the response, since glia are not destroyed by ibotenate (see Section 7.4.1).

We are thus left with the problem of how to reconcile these results with the "textbook" nerve-ending preparation whose contents are separated from the postsynaptic cell by the synaptic cleft. A possible explanation is offered in Figure 7.3, where A is a cholinergic nerve ending, B is a nerve ending derived from an intrinsic neuron within the hippocampus that makes an axoaxonal synaptic connection with A, and C is a dendritic process from a postsynaptic cell. The particles are presumed to fragment and reseal upon homogenization at sites indicated by the dotted lines. Since the fimbrial lesion has no effect on stimulated PA and PI turnover while ibotenate does, the muscarinic receptors must reside in either neuron B or C. Is there any evidence to favor a dendritic rather than a "synaptosomal" location for these receptors? In an autoradiographic study (Kuhar and Yamamura, 1976) muscarinic receptors were found to be especially concentrated over dendritic fields. This raises the possibility that dendrites break off during homogenization of the hippocampus to form "dendrosomes," and these resealed structures account for the presence of the muscarinic receptors in nerve-ending fractions that are coupled to phospholipid turnover. The formation of "dendrosomes" has previously been observed in the substantia nigra (Hefti and Lichtensteiger, 1978). Muscarinic receptors are also thought to exist (as typified by neuron B) on noradrenergic, serotonergic, and dopaminergic nerve endings (Gior-

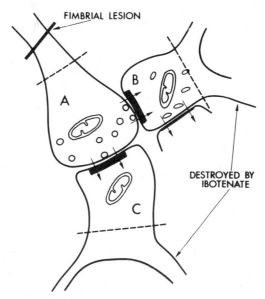

FIGURE 7.3 Synaptic interrelationships in the hippocampus may explain the results of lesions on stimulated labeling in nerve-ending fractions. (A) A cholinergic nerve terminal whose cell body is outside of the hippocampus. It forms a synapse with intrinsic neurons of the hippocampus axoaxonally (B) or axodendritically (C). On homogenization these fragments break off and are resealed, as indicated by the dashed lines. See test.

guieff et al., 1977; Hery et al., 1977; de Belleroche and Bradford, 1978; Ganguly and Das, 1979). However, both the previous demonstrations of an extrinsic origin for noradrenergic and serotonergic fiber tracts in the hippocampus (Storm-Mathisen and Guldberg, 1974; Schwarcz et al., 1979) and the location of muscarinic receptors to intrinsic cells from ibotenate lesion experiments imply that muscarinic receptors are not present to a significant extent on nerve endings derived from these tracts. At present the explanation most consistent with our results is that muscarinic receptors coupled to phospholipid turnover are present on resealed dendritic fragments. In any case, it may be concluded that the physiological significance of stimulated phospholipid labeling by muscarinic agonists is related to events that directly mediate or modulate the activity of cholinoceptive neurons.

7.5   FUNCTIONAL SIGNIFICANCE OF ENHANCED PHOSPHOLIPID TURNOVER

While there is overwhelming evidence that enhanced labeling of PA and PI reflects a receptor–ligand interaction, it is by no means established

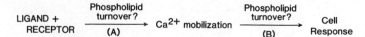

FIGURE 7.4 Possible sequential relationships between stimulated phospholipid turnover, Ca^{2+} mobilization, and cellular responses. Stimulated phospholipid turnover may (A) precede Ca^{2+} mobilization (Michell, 1975), (B) result from an increase in intracellular Ca^{2+} concentration (Cockcroft et al., 1981), or alternatively, not be a causally related concomitant of receptor activation or of Ca^{2+} mobilization.

whether the phenomenon plays an obligatory role in the physiological consequences of receptor occupancy. Current hypotheses on the function of stimulated labeling are based primarily on the extraneural systems emphasized in this section.

7.5.1 Does Stimulated Turnover Regulate a Calcium Gate or Is It the Result of Calcium Mobilization—or Neither?

In 1975 Michell proposed a hypothesis that ascribed a common biochemical function to the enhanced phospholipid turnover demonstrable in a diverse range of tissues (see Fig. 7.4). Included in his compendium were examples of stimulated PI and PA labeling from $^{32}P_i$, of [^{3}H]*myo*-inositol incorporation into PI, and of changes in the measured amounts of PI and PA observed in the absence of added radioactive precursors. He observed that the various responses were often triggered by receptors whose activation controls a rise in intracellular Ca^{2+}, whereas other receptors linked to different effector systems (e.g., β-adrenergic receptors and adenylate cyclase) do not elicit increased phospholipid turnover. In the tissues originally investigated both PI labeling and breakdown were found to be considerably less sensitive to Ca^{2+} depletion or addition than the attendant physiological responses, e.g., secretion or contraction (Michell, 1979). Similarly, the concentrations of agonist required for maximal PI turnover were considerably higher than those needed to induce the full physiological effect. These high concentrations were similar to those required for full occupancy of the receptor by the agonist (Michell et al., 1976; Fig. 7.5). The observation of maximal physiological response at a fractional occupancy of the receptor population is indicative of the regulatory properties of second messenger systems (Berridge, 1981). From this Michell proposed that phospholipid turnover precedes Ca^{2+} influx and constitutes a biochemical mechanism responsible for Ca^{2+} gating at the plasma membrane. How has this hypothesis fared since 1975? There has been both supportive and contradictory evidence. In preparations derived from such tissues as the insect salivary gland, lacrimal gland,

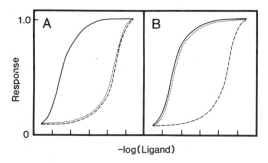

FIGURE 7.5 Diagrammatic representations of differences in receptor occupancy require-ments for stimulated labeling. (*a*) A tissue in which receptor occupancy and phospholipid turnover are closely correlated (e.g., muscarinic stimulation of PI turnover in the ileum) and (*b*) one in which it is not (e.g., neutrophils stimulated by chemotactic peptide): ——, physiological response (contraction, secretion, etc.); -----, receptor occupancy curve; . . . . ., stimulated phospholipid turnover (breakdown or labeling).

parotid, and ileum as well as in the hepatocyte, receptor-linked changes in PI turnover are claimed to be relatively independent of Ca^{2+} availability (Michell, 1979; Michell and Kirk, 1981). Ca^{2+} insensitivity, often taken as support for the Ca^{2+} gating hypothesis, is not always demonstrable (Cockcroft, 1981; Prpić et al., 1982). The hypothesis also predicts that the agonist concentration requirement for enhanced PI turnover should closely match that for receptor occupancy, but this too is not observed invariably (Michell et al., 1976; Kirk et al., 1981b; Weiss and Putney, 1981). Perhaps the most direct support of the hypothesis comes from the demonstration that the ability of the insect salivary gland to gate Ca^{2+} is directly related to the content of membrane PI (Berridge and Fain, 1979; Fain and Berridge, 1979).

In pancreas (Farese et al., 1980, 1982), iris smooth muscle (Akhtar and Abdel-Latiff, 1980), and neutrophils (Cockcroft et al., 1980a,b, 1981), enhanced phospholipid turnover is dependent on the presence of extra-cellular Ca^{2+} and can be mimicked by addition of divalent cation ion-ophores such as A23187 or ionomycin. There is also evidence that for neutrophils stimulated by the chemotactic peptide f-met-leu-phe, en-hanced phospholipid turnover shows "receptor reserve," which would not be expected were stimulated phospholipid turnover intrinsic to the consequence of occupation of these receptors (Cockcroft et al., 1981b; Fig. 7.5b). In these tissues, then, the alterations of PA and PI turnover could be construed to result from Ca^{2+} mobilization rather than the re-verse. It now seems unlikely that there is a single causal relationship between phospholipid labeling and Ca^{2+} entry into cells, even though it may prove ultimately to be the case in some tissues (see Hawthorne and Pickard, 1979; Hawthorne, 1982; and Michell, 1982).

The possible role of Ca^{2+} in stimulated phospholipid labeling in the nervous system has been extensively investigated in isolated nerve-ending preparations. Although added Ca^{2+} is not required for demonstration of the muscarinic stimulation of PA and PI labeling, removal of endogenous Ca^{2+} with a chelator such as EDTA or EGTA severely inhibits or abolishes the response to added Ach (Schacht and Agranoff, 1972; Griffin et al., 1979; Fisher and Agranoff, 1980). Moreover, addition of A23187 or ionomycin, both of which can raise intracellular Ca^{2+}, results in a selective stimulation of PA and PI labeling comparable in magnitude to that resulting from Ach addition (Griffin and Hawthorne, 1978; Fisher and Agranoff, 1980, 1981). Although these results might be interpreted to mean that muscarinic receptors in the CNS (like many outside the CNS) are coupled to Ca^{2+} influx and that the rise in intracellular Ca^{2+} leads to stimulated phospholipid labeling, there are other possible explanations. First, in addition to reducing the availability of extracellular Ca^{2+}, EGTA may deplete nerve-ending preparations of intracellular Ca^{2+} stores. It is thus uncertain whether the requirement for Ca^{2+} in stimulated labeling is intra- or extracellular (I. D. Scott et al., 1980). The concentration of Ca^{2+} required for measurable enhanced phospholipid labeling inferred from EDTA or EGTA-Ca^{2+} buffer mixtures is less than 10^{-6} M (see Section 7.3.3). This concentration of Ca^{2+} approximates that found in the cytosol and is considerably lower than that required for elicitation of stimulated phospholipid turnover in iris smooth muscle (Akhtar and Abdel-Latif, 1980), pancreas (Farese et al., 1980), or neutrophils (Cockcroft et al., 1980a,b, 1981). Second, there is as yet no direct evidence that muscarinic receptors in excitable tissues are linked to Ca^{2+} influx (Snider et al., 1984). Sokolovsky and Bartfai (1981) also found no link between activation of muscarinic receptors in *Torpedo* synaptosomes and Ca^{2+} influx, and we have been unable to find such evidence in nerve-ending preparations from mammalian brain (L. A. A. Van Rooijen and B. W. Agranoff, submitted). Similarly, the muscarinic stimulation of PA and PI turnover in adrenal medulla does not require added Ca^{2+}, even though the response is strongly inhibited by addition of EGTA (Trifaro, 1969b; Fisher et al., 1981; Azila and Hawthorne, 1982). In this tissue nicotinic (and not muscarinic) receptors are linked to Ca^{2+} influx, not stimulated phospholipid labeling (Kilpatrick et al., 1980; Fisher et al., 1981a). Furthermore, muscarinic receptor activation in the bovine adrenal medulla results in an inhibition of stimulated catecholamine release (Swilem et al., 1983). Taken together, the results from nerve-ending and adrenal medulla preparations indicate that the maintenance of some minimal level of intracellular Ca^{2+} is necessary for evocation of stimulated phospholipid labeling, but there is little reason at present to suggest that the response in these tissues is dependent on calcium influx or mobilization.

7.5.2 Production of Phosphatidate: An Endogenous Calcium Ionophore?

Of possible relevance to the significance of stimulated phospholipid labeling is the suggestion that PA is an endogenous Ca^{2+} ionophore and might mediate Ca^{2+} mobilization in those tissues in which phospholipid turnover appears to be followed by Ca^{2+} influx. PA has been shown to function as a Ca^{2+} ionophore in Pressman chamber experiments (Tyson et al., 1976) and in multilamellar liposomes (Serhan et al., 1981). Recent evidence indicates a role for PA in cellular Ca^{2+} translocation. Salmon and Honeyman (1980) found that when Ach was added to smooth muscle cells, there was a measurable increase in the chemical amount of PA within 10 s and that the contractile response of the cells could be mimicked by exogenously applied PA (10^{-8}–10^{-6} M). Experiments performed with the rat parotid gland provide additional support. Putney et al. (1980) found that added PA (10^{-5} M) stimulates Ca^{2+}-dependent $^{86}Rb^+$ release in a manner analogous to that of Ach, with the exception that the effect of PA is independent of the muscarinic receptor and is not blocked by inclusion of atropine. PA has no effect on $^{86}Rb^+$ release when Ca^{2+} is omitted. The effects of several Ca^{2+} antagonists on PA-dependent partitioning of $^{45}Ca^{2+}$ from an aqueous to an organic phase was also examined. Calculation of the effectiveness of these antagonists in blocking the binding of Ca^{2+} to the negatively charged headgroup of PA gives values that strongly correlate with pharmacological estimates of the dissociation constants of these antagonists for cholinergically activated Ca^{2+} channels (Putney et al., 1980). There is also evidence that PA can act as a Ca^{2+} ionophore in neural preparations. Harris et al. (1981) found that added PA (but not other phospholipids) stimulates both the uptake of $^{45}Ca^{2+}$ by nerve terminals isolated from striatum and the release of [^{3}H]dopamine. From these results they suggest that PA may act as a Ca^{2+} ionophore and serve as a link between depolarization and neurotransmitter release. Exogenously added PA also results in a stimulation of Ca^{2+} influx and cGMP accumulation, when applied to neuroblastoma N1E115 cells (Ohsako and Deguchi, 1981). While the hypothesis that PA serves as a biological ionophore is attractive and might be considered to provide support for the Ca^{2+} gating hypothesis, certain difficulties exist. First, the effects of exogenously added PA are often unpredictable. For example, PA addition does not activate K^+ release from lacrimal gland slices (Putney, 1981), nor does it cause intact platelets to aggregate (Gerrard et al., 1978). Second, in some instances enhanced PA labeling is not paralleled by an increase in its *chemical* amount, for example, in nerve-ending preparations, iris smooth muscle, and adrenal medulla. For these tissues a highly localized increase in PA content within the membrane must be envisaged for the hypothesis to be tenable. Third, PA production in response to f-met-leu-phe addition to neutrophils occurs too slowly to account for the onset of Ca^{2+}-activated lysosomal enzyme release (Cockcroft et al., 1980b).

7.5.3   Generation of Inositol Trisphosphate: An Intracellular Second Messenger?

An attractive hypothesis that seeks to explain the close association between calcium mobilization and stimulated inositol lipid turnover invokes a product of PIP_2 breakdown—inositol trisphosphate. Streb et al. (1983) have shown that the addition of micromolar concentrations of inositol trisphosphate to pancreatic acinar cells made "leaky" by washing in a Ca^{2+}-free buffer stimulates the efflux of intracellular calcium from nonmitochondrial sources. Only inositol trisphosphate acts to release intracellular Ca^{2+}; inositol mono- and bisphosphate are ineffective, while chemically induced randomization of the phosphate groups on the inositol ring of inositol trisphosphate markedly reduces efficacy. Similar results have been obtained from saponin-permeabilized hepatocyte preparations (Joseph et al., 1984). Given the rapid release and degradation of inositol trisphosphate in hormonally stimulated cells (Berridge, 1983) and its specificity of action, the role of inositol trisphosphate as a second messenger in calcium mobilization will undoubtedly attract further investigation.

7.5.4   Does Inositol Phospholipid Hydrolysis Modulate the Activities of Enzymes in the Plasma Membrane?

There is increasing evidence that some muscarinic receptors are not coupled to Ca^{2+} fluxes but appear to modulate the activity of adenylate cyclase, an enzyme regulated by other receptor–ligand activations (Berridge, 1980; Jacobs et al., 1980). Cockcroft (1982) has suggested that this inhibition of adenylate cyclase might be accomplished through the hydrolysis of PI, which is thought to anchor the cyclase within the membrane. PI-phospholipase C treatment of membranes has indeed been shown to result in a selective loss of certain enzymes (Low and Finean, 1978; Low and Zilversmit, 1980), and Panagia et al. (1981) demonstrated a loss of adenylate cyclase activity following PI hydrolysis in heart sar-

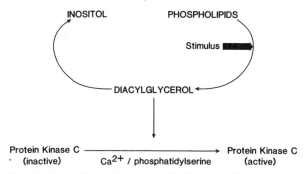

FIGURE 7.6 Possible interrelationship between lipid and protein phosphorylation. See text.

colemmal membranes as well as restoration of activity when PI-depleted membranes were recombined with supernatant.

7.5.5 Production of Diacylglycerol: A Link between Lipid and Protein Phosphorylation?

In many tissues in which cell surface receptors are coupled to increased PA and PI labeling, there is an increase in the phosphorylation of specific proteins. Thus, the demonstration in several tissues of a novel protein kinase (protein kinase C) that is Ca^{2+} dependent ($K_a = 10^{-5}\,M$) and also requires the presence of membrane lipid to become fully active was of particular interest (Takai et al., 1979a,b; Minakuchi et al., 1981; Tanigawa et al., 1982; Nishizuka, 1983). Phosphatidylserine is an effective activator, and the additional presence of diacylglycerol with at least one unsaturated fatty acid in either the C1 or C2 position is also required for full expression (Mori et al., 1982). Diacylglycerol is difficult to detect in resting cells, but a variety of ligands that initiate the breakdown of inositol phospholipids presumably result in a transient increase in diacylglycerol availability. Increases in diacylglycerol have been reported in platelets (Rittenhouse-Simmons, 1979), pancreas (Banschbach et al., 1981), and mast cells (Kennerly et al., 1979a). A sequence of events can be proposed to link initial changes in inositol phospholipid turnover with subsequent alterations in protein phosphorylation (see Fig. 7.6). In the platelet thrombin activation results in a selective phosphorylation of a 40,000 molecular weight polypeptide following an initial accumulation of diacylglycerol (Kawahara et al., 1980). However, in other tissues, such as nerve endings, neither Ach nor norepinephrine addition result in an increase in protein phosphorylation (Krueger et al., 1977). Similarly, in dissociated avian salt gland cells muscarinic receptor activation results in a marked increase in

PA labeling but has no detectable effect on protein phosphorylation (Fisher et al., 1983b).

7.5.6   Does Polyphosphoinositide Turnover Mediate Ion Fluxes at the Plasma Membrane?

In brain polyphosphoinositides are believed to be present exclusively in plasma membrane fractions, including the myelin membrane. The myelin pool appears to be relatively stable while that in the remaining plasma membrane disappears rapidly postmortem (Eichberg and Hauser, 1973) and may constitute a fraction of the polyphosphoinositides under neuroeffector control (see Section 7.3.3). PIP and PIP_2 have been suggested as mediators of the propagation of the nerve action potential based on their plasma membrane location and the observation that both bind considerable amounts of divalent cations, especially Ca^{2+} (Kerr et al., 1964; Eichberg and Dawson, 1965). PIP–PIP_2 interconversions could regulate the amount of Ca^{2+} bound to a specific membrane site and thus affect the opening and closing of Na^+ and K^+ channels. In support of this is the calculation by Hendrickson and Reinertsen (1971) that conversion of PIP_2 to PIP would result in the release of 70% of plasma membrane–bound Ca^{2+}. Hawthorne and Kai (1970) proposed a model whereby changes in the $PIP_2 \rightleftharpoons PIP \rightleftharpoons PI$ equilibrium would result in an altered ion permeability of the membrane. The key transformation was thought to be conversion of either PIP_2 or PIP, both having high affinity for Ca^{2+} to PI, a lipid with low Ca^{2+} affinity. Ca^{2+} would form a bridge between molecules of PIP and/or PIP_2, and its removal (following phosphomonesteratic or phosphodiesteratic cleavage of these lipids) would result in the opening of a channel. There seems little doubt that inositol phospholipid interconversions can lead to changes in Ca^{2+} binding by membranes, as has been shown in erythrocyte preparations (Buckley and Hawthorne, 1972), in which the amount of Ca^{2+} bound to erythrocyte membranes increased in parallel with the incorporation of $^{32}P_i$ into the polyphosphoinositides. There remains the question of how responsive the polyphosphoinositides are to nerve conduction. Results from studies employing electrical stimulation techniques yield conflicting results. Thus, on electrical stimulation of the vagus nerve, PIP_2 labeling is reported to increase (White et al., 1974), decrease (White and Larrabee, 1973), or remain unchanged (Salway and Hughes, 1972). Birnbirger et al. (1971) observed a loss of label from PIP_2 on electrical stimulation of lobster nerves, while Tret'jak et al. (1977) noted an increase in PIP_2 labeling after stimulation of crab nerve fibers. Recently evidence in favor of a role for PIP and PIP_2 in impulse conduction has emerged from studies with an unusual tissue—the auditory organ of the noctuid moth. Kilian and Schacht (1979) found that both the scoloparium (sensory cells) and the nodular sclerite (strip of cuticle adjacent to the tympanic membrane) rapidly incorporate $^{32}P_i$ into PIP and PIP_2, with considerably less incorporation into other phospholipids. When "labeled moths" were stimulated with a pulse-tone signal (40 kHz, 75 dB), $^{32}P_i$ incorporation into both PIP and PIP_2 increased in the scoloparium but not in the nodular sclerite. The application of a continuous tone, which results in a rapid adaptation of spike activity, did not increase $^{32}P_i$ incorporation, indicating that the alterations of poly-phosphoinositide labeling correlate with the propagation of action potentials.

Additional evidence to suggest a role for the polyphosphoinositides in nerve conduction comes from studies on sciatic nerves of diabetic rats treated with streptozotocin. Human diabetic neuropathy is characterized by a reduction in nerve conduction velocity, segmental demyelination, and axonal loss. Most, if not all, of these characteristics have also been observed in chemically induced diabetes. Possible involvement of PI turnover in this deficiency has been considered (Palmano et al., 1977; Whiting et al., 1979). Natarajan et al. (1981) observed that sciatic nerves derived from streptozotocin-treated rats incorporated substantially less $^{32}P_i$ into PIP_2, PIP, and PI than the controls, although somewhat different results were obtained by Bell et al. (1982).

7.5.7 Is Enhanced Phospholipid Labeling Related to Arachidonate Metabolism?

The bulk of arachidonate in mammalian cells is located in the 2-acyl position of phospholipids, and virtually none is in the free state (Bills et al., 1977; Wolfe, 1982). In PI the fatty acid at C1 is usually stearate when arachidonate is at C2. PI shows the greatest enrichment of arachidonate on a mole-fraction basis, while the largest *amounts* of cellular arachidonate are in the three other phospholipids, phosphatidylcholine, phosphatidylethanolamine, and its plasmalogen form. Because of its enrichment in arachidonate, it is not surprising that stimulated PI turnover has been implicated in the release of this fatty acid, and its subsequent conversion into prostaglandins, thromboxanes, and leukotrienes (Bell et al., 1979). Deacylation is considered to be rate limiting in prostanoid synthesis (Irvine, 1982) and may occur either by means of phospholipase A_2 action on PI (Bills et al., 1977) or via the action of either diacylglycerol lipase following phosphodiesteratic cleavage of PI to diacylglycerol (Bell et al., 1979) or PA-specific phospholipase A_2 (Billah et al., 1981) following conversion of the released diacylglycerol to PA. PI hydrolysis may thus play an important role in the regulation of synthesis of prostaglandins and related metabolites. In several secretory tissues arachidonate-derived metabolites are released in response to activation of the same receptor class that elicits an increased PI turnover, for example, muscarinic cholinergic in the pancreas (Banschbach and Hokin-Neaverson, 1980; Marshall et al., 1981), thrombin in platelets (Lapetina and Cuatrecasas, 1979), f-met-leu-phe in neutrophils (Cockcroft et al., 1980a,b, 1981; Walsh et al., 1981), and anti-IgE in mast cells (Kennerly et al., 1979b,c; Schellenberg, 1980; Stenson et al., 1980). While circumstantial evidence has led to the suggestion that arachidonate release and prostaglandin formation are a causal link between receptor–ligand-mediated phospholipid turnover and stimulus–secretion coupling (Marshall et al., 1981), a number of counterarguments can be raised (Cockcroft, 1981; Putney, 1981; Irvine, 1982; Neufeld and Majerus, 1983). A major objection is that the amount of PI broken down in both thrombin-stimulated platelets and muscarinic stimulation of pancreas is compensated for by a near-quantitative increase in the amount of PA and/or diacylglycerol produced (Geison et al., 1976; Rittenhouse-Simmons, 1979; Bell and Majerus, 1979; Broekman et al., 1980; Prescott and Majerus, 1981). The conservation predicted by a PA-PI cycle was convincingly demonstrated by Broekman et al. (1981) who compared the amounts of fatty acids in the individual lipids with that liberated after application of thrombin to platelets. At a time during which arachidonate release was clearly observed, no *net* loss of arachidonate was observed from PA + PI. Also, in macrophages the arachidonate present in PI is insufficient to account for the amount of arachidonate mobilized (W. A. Scott et al., 1980; Cockcroft, 1981). In both platelets and neutrophils arachidonate is lost from phosphatidylcholine and phosphatidylethanolamine, two lipids that do not participate in enhanced phospholipid turnover (Walsh et al., 1981; Broekman et al., 1981; McKean et al., 1981). It can be concluded from these experiments that the principal phospholipid reservoir of arachidonate in thrombin-stimulated platelets may not be PI. In any event, arachidonate release does not appear to be the sole purpose of stimulated phospholipid turnover. In the pancreas, for example, PI breakdown exceeds prostaglandin formation by more than three orders of magnitude (Banschbach and Hokin-Neaverson, 1980). It remains possible that phosphoinositide breakdown initiates a metabolic cascade that eventually calls on arachidonate in other lipids, for example by activating phospholipase A_2 with Ca^{2+}.

While stimulation of platelet receptors results in the formation of prostaglandins and thromboxanes, and application of the latter can mimic receptor activation with regard to secretion, there is no parallel relationship between pharmacological inhibition of arachidonate metabolism and inhibition of the appropriate cellular response. In the platelet 20 μM eicosatetraynoic acid (ETYA) does not affect the secretion of serotonin induced by thrombin but totally blocks arachidonate metabolism at both cyclooxygenase and lipoxygenase stages (Lapetina and Cuatrecasas, 1979). Furthermore, ETYA is relatively ineffective against f-met-leu-phe-induced secretion and totally ineffective against that induced by the complement fragment $C5_a$ (Naccache et al., 1979).

7.6 SUMMARY

The biochemical basis of neurotransmitter-induced stimulation of phosphoinositide turnover in the nervous system and its possible functional significance has been evaluated in the context of current progress and in the understanding of similar processes in nonneural systems. The enhanced incorporation of $^{32}P_i$ into PA and PI is observed in response to the occupancy of a large number of pharmacologically distinct receptor types in several neural preparations and appears to be the function of neuronal rather than glial elements. Recent evidence suggests that the receptor–ligand interaction results in the phosphodiesteratic cleavage of one or both polyphosphoinositides with the concomitant formation of diacylglycerol. The latter is rapidly phosphorylated in the presence of $[^{32}P]ATP$ to labeled PA and subsequently to PI. The increased turnover of the phosphorylinositol moiety of the inositol lipids occurs in the absence of significant changes in the glycerol backbone.

An important question that remains unanswered relates to the physiological significance of these biochemical events in the nervous system. Although a strong correlation exists in certain nonneural tissues between stimulated PA and phosphoinositide turnover and calcium mobilization, such a link is not yet readily apparent in the nervous system. For example, muscarinic receptor activation has yet to be shown to be linked to either Ca^{2+} influx or intracellular calcium mobilization. Also, while stimulated PA and phosphoinositide turnover requires the maintenance of a minimal concentration of Ca^{2+}, it is unlikely to be regulated by the changes in intracellular Ca^{2+} concentrations that pertain to physiological stimulation. One possibility that merits further attention is that the phosphodiesteratic breakdown of PIP and PIP_2 provides the diacylglycerol component for the full activation of a protein kinase C. The latter enzyme is present in high concentrations in brain and may provide an important link between lipid and protein phosphorylation.

The use of Li^+ to inhibit the breakdown of water-soluble inositol phosphates that accumulate following receptor activation has provided an important technical advance in the study of inositol lipids. Its use has furnished direct evidence for the stimulated phosphodiesteratic cleavage of inositol lipids and, because it affords increased sensitivity, has led to the identification of a class of neuropeptides that increase inositol lipid turnover. The use of such technical advances, together with a better understanding of the regulation of polyphosphoinositide metabolism, will undoubtedly shed much light in the future on the role of stimulated phospholipid turnover in cell–cell communication in the nervous system.

REFERENCES

Abdel-Latif, A.A., Yau, S.-J., and Smith, J.P., *J. Neurochem.*, *22*, 383–393 (1974).

Abdel-Latif, A.A., Akhtar, R.A., and Hawthorne, J.N., *Biochem. J.*, *162*, 61–73 (1977).

Agranoff, B.W., *Trends Biochem. Sci.*, *3*, N283–N285 (1978).

Agranoff, B.W., and Bleasdale, J.E., in W. W. Wells and F. Eisenberg, Eds., *Cyclitols and Phosphoinositides*, Academic Press, New York, 1978, pp. 105–120.

Agranoff, B.W., Bradley, R.M., and Brady, R.O., *J. Biol. Chem.*, *233*, 1077–1083 (1958).

Agranoff, B.W., Murthy, P., and Seguin, E.B., *J. Biol. Chem.*, *258*, 2076–2078 (1983).

Akhtar, R.A., and Abdel-Latif, A., *J. Pharmacol. Exp. Ther.*, *204*, 655–668 (1978).

Akhtar, R.A., and Abdel-Latif, A.A., *Biochem. J.*, *192*, 783–791 (1980).

Althaus, H.H., Neuhoff, V., and Osborne, N.N., *Experientia*, *31*, 266–268 (1975).

Aly, M.I., and Abdel-Latif, A.A., *Neurochem. Res.*, *7*, 159–169 (1982).

Anderson, R.E., and Hollyfield, J.G., *Biochim. Biophys. Acta*, *665*, 619–622 (1981).

Azila, N., and Hawthorne, J.N., *Biochem. J.*, *204*, 291–299 (1982).

Banschbach, M.W., and Hokin-Neaverson, M., *FEBS Lett.*, *117*, 131–133 (1980).

Banschbach, M.W., Geison, R.L., and Hokin-Neaverson, M., *Biochim. Biophys. Acta*, *663*, 34–45 (1981).

Bell, R.L., and Majerus, P.W., *J. Biol. Chem.*, *255*, 1790–1792 (1979).

Bell, R.L., Kennerly, D.A., Stanford, N., and Majerus, P.W., *Proc. Nat. Acad. Sci.*, *76*, 3238–3241 (1979).

Bell, M.E., Peterson, R.G., and Eichberg, J., *J. Neurochem.*, *39*, 192–200 (1982).

Benjamins, J.A., and Agranoff, B.W., *J. Neurochem.*, *16*, 513–527 (1969).

Berg, G.R., and Klein, D.C., *J. Neurochem.*, *19*, 2519–2532 (1972).

Berridge, M.J., *Trends Pharmacol. Sci.*, *1*, 419–424 (1980).

Berridge, M.J., *Mol. Cell. Endocrinol.*, *24*, 115–140 (1981).

Berridge, M.J., *Biochem. J.*, *212*, 849–858 (1982).

Berridge, M.J., and Fain, J.N., *Biochem. J.*, *178*, 59–69 (1979).

Berridge, M.J., Downes, C.P., and Hanley, M.R., *Biochem. J.*, *206*, 587–595 (1982).

Berridge, M.J., Dawson, R.M.C., Downes, C.P., Heslop, J.H., and Irvine, R.F., *Biochem. J.*, *212*, 473–482 (1983).

Billah, M.M., and Michell, R.H., *Biochem. J.*, *182*, 661–668 (1979).

Billah, M.M., Lapetina, E.G., and Cuatrecasas, P., *J. Biol. Chem.*, *256*, 5399–5403 (1981).

Bills, T.K., Smith, J.B., and Silver, M.J., *J. Clin. Invest.*, *60*, 1–6 (1977).

Birdsall, N.J.M., Burgen, A.S.V., and Hulme, E.C., *Mol. Pharmacol.*, *14*, 723–736 (1978).

Birnbirger, A.C., Birnbirger, K.L., Eliasson, S.G., and Simpson, P.C., *J. Neurochem.*, *18*, 1291–1298 (1971).

Bleasdale, J.E., and Hawthorne, J.N., *J. Neurochem.*, *24*, 373–379 (1975).

Bleasdale, J.E., Hawthorne, J.N., Widlund, L., and Heilbronn, E., *Biochem. J.*, *158*, 557–565 (1976).

Bostwick, J.R., and Eichberg, J., *Neurochem. Res.*, *6*, 1053–1065 (1981).

Broekman, M.J., Ward, J.W., and Marcus, A.J., *J. Clin. Invest.*, *66*, 275–283 (1980).

Broekman, M.J., Ward, J.W., and Marcus, A.J., *J. Biol. Chem.*, *256*, 8271–8274 (1981).

Brown, D.A., Fatherazi, S., Garthwaite, J., and White, R.D., *Br. J. Pharmac.*, *70*, 577–592 (1980).

Brown, E., and Nahorski, S.R., *Br. J. Pharmac.*, *78*, 108P (1983).

Buckley, J.T., and Hawthorne, J.N., *J. Biol. Chem.*, *247*, 7218–7223 (1972).

Burt, D.R., and Larrabee, M.G., *J. Neurochem.*, *21*, 255–272 (1973).

Canessa de Scarnati, O., Sato, M., and De Robertis, E., *J. Neurochem.*, *27*, 1575–1577 (1976).

Canessa de Scarnati, O., Sato, M., and De Robertis, E., *Neurochem. Res.*, *7*, 213–219 (1982).

Carter, J.R., Kennedy, E.P., *J. Lipid Res.*, *7*, 678–683 (1966).

Cockcroft, S., *Trends in Pharm. Sci.*, *2*, 340–342 (1981).

Cockcroft, S., *Trends in Pharm. Sci.*, *3*, 139 (1982).

Cockcroft, S., Bennett, J.P., and Gomperts, B.D., *FEBS Lett.*, *110*, 115–116 (1980a).

Cockcroft, S., Bennett, J.P., and Gomperts, D.B., *Nature*, *288*, 275–277 (1980b).

Cockcroft, S., Bennett, J., and Gomperts, B., *Biochem. J.*, *200*, 501–508 (1981).

Cohen, M.M., Schmidt, D.M., McGlennen, R.C., and Klein, W.L., *J. Neurochem.*, *40*, 547–554 (1983).

Colodzin, M., and Kennedy, E.P., *J. Biol. Chem.*, *240*, 3771–3780 (1965).

Cotman, C.W., McCaman, R.E., and Dewhurst, S.A., *Biochim. Biophys. Acta*, *249*, 395–405 (1971).

Cragg, B.G., in A.N. Davison and J. Dobbing, Eds., *Applied Neurochemistry*, Blackwell, Oxford, 1968, p. 34.

Daum, P.R., Downes, C.P., and Young, J.M., *Eur. J. Pharmac.*, *87*, 497–498 (1983).

Dawson, R.M.C., *Biochim. Biophys. Acta*, *33*, 68–77 (1959).

Dawson, R.M.C., and Eichberg, J., *Biochem. J.*, *96*, 634–643 (1965).

Dawson, R.M.C., and Thompson, W., *Biochem. J.*, *91*, 244–250 (1964).

Dawson, R.M.C., Hemington, N., and Irvine, R.F., *Eur. J. Biochem.*, *112*, 33–38 (1980).

de Belleroche, J., and Bradford, H.F., *Brain Res.*, *142*, 53–68 (1978).

Dennis, S.G., *Neurosci. Res. Prog. Bull.*, *20*, 350–353 (1982).

Derome, G., Tseng, R., Mercier, P., Lemaire, I., and Lemaire, S., *Biochem. Pharmacol.*, *30*, 855–860 (1981).

Deshmukh, D.S., Kuizon, S., Bear, W.D., and Brockerhoff, H., *Neurochem. Res., 7*, 617–626 (1982).

Downes, C.P., *Trends in Neurosci., 6*, 313–316 (1983).

Downes, C.P., and Wusteman, M.M., *Biochem. J., 216*, 633–640 (1983).

Durell, J., and Sodd, M., *J. Biol. Chem., 239*, 747–752 (1964).

Durell, J., Garland, J.T., and Friedel, R.O., *Science, 165*, 862–866 (1969).

Eichberg, J., and Dawson, R.M.C., *Biochem. J., 96*, 644–650 (1965).

Eichberg, J., and Hauser, G., *Biochim. Biophys. Acta, 326*, 210–223 (1973).

Eichberg, J., Shein, H.M., and Hauser, G., *Biochem. Soc. Trans., 1*, 352–359 (1973).

Eisenberg, F., and Hasegawa, R., *Trends in Biochem. Sci., 6*, ix (1981).

Fain, J.N., and Berridge, M.J., *Biochem. J., 178*, 45–58 (1979).

Farese, R.V., Larson, R.E., Sabir, M.A., *Biochim. Biophys. Acta, 633*, 479–484 (1980).

Farese, R.V., Larson, R.E., and Sabir, M., *Biochim. Biophys. Acta, 710*, 391–399 (1982).

Fisher, S.K., and Agranoff, B.W., *J. Neurochem., 34*, 1231–1240 (1980).

Fisher, S.K., and Agranoff, B.W., *J. Neurochem., 37*, 968–977 (1981).

Fisher, S.K., Boast, C.A., and Agranoff, B.W., *Brain Res., 189*, 284–288 (1980).

Fisher, S.K., Holz, R.W., and Agranoff, B.W., *J. Neurochem., 37*, 491–497 (1981a).

Fisher, S.K., Frey, K.A., and Agranoff, B.W., *J. Neurosci., 1*, 1407–1413 (1981b).

Fisher, S.K., Klinger, P.D., and Agranoff, B.W., *J. Biol. Chem., 258*, 7358–7363 (1983a).

Fisher, S.K., Hootman, S.R., Heacock, A.M., Ernst, S.A., and Agranoff, B.W., *FEBS Lett., 155*, 43–46 (1983b).

Fisher, S.K., Van Rooijen, L.A.A., and Agranoff, B.W., *Trends in Biochem. Sci., 9*, 53–56 (1984).

Fisher, S.K., Figueiredo, J.C., and Bartus, R.T., *J. Neurochem., 43*, 1171–1179 (1984).

Fried, R.L., and Blaustein, M.P., *Nature, 261*, 255–256 (1973).

Friedel, R.O., and Schanberg, S.M., *J. Pharmacol. Exp. Ther., 183*, 326–332 (1972).

Friedel, R.O., and Schanberg, S.M., *J. Neurochem., 24*, 819–820 (1975).

Friedel, R.O., Brown, J.D., and Durell, J., *J. Neurochem., 16*, 371–378 (1969).

Friedel, R.O., Johnson, J.R., and Schanberg, S.M., *J. Pharmacol. Exp. Ther., 184*, 583–589 (1973).

Friedel, R.O., Berry, D.E., and Schanberg, S.M., *J. Neurochem., 22*, 873–875 (1974).

Friedel, R.O., Slotnick, R.N., and Bombardt, P.A., *Life Sci., 20*, 235–242 (1977).

Ganguly, D.K., and Das, M., *Nature, 278*, 645–646 (1979).

Geison, R.L., Banschbach, M.W., Sadeghian, K., and Hokin-Neaverson, M., *Biochem. Biophys. Res. Commun., 68*, 343–349 (1976).

Gerrard, S.M., Butler, A.M., Peterson, D.A., and White, J.G., *Prostaglandins and Medicine, 1*, 387–396 (1978).

Giorguieff, M.F., Le Floc'h, M.L., Glowinski, J., and Besson, M.J., *J. Pharmacol. Exp. Ther., 200*, 535–544 (1977).

Goracci, G., Blomstrand, C., Arienti, G., Hamberger, A., and Porcellati, G., *J. Neurochem., 20*, 1167–1180 (1973).

Griffin, H.D., and Hawthorne, J.N., *Biochem. J., 176*, 541–552 (1978).

Griffin, H.D., Hawthorne, J.N., Sykes, M., and Orlacchio, A., *Biochem. Pharmacol., 28*, 1143–1147 (1979).

Hallcher, L.M., and Sherman, W.R., *J. Biol. Chem.*, *255*, 10,896–10,901 (1980).

Harris, R.A., Schmidt, J., Hitzemann, B.A., and Hitzemann, R.J., *Science, 212*, 1290–1291 (1981).

Harwood, J.L., and Hawthorne, J.N., *J. Neurochem.*, *16*, 1377–1387 (1969).

Hauser, G., and Eichberg, J., *J. Biol. Chem.*, *250*, 105–112 (1975).

Hauser, G., and Parks, J.M., *J. Neurosci. Res.*, *10*, 295–302 (1983).

Hauser, G., Shein, H.M., and Eichberg, J., *Nature*, *252*, 482–483 (1974).

Hauser, G., Nijjar, M.S., Smith, T.L., and Eichberg, J., in W.W. Wells and F. Eisenberg, Eds., *Cyclitols and Phosphoinositides*, Academic Press, New York, 1978, pp. 167–182.

Hawthorne, J.N., *Nature, 295*, 281–282 (1982).

Hawthorne, J.N., and Kai, M., in A. Lajtha, Ed., *Handbook of Neurochemistry*, Vol. 3, Plenum Press, New York, 1970, pp. 491–508.

Hawthorne, J.N., and Pickard, M.R., *J. Neurochem.*, *32*, 5–14 (1979).

Hefti, F., and Lichtensteiger, W., *J. Neurochem.*, *30*, 1217–1230 (1978).

Hendrickson, H.S., and Reinertsen, J.L., *Biochem. Biophys. Res. Commun.*, *44*, 1258–1264 (1971).

Hery, F., Bourgoin, S., Hamon, M., Ternaux, J., and Glowinski, J., *Naunyn-Schmiedebergs Arch. Pharmacol.*, *296*, 91–97 (1977).

Hirasawa, K., Irvine, R.F., and Dawson, R.M.C., *Biochem. J.*, *193*, 607–614 (1981a).

Hirasawa, K., Irvine, R.F., and Dawson, R.M.C., *Eur. J. Biochem.*, *120*, 53–58 (1981b).

Hokin, L.E., *Proc. Nat. Acad. Sci.*, *53*, 1369–1376 (1965).

Hokin, L.E., *J. Neurochem.*, *13*, 179–184 (1966).

Hokin, L.E., and Hokin, M.R., *Biochim. Biophys. Acta*, *18*, 102–110 (1955).

Hokin, L.E., and Hokin, M.R., *J. Biol. Chem.*, *233*, 800–804 (1958a).

Hokin, L.E., and Hokin, M.R., *J. Biol. Chem.*, *233*, 818–821 (1958b).

Hokin, L.E., and Hokin, M.R., *J. Biol. Chem.*, *233*, 822–826 (1958c).

Hokin, L.E., and Hokin, M.R., *J. Biol. Chem.*, *234*, 1387–1390 (1959).

Hokin, M.R., *J. Neurochem.*, *16*, 127–134 (1969).

Hokin, M.R., *J. Neurochem.*, *17*, 357–364 (1970).

Hokin, M.R., and Hokin, L.E., *J. Biol. Chem.*, *209*, 549–558 (1953).

Hokin, M.R., and Hokin, L.E., *J. Biol. Chem.*, *234* 1381–1386 (1959).

Hokin, M.R., and Hokin, L.E., *J. Gen. Physiol.*, *50*, 793–811 (1967).

Hokin, M.R., Hokin, L.E., and Shelp, W.D., *J. Gen. Physiol.*, *44*, 217–226 (1960).

Hokin-Neaverson, M., *Adv. Exp. Med. Biol.*, *83*, 429–446 (1977).

Hokin-Neaverson, M.R., *Biochem. Pharmacol.*, *29*, 2697–2700 (1980).

Horwitz, J., Tsymbalov, S., and Perlman, R.L., *J. Pharmacol. Exp. Ther.*, *229*, 577–582 (1984).

Irvine, R.F., *Biochem. J.*, *204*, 3–16 (1982).

Irvine, R.F., and Dawson, R.M.C., *J. Neurochem.*, *31*, 1427–1434 (1978).

Irvine, R.F., Hemington, N., and Dawson, R.M.C., *Biochem. J.*, *164*, 277–280 (1977).

Irvine, R.F., Hemington, N., and Dawson, R.M.C., *Biochem. J.*, *176*, 475–484 (1978).

Irvine, R.F., Hemington, N., and Dawson, R.M.C., *Eur. J. Biochem.*, *99*, 525–530 (1979).

Jacobs, K.H., Aktories, K., Lasch, P., Saur, W., and Schultz, G., *Hormone Cell Regulation*, *4*, 89–106 (1980).

Jolles, J., Wirtz, K.W.A., Schotman, P., and Gispen, W.H., *FEBS Lett.*, *105*, 110–114 (1979).

Jolles, J., Zwiers, H., Vandongen, C.J., Schotman, P., Wirtz, K.W.A., and Gispen, W.H., *Nature*, *286*, 623–625 (1980).

Jolles, J., Bar, P.R., and Gispen, W.H., *Brain Res.*, *224*, 315–326 (1981a).

Jolles, J., Schrama, L.H., and Gispen, W.H., *Biochim. Biophys. Acta*, *666*, 90–98 (1981b).

Jolles, J., Zwiers, H., Dekker, A., Wirtz, K.W.A., and Gispen, W.H., *Biochem. J.*, *194*, 283–291 (1981c).

Jones, L.M., and Michell, R.H., *Biochem. J.*, *148*, 479–485 (1975).

Jones, L.M., Cockcroft, S., and Michell, R.H., *Biochem. J.*, *182*, 669–676 (1979).

Joseph, S.K., Thomas, A.P., Williams, R.J., Irvine, R.F., and Williamson, J.R., *J. Biol. Chem.*, *259*, 3077–3081 (1984).

Kai, M., White, G.L., and Hawthorne, J.N., *Biochem. J.*, *101*, 328–337 (1966).

Kai, M., Salway, J.G., and Hawthorne, J.N., *Biochem. J.*, *106*, 791–801 (1968).

Kawahara, Y., Takai, Y., Minakuchi, R., Sano, K., and Nishizuka, Y., *Biochem. Biophys. Res. Commun.*, *97*, 309–317 (1980).

Kennerly, D.A., Parker, C.W., and Sullivan, T.J., *Fed. Proc.*, *38*, 1018 (1979a).

Kennerly, D.A., Secosan, C.J., Parker, C.W., and Sullivan, T.J., *J. Immunol.*, *123*, 1519–1524 (1979b).

Kennerly, D.A., Sullivan, T.J., and Parker, C.W., *J. Immunol.*, *122*, 152–159 (1979c).

Keough, K.M.W., and Thompson, W., *J. Neurochem.*, *17*, I–II (1970).

Keough, K.M.W., and Thompson, W., *Biochim. Biophys. Acta*, *270*, 324–336 (1972).

Keough, K.M.W., MacDonald, G., and Thompson, W., *Biochim. Biophys. Acta*, *270*, 337–347 (1972).

Kerr, S.E., Kfoury, G.A., and Djibelian, L.G., *J. Lipid Res.*, *5*, 481–483 (1964).

Kilian, P.L., and Schacht, J., *J. Neurochem.*, *32*, 247–248 (1979).

Kilian, P.L., and Schacht, J., *J. Neurochem.*, *34*, 709–712 (1980).

Kilpatrick, D.L., Ledbetter, F.H., Carson, K.A., Kirshner, A.G., Slepetis, R., and Kirshner, N., *J. Neurochem.*, *35*, 679–692 (1980).

Kirk, C.J., Michell, R.H., and Hems, D.A., *Biochem. J.*, *194*, 155–165 (1981a).

Kirk, C.J., Creba, J.A., Downes, C.P., and Michell, R.H., *Biochem. Soc. Trans.*, *9*, 377–379 (1981b).

Krueger, B.K., Forn, J., and Greengard, P., *J. Biol. Chem.*, *252*, 2764–2773 (1977).

Kuhar, M.J., and Yamamura, H.I., *Brain Res.*, *110*, 229–243 (1976).

Lakshmanan, J., *Biochem. Biophys. Res. Commun.*, *82*, 767–775 (1978a).

Lakshmanan, J., *FEBS Lett.*, *92*, 159–162 (1978b).

Lakshmanan, J., *J. Neurochem.*, *32*, 1599–1601 (1979).

Lapetina, E.G., and Cuatrecasas, P., *Biochim. Biophys. Acta*, *573*, 394–402 (1979).

Lapetina, E.G., and Hawthorne, J.N., *Biochem. J.*, *122*, 171–179 (1971).

Lapetina, E.G., and Michell, R.H., *Biochem. J.*, *126*, 1141–1147 (1972).

Lapetina, E.G., and Michell, R.H., *Biochem. J.*, *131*, 433–442 (1973).

Lapetina, E.G., and Michell, R.H., *J. Neurochem.*, *23*, 283–287 (1974).

Lapetina, E.G., Brown, W.E., and Michell, R.H., *J. Neurochem.*, *26*, 649–651 (1976).

Larrabee, M.G., *J. Neurochem.*, *15*, 803–808 (1968).

Larrabee, M.G., and Leicht, W.S., *J. Neurochem.*, *12*, 1–13 (1965).

Low, M.G., and Finean, J.B., *Biochim. Biophys. Acta*, *508*, 565–570 (1978).

Low, M.G., and Zilversmit, D.B., *Biochemistry*, *19*, 3913–3918 (1980).

Lunt, G.G., and Pickard, M.R., *J. Neurochem.*, *24*, 1203–1208 (1975).

McKean, M.L., Smith, J.B., and Silver, M.J., *J. Biol. Chem.*, *256*, 1522–1524 (1981).

Marshall, P.J., Boatman, D.E., and Hokin, L.E., *J. Biol. Chem.*, *256*, 844–847 (1981).

Martin, T.F.J., *J. Biol. Chem.*, *24*, 14816–14822 (1983).

Matsuzawa, Y., and Hostetler, K.Y., *J. Biol. Chem.*, *255*, 646–652 (1980).

Michell, R.H., *Biochim. Biophys. Acta*, *415*, 81–147 (1975).

Michell, R.H., *Trends in Biochem. Sci.*, *4*, 128–131 (1979).

Michell, R.H., *Nature*, *296*, 492–493 (1982).

Michell, R.H., and Kirk, C.J., *Trends in Pharmacol. Sci.*, *2*, 86–89 (1981a).

Michell, R.H., and Kirk, C.J., *Biochem. J.*, *198*, 247–248 (1981b).

Michell, R.H., and Lapetina, E.G., *Nature, New Biol.*, *240*, 258–260 (1972).

Michell, R.H., Jafferji, S.S., and Jones, L.M., *FEBS Lett.*, *69*, 1–5 (1976).

Michell, R.H., Kirk, C.J., Jones, L.M., Downes, C.P., and Creba, J.A. *Phil. Trans. Roy. Soc. Lond. B*, *296*, 123–137 (1981).

Michell, R.H., Bone, E.A., Fretten, P., Palmer, S., Kirk, C.J., Hanley, M.R., Benton, H., Lightman, S.L., and Todd, K. in J.E. Bleasdale, J. Eichberg, and G. Hauser, eds., *Inositol and Phosphoinositides: Metabolism and Biological Regulation*, Humana Press, Clifton, N.J. (1985) pp. 221–236.

Miller, J.C., *Biochem. J.*, *168*, 549–555 (1977).

Minakuchi, R., Takai, Y., Yu, B., and Nishizuka, Y., *J. Biochem. (Tokyo)*, *89*, 1651–1654 (1981).

Mohd.Adnan, N.A., and Hawthorne, J.N., *J. Neurochem.*, *36*, 1858–1860 (1981).

Mori, T., Takai, Y., Yu, B., Takahashi, J., Nishizuka, Y., and Fujikara, T., *J. Biochem.*, *91*, 427–431 (1982).

Naccache, P.H., Showell, H.J., Becker, E.L., and Sha'afi, R.I., *Biochem. Biophys. Res. Commun.*, *87*, 292–299 (1979).

Natarajan, V., Dyck, P.J., and Schmid, H.H.O., *J. Neurochem.*, *36*, 413–419 (1981).

Neufeld, E.J., and Majerus, P.W., *J. Biol. Chem.*, *258*, 2461–2467 (1983).

Nijjar, M.S., and Hawthorne, J.N., *Biochim. Biophys. Acta*, *480*, 390–392 (1977).

Nijjar, M.S., Smith, T.L., and Hauser, G., *J. Neurochem.*, *34*, 813–821 (1980).

Nishizuka, Y., *Trends in Biochem. Sci.*, *8*, 13–16 (1983).

Ohsako, S., and Deguchi, T., *J. Biol. Chem.*, *256*, 10945–10948 (1981).

Ohsako, S., and Deguchi, T., *FEBS Lett.*, *152*, 62–66 (1983).

Palmano, K.P., Whiting, P.H., and Hawthorne, J.N., *Biochem. J.*, *167*, 229–235 (1977).

Palmer, F.B., and Rossiter, R.J., *Can. J. Biochem.*, *43*, 671–683 (1965).

Panagia, V., Michiel, D.F., Dhalla, K.S., Nijjar, M.S., and Dhalla, N.S., *Biochim. Biophys. Acta*, *676*, 395–400 (1981).

Paulus, H., and Kennedy, E.P., *J. Biol. Chem.*, *235*, 1303–1311 (1960).

Petzold, G.L., and Agranoff, B.W., *Fed. Proc.*, *24*, 476 (1965).

Petzold, G.L., and Agranoff, B.W., *J. Biol. Chem.*, *242*, 1187–1191 (1967).

Pickard, M.R., and Hawthorne, J.N., *J. Neurochem.*, *30*, 145–155 (1978).

Pickard, M.R., Hawthorne, J.N., Hayashi, E., and Yamada, S., *Biochem. Pharmacol. 26*, 448–450 (1977).

Poggioli, J., Weiss, S.J., McKinney, J.S., and Putney, J.W., Jr., *Mol. Pharmacol., 23*, 71–77 (1983).

Prescott, S.M., and Majerus, P.W., *J. Biol. Chem., 256*, 579–582 (1981).

Prpić, V., Blackmore, P.F., and Exton, J.H., *J. Biol. Chem., 257*, 11,323–11,331 (1982).

Putney, J.W., Jr., *Life Sci., 29*, 1183–1194 (1981).

Putney, J.W., Jr., Weiss, S.J., Van de Walle, C.M., and Haddas, R.A., *Nature, 284*, 345–347 (1980).

Raetz, C.R.H., Hirschberg, C.B., Dowhan, W., Wickner, W.T., and Kennedy, E.P., *J. Biol. Chem., 247*, 2245–2247 (1972).

Raetz, C.R.H., Dowhan, W., and Kennedy, E.P., *J. Bacteriol., 125*, 855–863 (1976).

Reddy, P.V., and Sastry, P.S., *Brain Res., 168*, 287–298 (1979).

Redman, C.M., and Hokin, L.E., *J. Neurochem., 11*, 155–163 (1964).

Rhodes, D., Prpić, V., Exton, J.H., and Blackmore, P.F., *J. Biol. Chem., 258*, 2770–2773 (1983).

Rittenhouse, H.G., Seguin, E.B., Fisher, S.K. and Agranoff, B.W., *J. Neurochem., 36*, 991–999 (1981).

Rittenhouse-Simmons, S., *J. Clin. Invest., 63*, 580–587 (1979).

Salmon, D.M., and Honeyman, T.W., *Nature, 284*, 344–345 (1980).

Salway, J.G., and Hughes, I.E., *J. Neurochem., 19*, 1233–1240 (1972).

Salway, J.G., Kai, M., and Hawthorne, J.N., *J. Neurochem., 14*, 1013–1024 (1967).

Schacht, J., and Agranoff, B.W., *J. Biol. Chem., 247*, 771–777 (1972).

Schacht, J., and Agranoff, B.W., *J. Biol. Chem., 249*, 1551–1557 (1974).

Schacht, J., Neale, E.A., and Agranoff, B.W., *J. Neurochem., 23*, 211–218 (1974).

Schellenberg, R.R., *Immunology, 41*, 123–129 (1980).

Schwarcz, R., Hokfelt, T., Fuxe, K., Jonsson, G., Goldstein, M., and Terenius, L., *Exp. Brain Res., 37*, 199–216 (1979).

Scott, I.D., Akerman, K.E.O., and Nicholls, D.G., *Biochem. J., 192*, 873–880 (1980).

Scott, W.A., Zrike, J., Hamill, A.L., Kempe, J., and Cohn, Z.A., *J. Exp. Med., 152*, 324–335 (1980).

Serhan, C., Anderson, P., Goodman, E., Dunham, P., and Weissmann, G., *J. Biol. Chem., 256*, 2736–2741 (1981).

Sheltawy, A., Brammer, M., and Borrill, D., *Biochem. J., 128*, 579–586 (1972).

Siman, R.G., and Klein, W.L., *J. Neurochem., 37*, 1099–1108 (1981).

Slotkin, T.A., Weigel, S.J., Whitmore, W.L., and Seidler, F.J., *Biochem. Pharmac., 31*, 1899–1902 (1982).

Smith, T.L., Eichberg, J., and Hauser, G., *Life Sci., 24*, 2179–2184 (1979).

Sneddon, J.M., and Keen, P., *Biochem. Pharmacol., 19*, 1297–1306 (1970).

Snider, R.M., McKinney, M., Forray, C., and Richelson, E., *Proc. Natl. Acad. Sci. USA 81*, 3905–3909 (1984).

Sokolovsky, M., and Bartfai, T., *Trends in Biochem. Sci., 6*, 303–305 (1981).

Soukup, J.F., Friedel, R.O., and Schanberg, S., *Biochem. Pharmacol. 27*, 1239–1243 (1978).

Stenson, W.F., Parker, C.W., and Sullivan, T.J., *Biochem. Biophys. Res. Commun.*, 96, 1045–1052 (1980).

Storm-Mathisen, J., and Guldberg, H.C., *J. Neurochem.*, 22, 793–803 (1974).

Streb, H., Irvine, R.F., Berridge, M.J., and Schulz, I., *Nature*, 306, 67–69 (1983).

Subramanian, N., Whitmore, W.L., Seidler, F.J., and Slotkin, T.A., *Life Sci.*, 27, 1315–1319 (1980).

Subramanian, N., Whitmore, W.L., Seidler, F.J., and Slotkin, T.A., *J. Neurochem.*, 36, 1137–1141 (1981).

Swilem, A.-M.F., Hawthorne, J.N., and Azila, N., *Biochem. Pharmacol.*, 32, 3873–3874 (1983).

Takai, Y., Kishimoto, A., Iwasa, Y., Kawahara, Y., Mori, T., and Nishizuka, Y., *J. Biol. Chem.*, 254, 3692–3695 (1979a).

Takai, Y., Kishimoto, A., Kikkawa, U., Mori, T., and Nishizuka, Y., *Biochem. Biophys. Res. Commun.*, 91, 1218–1224 (1979b).

Takenawa, T., Saito, M., Nagai, Y., and Egawa, K., *Arch. Biochem. Biophys.*, 182, 244–250 (1977).

Tanigawa, K., Kuzuya, H., Imura, H., Taniguchi, H., Baba, S., Takai, Y., and Nishizuka, Y. *FEBS Lett.*, 138, 183–186 (1982).

Thompson, W., *Can. J. Biochem.*, 45, 853–861 (1967).

Traynor, A.E., Schubert, D., and Allen, W.R., *J. Neurochem.*, 39, 1677–1683 (1982).

Tret'jak, A.G., Limarenko, I.M., Kossova, G.V., Gulak, P.V., and Kozlov, Y.P., *J. Neurochem.*, 28, 199–205 (1977).

Trifaro, J.M., *Mol. Pharmacol.*, 5, 382–393 (1969a).

Trifaro, J.M., *Mol. Pharmacol.*, 5, 424–427 (1969b).

Tyson, C.A., Zande, H.V., and Green, D.E., *J. Biol. Chem.*, 251, 1326–1332 (1976).

Van Rooijen, L.A.A., Seguin, E.B., and Agranoff, B.W., *Biochem. Biophys. Res. Comm.*, 112, 919–926 (1983).

Vickers, J.D., Kinlough-Rathbone, R.L., and Mustard, J.F., *Blood*, 60, 1247–1250 (1982).

Walsh, C.E., Dechatelet, L.R., Thomas, M.J., O'Flaherty, J.T., and Waite, M., *Lipids*, 16, 120–124 (1981).

Watson, S.P., and Downes, C.P., *Eur. J. Pharmacol.*, 93, 245–253 (1983).

Weiss, S.J., and Putney, J.W., *Biochem. J.*, 194, 463–468 (1981).

Weiss, S.J., McKinney, J.S., and Putney, J.W., Jr., *Biochem. J.*, 206, 555–560 (1982).

White, G.L., and Larrabee, M.G., *J. Neurochem.*, 20, 783–798 (1973).

White, G.L., Schellhase, H.U., and Hawthorne, J.N., *J. Neurochem.*, 22, 149–158 (1974).

Whiting, P.H., Palmano, K.P., and Hawthorne, J.N., *Biochem. J.*, 179, 549–553 (1979).

Woelk, H., Kanig, K., and Peiler-Ichikawa, K., *J. Neurochem.*, 23, 1057–1063 (1974).

Wolfe, L.S., *J. Neurochem.*, 38, 1–14 (1982).

Yagihara, Y., and Hawthorne, J.N., *J. Neurochem.*, 19, 355–367 (1972).

Yagihara, Y., Bleasdale, J.E., and Hawthorne, J.N., *J. Neurochem.*, 21, 173–190 (1973).

Yandrasitz, J.R., and Segal, S., *FEBS Lett.*, 108, 279–282 (1979).

Young, P.W., Bicknell, R.J., and Schofield, J.G., *J. Endocrinol.*, 80, 203–213 (1979).

Zeleznikar, R.J., Jr., Quist, E.E., and Drewes, L.R., *Mol. Pharmacol.*, 24, 163–167 (1983).

=eight

PHOSPHOLIPIDS IN DISORDERS OF THE NERVOUS SYSTEM

JOHN CALLAHAN

Research Institute
The Hospital for Sick Children
Toronto, Ontario, Canada

CONTENTS

8.1   INTRODUCTION   298

8.2   SPHINGOMYELIN LIPIDOSES: PRIMARY DEFECTS OF
        PHOSPHOLIPID METABOLISM   299
        8.2.1   Clinical Heterogeneity, 299
        8.2.2   Sphingomyelin Storage in the Brain, 300
        8.2.3   Bis(monoacylglycero)phosphate Storage, 301
        8.2.4   Sphingomyelin, Glycerophospholipids, and the
                  Sphingomyelinases, 303

8.3   NEUROLOGICAL DISORDERS WITH SECONDARY
        INVOLVEMENT OF PHOSPHOLIPIDS   307
        8.3.1   Disorders of the Basal Ganglia, 307
        8.3.2   Multiple Sclerosis, 312
        8.3.3   Other Diseases, 313

8.4   ANIMAL MODELS OF PHOSPHOLIPID DISORDERS   313
        8.4.1   Sphingomyelin Lipidosis as a Primary Defect, 313
        8.4.2   Secondary Forms of Phospholipid Abnormalities, 314

        REFERENCES   314

8.1   INTRODUCTION

The quantity of subject matter that could be included in this chapter is far too vast to be covered in any comprehensive way within a limited space. Indeed, a great many diseases that either primarily affect the nervous system or manifest major neurological complications can involve changes in phospholipid composition and metabolism. This is to be expected since the metabolic pathways altered in a number of these disorders are critically related to those of phospholipids. Thus, considering the abundance of phospholipids, an abnormality in one aspect of cell metabolism may well influence the status of these lipids, although such effects may be far removed from the principal defect responsible for the disorder.

In view of the plethora of information available, a decision has been made to emphasize lipidoses for which there is good evidence that abnormal phospholipid metabolism is the primary cause and then to consider more briefly a variety of neurological diseases, mainly degenerative, in which secondary phospholipid involvement is either known or suspected.

8.2 SPHINGOMYELIN LIPIDOSES: PRIMARY DEFECTS OF PHOSPHOLIPID METABOLISM

8.2.1 Clinical Heterogeneity

The only known diseases resulting from a primary defect in phospholipid metabolism are the sphingomyelin storage disorders. The original reports, early in this century, described the clinical, histological, and pathological hallmarks of the infantile form, called Niemann-Pick disease to this day. (For a review see Brady, 1983.) The major storage compound in these patients was identified as sphingomyelin in 1934 (Klenk, 1934). In the intervening years new and unusual variants of the classical disorder were reported. The largest group was included in the major work of Crocker and Farber (1958) who summarized the findings on 18 patients, the majority of whom had clinical presentations different from the descriptions of Niemann, Pick, and Videbaek (Videbaek, 1952). The patients displayed marked heterogeneity in age of onset, severity of neurological involvement, degree of visceromegaly, age at death, and course of the disorder (Crocker and Farber, 1958). The diseases spanned several cultural groups and involved both sexes. As a result of this work, a classification of these disorders grouped under the general heading of Niemann-Pick disease was proposed (Crocker, 1961). Type A is the acute, infantile neuronopathic (severe) form, while Type B is the nonneuronopathic, adult, and relatively benign form. A later-onset chronic form reminiscent of Type A neurologically, but in which patients live longer (Type C), and a neurological form localized to the Acadian population in Nova Scotia (Type D) completed the classification.

In the intervening two decades to the present time the number of variants of these disorders has increased so that Crocker's grouping is clearly outdated. In 1973 Neville et al. summarized the experience at that time and divided the disorders into six distinct categories including the vertical gaze ophthalmoplegias, which have emerged as a separate clinical entity.

Since 1973 additional variants have been reported, and it is apparent that a further and more comprehensive organization of the disorders is required. At present the simplest classification is based on the enzymopathy, a deficiency of sphingomyelinase. Patients with abnormalities similar to those of Crocker's types A and B have markedly diminished sphingomyelinase activity while patients with Type C and related variants have apparently normal sphingomyelinase activity. A detailed classification of these disorders is beyond the scope of this article and readers are directed to other more comprehensive discussions (Brady, 1983). It has been agreed among most of the researchers studying these disorders that Niemann-Pick variants who do not have deficient sphingomyelinase activity be considered as examples of Type C until such time as the exact enzyme deficiency is identified (Elleder and Jirasek, 1983).

8.2.2 Sphingomyelin Storage in the Brain

The phospholipid composition of the brain and visceral tissues of patients with these diseases does not invariably include an accumulation of sphingomyelin (Crocker, 1961; Dunn and Sweeney, 1971; Kamoshita et al., 1969; Lowden et al., 1967; Neville et al., 1973; Oppenheimer et al., 1967; Philippart et al., 1969). Crocker (1961) found an elevation of sphingomyelin in gray matter of five patients but not in white matter in Type A and normal limits for this lipid in the other variants. Kamoshita et al. (1969) also found an increased content in the gray and white matter in the infantile form. Membranous inclusion bodies isolated from the brain of this patient contained a high content of sphingomyelin (47.9% of the lipid) whereas the sphingomyelin content of myelin was normal. It was noted that sphingomyelin deposition in these organelles was far higher than the overall accumulation in the brain, which in turn was low compared to the inclusions in spleen and liver, where the sphingomyelin content reflected the overall deposition in the tissue. Compared to the marked deposition of gangliosides in the gangliosidoses, however, sphingomyelin accumulation in the brain in Niemann-Pick Type A is quite low. The degree of accumulation is more like the variants of Gaucher disease, in which there is an abnormality of glucocerebroside metabolism (Brady and Barranger, 1983; Suzuki et al., 1969). There are virtually no data on the lipid composition of the brain in the nonneuronopathic adult form (Type B). There have been many reports on the variants, classified as Type C or C-like, including the vertical-gaze ophthalmoplegias and adult variants (Elfenbein, 1968; Harzer et al., 1978; Karpati et al., 1977; Neville et al., 1973; Silverstein et al., 1970; Wenger et al., 1977). Surprisingly, where studied, there is little or no deposition of sphingomyelin in the brain in these disorders. It is unfortunate that no one has attempted to duplicate the interesting studies of Kamoshita et al., (1969) with the brain from these variants. The results of these isolations could point to new understanding of the pathogenesis of these diseases. Elleder et al. (1980) using enzyme histochemistry and electron microscopy identified a regional pattern of deposition in lysosomes in biopsy specimens of liver from two siblings with a variant form of Type A which was significantly distinct and different from the involvement in several other cases. They pointed to a regional mode of expression of the lipid storage in the liver and postulated that this could explain some of the features of the Type C variants of the disorders. Although they did not report findings on the brain, their experience extends and reaffirms earlier data (Kamoshita et al., 1969).

In virtually every form of sphingomyelin storage disease where the patient manifests abnormal neurological traits, examination of the brain has revealed a loss of neuronal elements, ballooned neurons, glial proliferation, and a general shrinkage of the brain mass. These changes are difficult to reconcile with the degree of accumulation of sphingomyelin, which as mentioned above is abnormal only in the infantile form. Indeed the composition of other lipid classes such as the gangliosides and the neutral glycolipids is altered, and the reasons for this are unclear (Lowden et al., 1967; Neville et al., 1973; Philippart, 1972).

This contrasts with the experience in the reticuloendothelial system where sphingomyelin deposition is clearly demonstrable in virtually every patient. In Types A and B and variants where sphingomyelinase activity is deficient, massive accumulation of sphingomyelin is noted. Adult patients with Type C and other variants where the enzyme activity is within normal limits *in vitro* have a much reduced accumulation. As Elleder et al. (1980) noted, few studies have examined the depositions of lipids regionally. At present the enzyme defect(s) in this group remain unknown.

8.2.3   Bis(monoacylglycero)phosphate Storage

The majority of the reports on Niemann-Pick disease have included data on the concentration of the major glycerophospholipids in various tissues. In general, no significant abnormalities have been identified. However, elevated amounts of an unusual phospholipid, bis(monoacylglycero)phosphate, have consistently been reported since the original recognition of this lipid in 1968 by Rouser and colleagues (Rouser et al., 1968). They described isolation of an acid phospholipid, normally found in trace quantities, with a glycerol:phosphate mole ratio of 2 (Fig. 8.1). This lipid was elevated about 85-fold over normal (while the sphingomyelin elevation was only 59-fold) in liver from a patient with the infantile form of Niemann-Pick disease. Similar accumulations were noted in the heart, kidney, spleen, and lung. The lipid was elevated in an

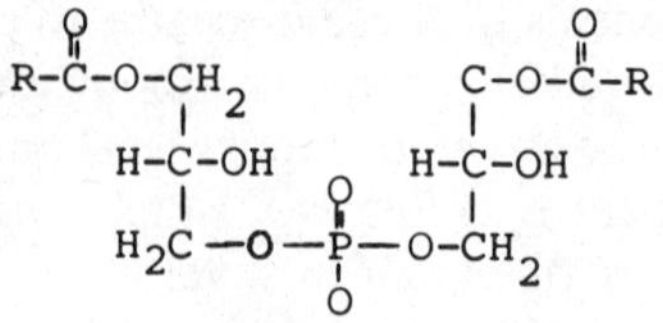

monoacylglycerol phosphomonoglyceride

lyso bis phosphatidic acid

bis(monoacylglycero)phosphate

bis(3-acyl-sn-glycerol-1)phosphate

FIGURE 8.1   Structure of bis(monoacylglycero)phosphate.

adult form of Niemann-Pick disease. Interestingly, this lipid did not accumulate in tissues from patients with infantile and chronic Gaucher disease, infantile metachromatic leukodystrophy, or in infantile G_{M2}-gan-
gliosidosis. However, accumulation of bis(monoacylglycero)phosphate
was recently described in muscle and urinary sediment from a patient
having mucolipidosis IV (Crandall et al., 1982). These findings have been
confirmed in several patients with other forms of Niemann-Pick disease
(Martin et al., 1972; Seng et al., 1971; Tjiong et al., 1973) and in patients
characterized by vertical-gaze paresis (Elleder et al., 1980; Harzer et al.,
1978; Karpati et al., 1977; Wenger et al., 1977). Some of the latter cases
have documented elevation of sphingomyelin in visceral tissues but no
abnormality in sphingomyelinase has been identified. The presence of
bis(monoacylglycero)phosphate in the human brain has not been extensively examined, but where analyses have been reported, this lipid has
not been detected (Martin et al., 1972). It is possible that its presence
could be verified with larger sample sizes. Reexamination of liver from
the case reported by Lowden et al. (1967) revealed a 35-fold accumulation
of bis(monoacylglycero)phosphate (J. W. Callahan, A. Poulos, and J. A.
Lowden, unpublished observations). The brain was not available for
analysis. This phospholipid also accumulated in the spleen of one of
the patients examined by Wenger et al. (1977) (case one; personal
communication) where an elevation of sphingomyelin was also observed and in which the residual activity of sphingomyelinase was 10–
40% of normal. Poulos et al. (1983a) found massive storage of
bis(monoacylglycero)phosphate such that it accounted for 23% of the total
phospholipid pool in the liver of a 72-year-old man who had no previous
history of hepatosplenomegaly. The liver biopsy had a content of sphingomyelin within normal limits with about 33% of the normal sphingo-

myelinase activity. The enzyme activity was even lower in leukocytes and cultured fibroblasts. The patient had been treated with furosemide, digoxin, and warfarin, drugs which could but are not known to affect bis(monoacylglycero)phosphate metabolism. Another adult case of bis(monoacylglycero)phosphate storage has been reported (Yamamoto et al., 1970), but no data on any medications or the level of sphingomyelinase were included. Comparisons have been made between these adult variants and the Sea Blue Histiocytosis Syndrome (Sawitsky et al., 1972; Silverstein and Ellefson, 1972; Silverstein et al., 1970). It is clear that some forms of the disease are due to abnormal sphingomyelinase and are clinically similar to the nonneuronopathic form of Niemann-Pick disease (Type B) whereas other cases appear to be different (Fried et al., 1978; Resner et al., 1970; Varela-Duran et al., 1980).

Bis(monoacylglycero)phosphate is produced from phosphatidylglycerol and acylphosphatidylglycerol (Poorthuis and Hostetler, 1975). Its synthesis is increased in humans and rats treated with the coronary vasodilator, 4,4-diethylaminoethoxyhexestrol (Yamamoto et al., 1971a,b) and in experimental animals treated with triparanol (Adachi et al., 1972), chloroquine (Tjiong and Debuch, 1978), and possibly gentamicin (Aubert-Tulkens et al., 1979). Wherrett and Huterer (1972) initially showed that this lipid was localized to lysosomes in rats treated with Triton WR1339. The bis(monoacylglycero)phosphate accumulated in rat liver tritosomes has a high content of $22:6$ fatty acid whereas the lipid isolated from liver of a patient who died with an undefined lipidosis (Wherrett and Huterer, 1973) and from a patient with the Type B form of Niemann-Pick disease (A. Poulos and J. W. Callahan, unpublished observations) had a high content of $18:1$.

8.2.4 Sphingomyelin, Glycerophospholipids, and the Sphingomyelinases

The biochemical basis for the several variants of sphingomyelin lipidoses and the relationship between sphingomyelin and bis(monoacylglycero)phosphate has been difficult to reconcile, but recent experiments have provided partial answers to this question (Huterer et al., 1983; Matsuzawa and Hostetler, 1980). Huterer et al. (1983) found that purified placental sphingomyelinase (Jones et al., 1981) hydrolyzes phosphatidylglycerol, the precursor of bis(monoacylglycero)phosphate. Normal human fibroblasts hydrolyzed phosphatidylglycerol into lysophosphatidylglycerol and di- and monoacylglycerols (Fig. 8.2). The data suggested that both phospholipids are substrates for sphingomyelinase. In addition, hydrolysis of phosphatidylglycerol was deficient in cultured fibroblasts derived from patients with types A and B and an adult variant of Niemann-

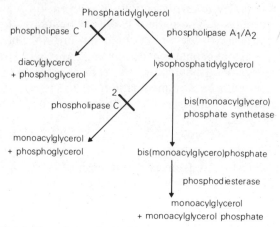

FIGURE 8.2   Metabolism of phosphatidylglycerol. Reactions 1 and 2 are blocked in Niemann-Pick disease variants characterized by a sphingomyelinase deficiency (Huterer et al., 1982).

Pick disease, while the activity was within normal limits in Type C and a case of vertical-gaze paresis. Bis(monoacylglycero)phosphate does not appear to be a substrate for sphingomyelinase. Taken together these results suggest that bis(monoacylglycero)phosphate may be the storage form of phosphatidylglycerol in those diseases characterized by a sphingomyelinase deficiency. Recent analyses by Poulos and Callahan (unpublished observations) failed to demonstrate any accumulation of phosphatidylglycerol in a variety of Niemann-Pick lipid extracts, a finding that is consistent with this view.

Hostetler and Hall (1980) recently demonstrated that hydrolysis of phosphatidylcholine occurred in rat tissues via a phospholipase C. Beaudet et al. (1980) showed a deficiency of phosphatidylcholine phospholipase C (which in this context is presumed to be sphingomyelinase) in cultured fibroblasts derived from Niemann-Pick patients. Appreciable hydrolysis of phosphatidylcholine in both studies required prolonged incubation periods compared to those required for phosphatidylglycerol (Huterer et al., 1983). However, more recent work has shown that phosphatidylcholine is rapidly hydrolyzed by purified sphingomyelinase and by extracts of cultured fibroblasts in the presence of sodium taurocholate (Wherrett and Huterer, 1983). Phosphatidylcholine is also metabolized by a phospholipase C that is distinct and separate from sphingomyelinase. A recent report (Edgar and Freysz, 1982) described this enzyme in rat brain. In all these experiments the rates of hydrolysis catalyzed by phospholipases C are influenced by the competing deacylation reactions brought about by phospholipases A_1 and A_2. Indeed, Kunze et al. (1982) recently showed that phosphatidylcholine and phosphatidylethanolamine are hydrolyzed preferentially by way of A_1 and A_2 in rat liver tritosomes with only minor contributions by phospholipase C and lysophospholipase C. These workers also suggested that the principal site of the hydrolysis of these lipids was in lysosomes.

Because sphingomyelinase is a major enzyme for sphingomyelin, phosphatidylglycerol, and phosphatidylcholine hydrolysis, we are forced to conclude that it is responsible for the storage of these compounds in patients with this lipidosis. However, the activity appears to be normal in many patients who manifest overt storage. Studies on the structural properties of sphingomyelinase indicate that the protein is microheterogeneous and a holopolymeric enzyme consisting of a single polypeptide chain. The apparent molecular mass for the purified brain enzyme is 180,000 daltons (Yamanaka and Suzuki, 1982). The apparent molecular mass of the carboxymethylated polypeptides as judged by SDS–polyacrylamide gels (89,000 daltons) (Jones et al., 1981) is the same as that obtained by irradiation (Maret et al., 1983) but is higher than that found for the brain enzyme (70,000 daltons) (Yamanaka and Suzuki, 1982). On isoelectric focusing, both the native enzyme and the carboxymethylated polypeptides display heterogeneous acidic isoelectric points of pI 4.6–5.0 (Jones et al., 1983). These studies have been complicated by the tendency of the protein to form aggregates and to alter its isoelectric properties in the presence of detergents such as Triton X100 (Besley, 1976; Callahan et al., 1981). Although the enzyme appears to possess significant hydrophobic character, its amino acid composition does not show a strikingly high content of hydrophobic or aromatic residues (Jones et al., 1983).

Earlier studies suggested that the Niemann-Pick variants characterized by near normal levels of enzyme were due to loss of a specific isoenzyme (Callahan et al., 1975). More recent studies by Besley and Moss (1983) and by Poulos et al. (1983b) using isoelectric focusing of enzyme obtained from cultured fibroblasts have led to conflicting conclusions, and it appears that we cannot show a consistent and reliable enzyme defect in this disorder. Although the data available on sphingomyelinase activity in patients with near normal levels of enzyme suggest that it is indeed normal, it has not been highly purified from these sources, and no direct studies of its structural properties have appeared (Muller and Harzer, 1980; Vanier et al., 1980). Other aspects of phospholipid hydrolases including sphingomyelinase are discussed in Chapter 2.

There is some evidence that activator proteins may be involved in the hydrolysis of sphingomyelin. Christomanou (1980) and Baraton and Revol (1977) have suggested that activator proteins are required for enzyme activity *in vivo* and that these proteins may be defective in some forms of Niemann-Pick disease. The fact that the purified placental enzyme and crude extracts of liver from Type C variants were able to hydrolyze liposomal sphingomyelin in the absence of detergents or exogenous activator proteins diminishes this as a potential answer to this problem (Huterer et al., 1983; Poulos et al., 1983c).

Recent experiments have analyzed the rates of uptake and the metabolism of exogenous radiolabeled sphingomyelin in intact cultured fibroblasts (Beaudet and Manschreck, 1982; Kudoh et al., 1983; Spence, 1982). For Niemann-Pick lines the data clearly demonstrate reduced metabolism in cells derived from Types A and B but nearly normal levels of conversion in Type C cells. Using this technique, Beaudet and Manschreck (1982) and Kudoh et al., (1983) could discriminate between Types A and B since the latter had higher residual enzyme activity in intact cells. The dilemma over the defect in Type C was not resolved using this technique, although recent studies of Gatt and Bierman (1980) and Alpert and Beaudet (1981) have suggested that a membrane system involving lipoprotein components may be involved in sphingomyelinase activity or sphingomyelin mobilization.

It is possible that enzymes other than lysosomal sphingomyelinase contribute to the pathogenesis of these diseases. Matsuzawa and Hostetler (1980) demonstrated a bis(monoacylglycero)phosphate synthetase localized in rat liver tritosomes, and if the enzyme is present in the human, this could explain the high content of bis(monoacylglycero)phosphate in liver of patients with no sphingomyelin storage since the levels of this enzyme would increase, along with an increase in the pool of lysosomes in the tissue. In addition, since the level of the synthetase can be modified, it is possible that altered sphingomyelin or phosphatidylglycerol content of tissues could increase further its level of activity. The donor of the fatty acid required for biosynthesis of bis(monoacylglycero)phosphate in this system has been identified as phosphatidylinositol (Matsuzawa et al., 1978), which does not appear to be a substrate for sphingomyelinase. Although a phosphodiesterase that hydrolyzes bis(monoacylglycero)-phosphate has been found in rat liver (Fig. 8.2), its activity toward this lipid appears to be sluggish (Matsuzawa and Hostetler, 1979).

Finally, it should be mentioned that the brain is rich in a sphingomyelinase localized in plasma membrane that is different from the lysosomal enzyme in that its activity requires a metal ion and is optimal at physiological pH values (Gatt, 1976; Rao and Spence, 1976). The enzyme is particularly high in neurones and neuronal elements, the testis, and the adrenal and is found in very low amounts in other extraneural tissues (Spence et al., 1981). The sphingomyelinase is stimulated by halothane and bee melittin (Pellkofer and Sandhoff, 1980; Pellkofer et al., 1982) in synaptosomal fractions, and it could play an important role in neural communication and endocytosis as a supplier of membrane ceramide in phospholipid base exchange and phospholipase C-like reactions at cell surfaces (Hebdon, 1982; Marggraf et al., 1981a,b). In the brains of patients with types A and C Niemann-Pick disease, the activity of this microsomal enzyme is near normal (Gatt et al., 1978).

8.3   NEUROLOGICAL DISORDERS WITH SECONDARY INVOLVEMENT OF PHOSPHOLIPIDS

8.3.1   Disorders of the Basal Ganglia

8.3.1.1   Clinical Correlations

The diseases correlated for purposes of this discussion include Huntington's, Parkinson's, Tardive Dyskinesia, and Alzheimer's disease, and the reader is directed to more comprehensive discussions of these disorders (Bird, 1978; Chase, 1975; Corkin, 1981; Cotzias et al., 1975; Spokes, 1981). Each is a separate disorder with its own clinical heterogeneity. Huntington's disease is characterized by choreiform movements with onset usually in midlife (30–50 years of age). The clinical course of this sex-linked disorder is variable, but progression is usually slow with death in the sixth or seventh decade. The disease is characterized by progressive dementia manifested by emotional and personality changes and loss of recent memory. The greatest degree of neuropathological abnormalities are noted in the caudate nucleus, putamen, globus pallidus, and zona reticulata of the substantia nigra. These structures occur within the basal ganglia and are involved in the coordination of movements.

Parkinson's disease is also a progressive condition characterized by dyskinesic movements, tremor, and rigidity. Bradykinesia contributes significantly to micrographia, facial masking, hypophonia, and intention tremor. These features are very variable in distribution and intensity. The disease symptoms are usually present in the aged population and have been treated with a variety of agents including L-dopa and more recently amantadine hydrochloride.

Alzheimer's disease can begin in middle life and is characterized by deficits in cognitive function including memory, language, sensorimotor, and perceptual capacities. These changes occur slowly and insidiously. The pathological hallmarks of this disease include the presence of senile plaques, bundles of paired helical fragments, progressive deterioration of dendritic processes, and degeneration of cytoplasmic vacuoles. The changes are bilateral and principally involve numerous brain regions, the cingulate gyrus, amygdala, hippocampus, hypothalamus, and other brain stem structures. The caudate nucleus, thalamus, and mamillary bodies are minimally involved.

In Tardive Dyskinesia the most notable features are involuntary movements including facial grimacing, chewing, and tongue writhing and choreoathetotic movements similar to those seen in Huntington's disease. This disorder occurs in about 15–25% of patients on long-term antipsychotic drug therapy and is more prevalent in the aged population. It displays a periodicity since it may disappear following withdrawal of drug treatment. Other variants such as acute dyskinesia occur in children and young adults but also appear related to drug therapy and are resolved with reductions of dosages or change in medications. Some forms of Tardive Dyskinesia do not respond to these manipulations and appear to be permanent abnormalities. Anti-Parkinsonian agents are ineffective and may aggravate the condition.

The common thread in all of these disorders is the involvement of the movement and coordination centers in the brain. However, the extrapyramidal system is closely interconnected with cortical centers and is dominated by cortical influences. Since the areas of the basal ganglia are involved simultaneously in the enhancement or suppression of certain muscle groups in order to facilitate coordination of movements, it is not hard to imagine how the levels of neurotransmitters can influence the concerted action of this system.

A recent retrospective study of 34 cases who met the neuropathological criteria of Parkinson's disease were reviewed to determine the extent of relationship to changes seen in Alzheimer's disease (Hakim and Mathieson, 1979). They found in 33 of these cases that some or all of the neuropathological changes of Alzheimer's disease were present. Nineteen of these had dementia. This correlation is quite striking and suggests that these two conditions might be causally related.

8.3.1.2 Phospholipid Composition of the Brain

There have been few analyses of the lipid composition of the brain in patients with these diseases. Of those that have been done, the findings are not particularly striking. Den Hartog Jager (1969, 1970) and Riekkinen et al. (1975) analyzed the phospholipid samples of composition from a total of five patients. Both studies reported a small increase in sphingomyelin content, the increase being particularly noteworthy in Lewy bodies of the substantia nigra and locus coeruleus. This was offset by a net decrease in phosphatidylethanolamine and phosphatidylcholine. Interestingly, similar sphingomyelin-containing inclusion bodies have also been noted in the adrenal medulla. The overall phospholipid composition of the brain was not different from controls, however, and the changes in the distribution were restored to normal in those patients on L-dopa therapy.

Analyses of brain biopsies from patients with Huntington's disease did not reveal any specific abnormalities of phospholipids. Although the total lipid composition was reduced, the distribution of phospholipid classes was not altered either in the basal ganglia or in erythrocytes (Norton et al., 1978; Zanella et al., 1980). Other lipid types such as the gangliosides were not markedly abnormal but were also decreased in total amounts. This reflects, as in the other extrapyramidal disorders, the neuropathological status of the patient rather than any specific metabolic abnormality. Goebel et al. (1978) carried out a series of investigations on a case of juvenile Huntington's disease. Again, the phospholipid composition was essentially normal, although some deposition of lipofuscin and a slightly abnormal fatty acid composition of sphingomyelin was found. These changes were nonspecific and considered to be related to the degree of neuronal loss and demyelination. Gray matter lipid composition was normal in adult Huntington's (Hooghwinkel et al., 1978). Borri et al. (1967) analyzed the caudate nucleus from three patients and observed a relative increase in sphingomyelin and a decline in phosphatidylcholine. The distortion of the sphingomyelin–phosphatidylcholine ratio is similar to that previously noted in Parkinson's patients. The fatty acid composition of all the phospholipids was entirely normal. Patients with Alzheimer's disease, where the neuronal involvement is usually more widespread than that in Huntington's or Parkinson's, have the same lipid status as the previous two disorders in spite of the difference in severity of the neuropathological lesions (Rouser et al., 1969; Suzuki et al., 1965).

8.3.1.3 *Biogenic Amines and Therapeutic Interventions*

Parkinson's, Alzheimer's, and Huntington's diseases are related with respect to their biochemical abnormalities in biogenic amine metabolism. The principal change in Parkinson's is a reduction in dopamine levels in the basal ganglia structures. Since this disease is localized principally to the aged population, this decline is partly related to normal aging of the brain. Animal experiments have shown that dopamine and norepinephrine are reduced in the brain of aged rats, and this decline is secondary to a reduction in tyrosine hydroxylase, the rate-controlling enzyme in the tyrosine metabolic pathway. This is also true in the human for both tyrosine hydroxylase and dopamine decarboxylase, the enzyme that converts dihydroxyphenylalanine to dopamine (Carlsson and Winblad, 1976; Finch, 1973; Gottfries, 1980).

In patients diagnosed as having Alzheimer's disease the changes seen in normal aging are more pronounced. Choline acetyltransferase activity is reduced up to 90% in the cortex and hippocampus, but the decrease is lower in the caudate nucleus. Dopamine, norepinephrine, and serotonin levels have been reported as normal or reduced depending on the brain region examined but in general levels are not as markedly nor as uniformly depressed as choline acetyltransferase, the enzyme that synthesizes acetylcholine (Gottfries, 1980; Perry et al., 1981; Terry and Davies, 1980).

Huntington's disease brain appears to be more severely affected in the nigrostriatal dopaminergic tracts. Here, the tyrosine hydroxylase activity is increased as is the level of dopamine and norepinephrine. Serotonin is probably normal, but choline acetyltransferase, acetylcholine, and γ-aminobutyric acid levels are depressed. The overall effect in this disease is an apparent increase in dopaminergic activity, which reflects a relative lack of modulation by several antagonistic influences, one of which is γ-aminobutyric acid. The level of glutamic acid decarboxylase, the GABA-forming enzyme, is markedly reduced (Bird, 1978; Spokes, 1981).

The role of lipids in the modulation of these effects is a subject of active research. There is ample evidence that lipid levels are influenced by the various amines. Acetylcholine, norepinephrine, and serotonin, for example, stimulate the incorporation of labeled inorganic phosphate into phosphatidic acid and phosphatidylinositol in brain slices (Hokin, 1969, 1970; Durell and Sodd, 1966). This effect is not uniform in all areas and varies with the concentration of neurotransmitter employed. These substances also seem to reduce the incorporation into other lipids such as phosphatidylcholine, phosphatidylserine, and phosphatidylethanolamine. In the corpus striatum of guinea pig brain, γ-aminobutyric acid reduced the level of incorporation into the polyphosphoinositides (Hokin, 1970). These experiments have been duplicated by several groups of workers (Arienti et al., 1976; Canessa de Scarnati et al., 1976; Yagihara and Hawthorne, 1972).

These data suggest that acetylcholine stimulation of phospholipid turnover is principally related to phosphatidylinositol. In the caudate nucleus this is mediated by muscarinic receptors (Canessa de Scarnati et al., 1976; Larrabee and Leicht, 1965). Because of the variable effects of the separate biogenic amines, it appears certain that central nervous system neurons are subjected to enhancement or depression depending on the viability of synaptic connections and the levels of the various enzyme systems. It can be seen then that the level of the various amines can influence the overall composition of the phospholipids at any given time. These bio-chemical interrelationships are dealt with in greater detail in other chapters in this volume. Since the lipids must be considered with respect to their roles in events at cell surfaces, the earlier views of Hokin have taken on much significance. Hokin (1969) previously suggested that alterations in phospholipid levels in response to various amines should be examined with respect to long-term changes of neurons such as in the early stages of memory or learning processes. This takes on special significance in evaluating the pathophysiology of the diseases of the basal ganglia.

Yagihara and Hawthorne (1972) suggested that at least a portion of the new phospholipid synthesis stimulated by acetylcholine and other amines reflected restorative changes in neuronal membranes following release of the neurotransmitters at nerve endings. Recent data show that considerable rearrangement of the phospholipid composition at the cell surface occurs (Gaito et al., 1974; Kanfer, 1972; Marggraf et al., 1981a,b) and add new meaning to the views of Hokin and Hawthorne. In addition, phospholipids influence the activity of enzymes critically involved in the biosynthesis and function of neurotransmitters and receptor-mediated signal transfer activities (Axelrod, 1982; Leon et al., 1978; Lloyd and Davidson, 1979; Michell, 1982). Aspects of these functions and possible control mechanisms are discussed in other chapters of this volume.

Significant increases in brain acetylcholine have accompanied dietary administration of choline and phospholipid mixtures in experimental animals. Choline is less effective since it is readily converted to trimethylamine by the intestinal flora (Hirsch and Wurtman, 1978). Dietary lecithin has been employed in the management of patients with Alzheimer's disease, Parkinson's disease, Huntington's disease, Tardive Dyskinesia, and Friedrich's Ataxia. Corkin (1981) recently summarized the experience in studies on 113 Alzheimer's disease patients. The studies included 4 double blind trials of 4–6 weeks duration in which two studies used lecithin and two choline salts. The patients showed mild to moderate dementia at the outset of the studies, and no significant changes were noted in the subjects at the end of the trials. Etienne et al. (1981) carried out a recent study of 11 Alzheimer's patients. In early stages of the illness the patients were given 10 g of a lecithin preparation (Lethicon) three times daily. Both placebo and lecithin were given for consecutive 3-month periods. The authors concluded that there were no measureable improvements in any patients at the end of the 12-week period. Since the latter study fits all the criteria set out by Corkin (1981) for an optimum evaluation of the drug's effectiveness, it appears that this form of therapy alone may be ineffective in the majority of cases. However, Corkin does point out that in combination with additional pharmacologic agents such as anticholinesterase agents, a more notable improvement might be possible. Recent studies on the effect of lecithin treatment on 21 Parkinson's patients did show improvement on psychological testing in some patients when the lipid was included with regular L-dopa therapy (Toffano and Battistin, 1980), although about 60% of patients showed no effect. Similarly, no consistent benefit has been noted in Huntington's patients treated with either free choline or lecithin (Barbeau, 1978; Spokes, 1981). The same principles have underlined the use of lecithin therapy in Tardive Dyskinesia and Friedrich's Ataxia. In Tardive Dyskinesia the use of lecithin appears to be of some benefit (Barbeau, 1978; Gelenberg et al., 1979; Jackson et al., 1979), but there does not appear to be any improvement in patients with Friedrich's Ataxia (Jackson et al., 1979; Walker et al., 1980).

The data available do indicate that dietary lecithin preparations are not deleterious and may eventually prove beneficial if combined with other regimes. The critical factor may be the stage of the disease at which trials are initiated since neuronal loss is more widespread in the later course of these diseases.

8.3.2 Multiple Sclerosis

Multiple sclerosis, a chronic disease of the brain and spinal cord, is characterized by visual loss, imbalance, and weakness of the extremities. It is episodic with frank attacks followed by variable periods of remission. The pathogenesis of the disease is not clearly understood, but there is good evidence for some degree of genetic predilection coupled with an environmental component. The disease is found in greater numbers in temperate climates, and both computer tomography and histocompatibility typing have proven reliable diagnostic aids (Mastaglia and Cala, 1980; Oger and Arnason, 1979).

There have been many investigations of the phospholipid composition of the brain and, in particular, the myelin of patients with multiple sclerosis. Many reports have shown small but clearly detectable alterations in the composition of myelin phospholipids, cerebrosides, gangliosides, and cholesterol (Boggs and Moscarello, 1980; Clausen and Hansen, 1970; Winterfeld and Debuch, 1977). However, other investigations have found no changes from normal either in the composition of phospholipids and their fatty acid distribution or in the composition and fatty acid distribution of other lipid classes (Fewster et al., 1976; Suzuki et al., 1973). While care was taken in these studies to dissect away any obvious areas of necrosis, doubt remains that minute foci were completely removed from samples.

Recent studies have suggested that small changes in the overall composition of myelin may have an important effect on the immunogenicity and functional capacity of myelin. Boggs and Moscarello (1980) have shown, for example, that the amount of protein in multiple sclerosis myelin is slightly changed in comparison to the amount of lipid. They postulate this could influence either the phase transition temperature or fluidity of the membrane. It could also affect either the overall stability of the membrane or its immunogenicity (Boggs et al., 1981; Wood et al., 1980). However, studies using fluorescence polarization or electron spin resonance techniques, which are very sensitive and have been used to detect small changes in fluidity, failed to detect any abnormality in myelin from patients with the disease (Boggs and Moscarello, 1980).

8.3.3   Other Diseases

There are many additional diseases in which abnormalities in the fatty acid composition of the phospholipid pool have been found. Since they are not primarily diseases of phospholipid metabolism, they will not be discussed here.

Recently Grey and co-workers (1980) reported interesting observations on myotonic muscular dystrophy, an autosomal dominant disorder. These investigators found that upon incubation, intact erythrocytes from nine patients displayed a marked and specific reduction in phosphatidic acid production as compared to cells from control individuals. Since the prevailing view has been that a generalized membrane defect exists, these data were very exciting since they suggested that an abnormality in membrane phospholipid metabolism might be characteristic of the disease. Meredith et al. (1982), however, found no defect in phosphatidylinositol phosphodiesterase activity in erythrocyte ghosts from 10 patients with the disease. While this argues against a phospholipase C–mediated mechanism of decreased phosphatidic acid formation, it is possible that an abnormal phospholipase D or diacylglycerol kinase could be responsible (Allan et al., 1980; Marggraf et al., 1981a,b).

8.4   ANIMAL MODELS OF PHOSPHOLIPID DISORDERS

8.4.1   Sphingomyelin Lipidosis as a Primary Defect

Two animal models of the human infantile form of sphingomyelin lipidosis (Type A, Niemann-Pick disease) have been discovered. Bundza et al. (1979) described a 5-month-old miniature poodle that presented with ataxia, loss of equilibrium, and head shaking. Sphingomyelin was accumulated in brain, liver, and kidney while ultrastructural deposits were identified in several additional tissues. Sphingomyelinase activity was almost totally absent in the brain. Wenger et al. (1980) described what appears to be the same disease in three unrelated litters of Siamese cats. Storage of sphingomyelin was found in the liver, and enzyme activity was virtually undetectable in the brain. The microsomal sphingomyelinase was unaffected. Neither study mentioned the presence of bis(monoacylglycero)phosphate.

Adachi et al. (1976) described accumulation of sphingomyelin and other phospholipids in the liver of an inbred strain of mice. Unfortunately, the disease is localized to the liver and is probably not related to a primary defect in sphingomyelinase. This disease is similar to the neuraminidase defect observed in the Sp strain of mice where the only abnormalities discernible involve the liver (Nilsson et al., 1981).

8.4.2 Secondary Forms of Phospholipid Abnormalities

There have been many descriptions of phospholipid diseases in experimental animals induced by administration of various drugs. Yamamoto and co-workers (1971a,b; Adachi et al., 1972) described accumulation of bis(monoacylglycero)phosphate in rats administered 4,4-diethylaminoethoxyhexestrol. This drug also produced the same lipidosis in humans. There was an overall increase in hepatic phospholipids, but bis(monoacylglycero)phosphate, which normally is found in trace quantities, increased up to 100-fold. As mentioned earlier, phospholipid abnormalities have also been associated with administration of triparanol, gentamicin, chloroquine, and AY9944 (Lullmann and Lullmann-Rauch, 1978; Nilsson et al., 1981; Sakuragawa et al., 1977). In none of the latter are the mechanisms leading to the sequelae of drug administration understood. These models may prove useful for studies of specific aspects of altered phospholipid metabolism, but much more work on the etiology of the disease process is needed before findings to date can be interpreted.

Finally, animal models of Huntington's and Parkinson's diseases and multiple sclerosis have been examined as analogs for the human condition (Harik et al., 1982; Marsden, 1979; Roth et al., 1982). None appear to fully express the constellation of features of the human diseases, and the role of the phospholipids is largely unknown.

REFERENCES

Adachi, S., Matsuzawa, Y., Yokomura, T., Ishikawa, K., Uhara, S., Yamamoto, A., and Nishikawa, M., *Lipids, 7*, 1–7 (1972).

Adachi, M., Volk, B.W., and Schneck, L., *Am. J. Pathol., 85,* 229–231 (1976).

Allan, D., Thomas, P., and Gatt, S., *Biochem. J., 191,* 669–672 (1980).

Alpert, A.J., and Beaudet, A.L., *J. Clin. Invest., 68,* 1592–1596 (1981).

Arienti, G., Corazzi, L., Woelk, H., and Porcellati, G., *J. Neurochem., 27,* 203–210 (1976).

Aubert-Tulkens, G., Van Hoof, F., and Tulkens, P., *Lab. Invest., 40,* 481–490 (1979).

Axelrod, J., *Neurosci. Res. Program Bull., 20,* 327–338 (1982).

Baraton, G., and Revol, A., *Clin. Chim. Acta, 76,* 339–343 (1977).

Barbeau, A., *Can. J. Neurol. Sci., 5,* 157–160 (1978).

Beaudet, A. L., Hampton, M. S., Patel, K., and Sparrow, J. T., *Clin. Chim. Acta, 108,* 403–414 (1980).

Beaudet, A. L., and Manschreck, A. A., *Biochem. Biophys. Res. Commun., 105,* 14–19 (1982).

Besley, G.T.N., *FEBS Lett., 80,* 71–74 (1977).

Besley, G.T.N., and Moss, S.E., *Biochim. Biophys. Acta, 752,* 54–64 (1983).

Bird, E.D., *Trends in Neurosci., 1,* 57–59 (1978).

Borri, P.F., Op den Velde, W.M., Hooghwinkel, G.J.M., and Bruyn, G.W., *Neurology, 17,* 172–178 (1967).

Boggs, J.M., and Moscarello, M.A., *Neurochem. Res., 5,* 329–336 (1980).

Boggs, J.M., Clement, I.R., Moscarello, M.A., Eylar, E. H., and Hashim, G., *J. Immunol., 126,* 1207–1211 (1981).

Brady, R.O., in J.B. Stanbury, J.B. Wyngaarden, D. S. Fredrickson, J.L. Goldstein, and M.S. Brown, Eds., *The Metabolic Basis of Inherited Disease,* McGraw-Hill, New York, 1983, pp. 831–841.

Brady, R.O., and Barranger, J.A., in J.B. Stanbury, J.B. Wyngaarden, D.S. Fredrickson, J.L. Goldstein and M.S. Brown, Eds., *Metabolic Basis of Inherited Disease,* McGraw-Hill, New York, 1983, pp. 842–856.

Bundza, A., Lowden, J.A., and Charlton, K.M., *Vet. Pathol., 16,* 530–538 (1979).

Callahan, J.W., Khalil, M.L., and Philippart, M., *Pediatr. Res., 9,* 909–913 (1975).

Callahan, J.W., Gerrie, J., Jones, C.S., and Shankaran, P., *Biochem. J., 193,* 275–283 (1981).

Canessa de Scarnati, O., Sata, M., and De Robertis, E., *J. Neurochem., 27,* 1575–1577 (1976).

Carlsson, A., and Winblad, B., *J. Neural. Transm., 38,* 271–276 (1976).

Chase, T.N., in T.N. Chase, Ed., *The Nervous System, Vol. 2,* Raven Press, New York, 1975, pp. 331–335.

Christomanou, H., *Z. Physiol. Chem., 361,* 1489–1502 (1980).

Clausen, J., and Hansen, I.B., *Acta Neurol. Scand., 46,* 1–17 (1970).

Cotzias, G.C., Papavasiliou, P.S., Ginos, J.Z., and Tolosa, F.S., in T.N. Chase, Ed., *The Nervous System, Vol. 2,* Raven Press, New York, 1975, pp. 323–329.

Corkin, S., *Trends in Neurosci., 4,* 287–290 (1981).

Crandall, B.F., Philippart, M., Brown, W.J., and Bluestone, D.A., *Amer. J. Med. Gen., 12,* 301–308 (1982).

Crocker, A.C., *J. Neurochem., 7,* 69–80 (1961).

Crocker, A.C., and Farber, S., *Medicine, 37,* 1–95 (1958).

den Hartog-Jager, W., *Arch. Neurol., 21,* 615–619 (1969).

den Hartog Jager, W., *Arch. Neurol., 23*, 528–533 (1970).

Dunn, H.C., and Sweeney, V.P., *Neurology, 21*, 442 (1971).

Durell, J., and Sodd, M.A., *J. Neurochem, 13*, 487–491 (1966).

Edgar, A.D., and Freysz, L., *Biochim. Biophys. Acta, 711*, 224–228 (1982).

Elfenbein, I.B., *Johns Hopkins Med. J., 123*, 205–211 (1968).

Elleder, M., and Jirasek, A., *Eur. J. Pediatr., 140*, 90–91 (1983).

Elleder, M., Smid, F., Harzer, K., and Cihula, J., *Virchows Arch. Pathol. Anat., 385*, 215–231 (1980).

Etienne, P., Dastoor, D., Gauthier, S., Ludwick, R., and Collier, B., *Neurology, 31*, 1552–1554 (1981).

Fewster, M.E., Hirono, H., and Mead, J.F., *J. Neurol., 213*, 119–131 (1976).

Finch, C.E., *Brain Res., 52*, 261–276 (1973).

Fried, K., Beer, S., Krespin, H.I., Leiba, H., Djaldetti, M., Zitman, D., and Klibansky, C., *Eur. J. Clin. Invest., 8*, 249–253 (1978).

Gaito, A., De Medio, G.E., Brunetti, M., Amaducci, L., and Porcellati, G., *J. Neurochem., 23*, 1153–1159 (1974).

Gatt, S., *Biochem. Biophys. Res. Commun., 68*, 235–241 (1976).

Gatt, S., and Bierman, E.L., *J. Biol. Chem., 255*, 3371–3376 (1980).

Gatt, S., Dinur, T., and Koplovic, J., *J. Neurochem., 31*, 547–550 (1978).

Gelenberg, A.J., Doller-Wojcik, J.C., and Growden, J.H., *Am. J. Psychiatr., 136*, 772–776 (1979).

Goebel, H.H., Heipertz, R., Scholz, W., Iqbal, K., and Tellez-Nagel, I., *Neurology, 28*, 23–31 (1978).

Gottfries, C.G., *Trends in Neurosci., 3*, 55–57 (1980).

Grey, J.E., Gitelman, H.J., and Roses, A.D., *J. Clin. Invest., 65*, 1478–1482 (1980).

Hakim, A.M., and Mathieson, G., *Neurology, 29*, 1209–1214 (1979).

Harik, S.I., La Mannco, J.C., Snyder, S., Wetherbee, J.R., and Rosenthal, M., *Neurology, 32*, 382–389 (1982).

Harzer, K., Schlote, W., Peiffer, J., Benz, H.U., and Anzil, A.P., *Acta Neuropathol., 43*, 97–104 (1978).

Hebdon, M., *Neurosci. Res. Program Bull., 20*, 321–327 (1982).

Hirsch, M.J., and Wurtman, R.J., *Science, 202*, 223–225 (1978).

Hokin, M., *J. Neurochem., 16*, 127–134 (1969).

Hokin, M., *J. Neurochem., 17*, 357–364 (1970).

Hooghwinkel, G.J.M., Bruyn, G.W., and de Rooj, R.E., *Neurology, 18*, 408–412 (1968).

Hostetler, K.Y., and Hall, L.B., *Biochem. Biophys. Res. Commun., 96*, 388–393 (1980).

Huterer, S., Wherrett, J.R., Poulos, A., and Callahan, J.W., *Neurology, 33*, 67–73 (1983).

Jackson, I.V., Nuttall, E.A., Ibe, I.D., and Perez-Cruet, J., *Amer. J. Psychiatry, 136*, 1458–1460 (1979).

Jones, C.S., Shankaran, P., and Callahan, J.W., *Biochem. J., 195*, 373–382 (1981).

Jones, C.S., Shankaran, P., Davidson, D.J., Poulos, A., and Callahan, J.W., *Biochem. J., 209*, 291–297 (1983).

Kamoshita, S., Aron, A.M., Suzuki, K., and Suzuki, K., *Amer. J. Dis. Child., 117*, 379–394 (1969).

Kanfer, J.N., *J. Lipid Res., 13*, 468–476 (1972).

Karpati, G., Carpenter, S., Wolfe, L.S., and Andermann, F., *Neurology, 27*, 32–42 (1977).

Klenk, E., Z. *Physiol. Chem., 229*, 151–156 (1934).

Kudoh, T., Velkoff, M.A., and Wenger, D.A., *Biochim. Biophys. Acta, 754*, 82–92 (1983).

Kunze, H., Hesse, B., and Bohn, E., *Biochim. Biophys. Acta, 711*, 10–18 (1982).

Larrabee, M.G., and Leicht, W.S., *J. Neurochem., 12*, 1–13 (1965).

Leon, A., Benvegnu, D., Toffano, G., Orlando, P., and Massari, P., *J. Neurochem., 30*, 23–26 (1978).

Lloyd, K.G., and Davidson, L., *Adv. Neurol., 23*, 705–716 (1979).

Lowden, J.A., LaRamee, M.A., and Wentworth, P., *Arch. Neurol., 17*, 230–237 (1967).

Lullmann, H., and Lullmann-Rauch, R., *Science, 200*, 568–569 (1978).

Maret, A., Potier, M., Salvayre, R., and Douste-Blazy, L., *FEBS Lett., 160*, 93–97 (1983).

Marggraf, W.D., Anderer, F.A., and Kanfer, J.N., *Biochim. Biophys. Acta, 661*, 61–73 (1981a).

Marggraf, W.D., Zertani, R., Anderer, F.A., and Kanfer, J.N., *Biochim. Biophys. Acta, 710*, 314–323 (1981b).

Marsden, C.D., *Adv. Neurol., 23*, 567–576 (1979).

Martin, J.J., Philippart, M., Van Hauwaert, J., Callahan, J.W., and Deberdt, R., *Arch. Neurol., 27*, 45–51 (1972).

Mastaglia, F.L., and Cala, L.A., *Trends in Neurosci., 3*, 16–20 (1980).

Matsuzawa, Y., and Hostetler, K.Y., *J. Biol Chem., 254*, 5997–6001 (1979).

Matsuzawa, Y., and Hostetler, K.Y., *J. Lipid Res., 21*, 202–214 (1980).

Matsuzawa, Y., Poorthuis, B.J.H.M., and Hostetler, K.Y., *J. Biol. Chem., 253*, 6650–6553 (1978)

Meredith, A.L., Harper, P.S., and Bradley, D.M., *Clin. Chim. Acta, 120*, 201–206 (1982).

Michell, R.H., *Neurosci. Res. Prog. Bull., 20*, 338–350 (1982).

Muller, H., and Harzer, K., *J. Neurochem., 34*, 446–448 (1980).

Neville, B.G.R., Lake, B.D., Stephens, R., and Sanders, M.D., *Brain, 96*, 97–120 (1973).

Nilsson, O., Fredman, P., Klinghardt, G.W., Dreyfus, H., and Svennerholm, L., *Eur. J. Biochem., 116*, 565–571 (1981).

Norton, W.T., Iqbal, K., Tiffany, C., and Tellez-Nagel, I., *Neurology, 28*, 812–816 (1978).

Oger, J.J.F., and Arnason, B.G.W., *Trends in Neurosci., 2*, 68–70 (1979).

Oppenheimer, D.R., Norman, R.M., Tingey, A.H., and Aherne, W.A., *J. Neurol. Sci., 5*, 575–588 (1967).

Pellkofer, R., and Sandhoff, K., *J. Neurochem, 34*, 988–992 (1980).

Pellkofer, R., Marsh, D., Hoffmann-Bleihauer, P., and Sandhoff, K., *J. Neurochem., 38*, 1230–1235 (1982).

Perry, E.K., Tomlinson, B.E., Blessed, G., Perry, R.H., Cross, A.J., and Crow, T.J., *J. Neurol. Sci., 51*, 279–287 (1981).

Philippart, M., in V. Zambotti, G. Tettamanti, and M. Arrigoni, Eds., *Glycolipids, Glycoproteins, and Mucopolysaccharides of the Nervous System*, Plenum, New York, 1972, pp. 231–254.

Philippart, M., Martin, L., Martin, J.J., and Menkes, J.H., *Arch. Neurol., 20*, 227–238 (1969).

Poorthuis, B.J.H.M., and Hostetler, K.Y., *J. Biol. Chem., 250,* 3297–3302 (1975).

Poulos, A., Beckman, K., Ellis, D.H., and Pollard, A.C., *Clin. Genet., 22,* 234–243 (1983a).

Poulos, A., Hudson, N., and Ranieri, E., *Clin Genet., 24,* 225–243 (1983b).

Poulos, A., Shankaran, P., Jones, C.S., and Callahan, J.W., *Biochim. Biophys. Acta, 751,* 428–431 (1983c).

Rao, B.G., and Spence, M.W., *J. Lipid Res., 17,* 506–515 (1976).

Resner, F., Kagen, M.D., and Dana, M., *N. Engl. J. Med., 282,* 1100–1101 (1970).

Riekkinen, P., Rinne, U.K., Pelliniemi, T.T., and Sonninen, V., *Arch. Neurol., 32,* 25–27 (1975).

Roth, G.A., Monferran, C.G., Maggio, B., and Cumar, F.A., *Life Sci., 30,* 859–866 (1982).

Rouser, G., Kritchevsky, G., Yamamoto, A., Knudson, A.G., and Simon, G., *Lipids, 3,* 287–290 (1968).

Rouser, G., Galli, C., Kritcher, G., *J. Am. Chem. Soc., 42,* 404–408 (1969).

Sakuragawa, N., Sakuragawa, M., Kuwabara, T., Pentchev, P.G., Barranger, J.A., and Brady, R.O., *Science, 196,* 317–319 (1977).

Sawitsky, A., Rosner, E., and Chodsky, S., *Sem. Hematol., 9,* 285–297 (1972).

Seng, P.N., Debuch, H., Witter, B., and Wiedemann, H.R., *Z. Physiol. Chem., 352,* 280–288 (1971).

Silverstein, M.N., and Ellefson, R.E., *Sem. Hematol., 9,* 299–307 (1972).

Silverstein, M.N., Ellefson, R.D., and Ahern, E.J., *N. Engl. J. Med., 282,* 1–4 (1970).

Spence, M.W., Clarke, J.T.R., and Cook, H.W., *J. Biol. Chem., 258,* 8595–8600 (1983).

Spence, M.W., Burgess, J.K., Sperker, E.R., Hamed, L., and Murphy, M.G., in J.W. Callahan and J.A. Lowden, Eds., *Lysosomes and Lysosomal Storage Diseases,* Raven Press, New York, 1981, pp. 219–228.

Spokes, E.G.S., *Trends in Neurosci., 4,* 115–118 (1981).

Suzuki, K., Katzman, R., and Korey, S.R., *J. Neuropathol. Exp. Neurol., 24,* 211–221 (1965).

Suzuki, K., Suzuki, K., and Kamoshita, S., *J. Neuropathol. Exp. Neurol., 28,* 25–73 (1969).

Suzuki, K., Kamoshita, S., Eto, Y., Tourtellotte, W.W., Gonatas, J.O., *Arch. Neurol., 28,* 293–297 (1973).

Terry, R.D., and Davies, P., *Ann. Rev. Neurosci., 3,* 77–95 (1980).

Tjiong, H.B., and Debuch, H., *Z. Physiol. Chem., 359,* 71–79 (1978).

Tjiong, H.B., Seng, P.N., Debuch, H., and Wiedemann, H.R., *J. Neurochem, 21,* 1475–1485 (1973).

Toffano, G., and Battistin, L., *Prog. Clin. Biol. Res., 39,* 205–214 (1980).

Vanier, M.T., Revol, A., and Fichet, M., *Clin. Chim. Acta, 106,* 257–267 (1980).

Varela-Duran, J., Roholt, P.C., and Ratcliff, N.B., *Arch. Pathol. Lab. Med., 104,* 30–34 (1980).

Videbaek, A., *Acta Paediat., 41,* 355–359 (1952).

Walker, J.L., Chamberlain, S., and Robinson, N., *J. Neurol. Neurosurg. Psych., 43,* 111–117 (1980).

Wenger, D.A., Barth, G., and Githens, J.H., *Am. J. Dis. Child., 131,* 955–961 (1977).

Wenger, D.A., Sattler, M., Kudoh, T., Snyder, S.P., and Kingston, R.S., *Science, 208,* 1471–1473 (1980).

Wherrett, J.R., and Huterer, S., *J. Biol. Chem.*, *247*, 4114–4120 (1972).

Wherrett, J.R., and Huterer, S., *Lipids*, *8*, 531–533 (1973).

Wherrett, J.R., and Huterer, S., *Neurochem Res.*, *8*, 89–98 (1983).

Winterfeld, M., and Debuch, H., *J. Neurol.*, *215*, 261–272 (1977).

Wood, D.D., Boggs, J.M., and Moscarello, M.A., *Neurochem. Res.*, *5*, 745–755 (1980).

Yagihara, Y., and Hawthorne, J.N., *J. Neurochem.*, *19*, 355–367 (1972).

Yamamoto, A., Adachi, S., Ishibe, T., Shinji, Y., Kaki-Uchi, Y., Seki, K.-I., and Kitani, T., *Lipids*, *5*, 566–571 (1970).

Yamamoto, A., Adachi, S., Kitani, T., Shinji, Y., Seki, K., Nasu, T., and Nishikawa, M., *J. Biochem.*, *69*, 613–615 (1971a).

Yamamoto, A., Adachi, S., Ishikawa, K., Yokomura, T., Kitani, T., Nasu, T., Imoto, T., and Nishikawa, M., *J. Biochem.*, *70*, 775–784 (1971b).

Yamanaka, T., and Suzuki, K., *J. Neurochem.*, *38*, 1753–1764 (1982).

Zanella, A., Izzo, C., Meola, G., Mariani, M., Colotti, M.T., Silano, V., Pellegata, G., and Scarlato, G., *J. Neurol. Sci.*, *47*, 93–103 (1980).

nine

ANIMAL MODELS OF NEUROLOGICAL DISORDERS: INSIGHT THROUGH STUDIES OF PHOSPHOLIPID METABOLISM

ROBERT M. GOULD

Institute for Basic Research in Developmental Disabilities
Staten Island, New York

CONTENTS

9.1   INTRODUCTION   322

    9.1.1   Phospholipids in Cell Membranes: Composition, 323
    9.1.2   Phospholipids in Cell Membranes: Dynamics, 324

9.2   PHOSPHOLIPID METABOLISM IN NEURONS AND GLIA   324

    9.2.1   Nervous System Barriers, 324
    9.2.2   Neuronal Lipid Metabolism, 325
    9.2.3   Glial Lipid Metabolism, 326

9.3   APPROACHES FOR STUDYING PHOSPHOLIPID
     METABOLISM IN ANIMALS   327

9.4   WALLERIAN DEGENERATION   328

    9.4.1   The Distal Nerve, 330
    9.4.2   The Retrograde Response, 339
    9.4.3   Nerve Regeneration, 342
    9.4.4   Myelination of Regenerating Axons, 343
    9.4.5   Degeneration of the CNS, 345

9.5   MODELS FOR DEMYELINATION AND
     HYPOMYELINATION   348

    9.5.1   Models of Demyelination, 348
    9.5.2   Mutants and Hypomyelination, 355

9.6   EXPERIMENTAL DIABETIC NEUROPATHY   361

9.7   CONCLUSIONS   367

    REFERENCES   367

9.1   INTRODUCTION

The major aims of this chapter are to review several of the simplest and
most popular animal models with nervous system impairment and discuss
ways in which changes in the nervous system phospholipids and their
metabolism could be relevant to the impairment. Brief introductory sec-

tions on the properties of phospholipids, the methods available for studying them, and application of these methods to phospholipid metabolism in neurons and glia are included as background.

9.1.1 Phospholipids in Cell Membranes: Composition

Phospholipids are a major structural component of all cell membranes, and physical and structural features of membranes are determined by these components (cf. Singer and Nicolson, 1972). Studies that compare the lipid and phospholipid compositions of normal and abnormal nervous tissues, isolated cells, and/or subcellular fractions would seem to be the most direct and straightforward way to relate lipids to the disorder. Phospholipid compositions from many preparations, including those of the nervous system, have been published (see White, 1973; Yao, 1984). Jungalwala (this volume) describes current methods for obtaining lipid composition data with limited quantities of biological sample.

The detection of compositional differences between normal and diseased tissue has been a key to characterizing enzymic defects in several lipid storage disease (Pentchev and Barranger, 1978; Brady, 1981, 1983; Stanbury et al., 1983). These disorders, however, rarely involve deficiency in specific enzymes involved in the synthesis or subsequent metabolism of phospholipids per se. It will be a rare circumstance that compositional studies pinpoint a neurological disorder to the lack of a specific enzyme of phospholipid metabolism. The human diseases in which phospholipid deficiencies have been found are Zellweger syndrome, a lethal hereditary disease in which plasmalogen is depleted (Borst, 1983; Heymans et al., 1983), Niemann-Pick disease, a sphingomyelin lipidosis (Brady, 1983), and possibly Refsum's syndrome, a phytanic acid storage disease (Steinberg, 1983). The defect in Zellweger syndrome is characterized by the absence of peroxisomes, the organelles where plasmalogen formation is localized (Hajra and Bishop, 1982).

Compositional approaches by themselves have had limited impact on gaining understanding of neurological disorders in animals and man for two reasons: (1) Nervous tissue is particularly heterogeneous and lipid composition data represent a mean from a multitude of membrane systems combined for the initial extraction. Alterations limited to a specific cell or a cellular specialization would only contribute in relation to that proportion of lipid of the cell or specialization present in the sample. Therefore, compositional changes produced repeatedly throughout a dominant membrane component, such as myelin sheaths, would be easy to elucidate, while those associated with less prominent membranes or with a limited proportion of dominant membranes would be difficult to detect.

(2) Biological membranes generally use the same phospholipids as building blocks, though diphosphatidyl glycerol is restricted to mitochondria (Hostetler, 1982). Differences in phospholipid composition in a malformed or malfunctioning membrane will possibly show up as subtle quantitative alterations rather than qualitative ones.

9.1.2   Phospholipids in Cell Membranes: Dynamics

Studies with radioactive precursors and fluorescent probes have shown that membrane lipids are dynamic both in their ability to move within and between membranes and in their metabolic turnover. The dynamic properties of membrane phospholipids are a very important facet of neuronal tissue metabolism, in part because neurons and glia must form and maintain extensive and highly specialized processes. A notable example is the myelin sheath elaborated by oligodendroglia and Schwann cells. Highlights of nervous tissues and lipid dynamics are considered elswhere (cf. Fisher and Agranoff, and Dawson, this volume).

A major theme of this chapter will be to consider how studies of lipid metabolism might provide important insights into understanding the neuropathological process, emphasizing impaired or altered membrane function. An increased susceptibility of neural tissue to physical and toxic injury is possibly due to the enormous dimensions of the specialized membranes of the neurons and glia cells. Before discussing diseases of nervous tissue, unique aspects of lipid metabolism in neurons and glia will be briefly considered (see also Ledeen, this volume).

9.2   PHOSPHOLIPID METABOLISM IN NEURONS AND GLIA

9.2.1   Nervous System Barriers

The central (CNS) and peripheral (PNS) nervous systems are separated from the rest of the body by the blood–brain and blood–nerve barriers, respectively (see Rapoport, 1976; Bradbury, 1979; and Katzman, 1981, for reviews). These barriers provide neural cells with special ionic and nutritive environments conducive to their viability and functional stability. Consequently, neural barriers influence the supply of metabolites, including precursors of lipid metabolism, to neural cells. Breakdown of the barriers will expose neurons and glia to less optimal and potentially deleterious environments that could compromise their metabolic and functional stability possibly through altering the influx of needed metabolites. Thus, the local tissue milieu is changed during ischemia, anoxia, edema, local inflammation, and other conditions in which the entry of blood-borne substances and cells occurs. Lipophilic agents, taken into an animal, readily penetrate blood–brain and/or blood–nerve barriers and interact with neural cell membranes. Diseases in which these barriers are compromised or bypassed are in general difficult to study with direct biochemical approaches, as there is usually wide variability in the development of the neurological condition (e.g., Section 9.5.1).

9.2.2 Neuronal Lipid Metabolism

The CNS and PNS are made up of neurons of varying shapes and sizes, having differing compositional and metabolic properties. While the functions, sizes, and geometries of neurons differ greatly, for the most part they maintain large amounts of their plasma membrane and cytoplasm, including internal membranous organelles, at considerable distances from their soma. A comprehensive understanding of neuronal lipid disposition and metabolism requires knowledge of metabolism as it occurs both in the perikarya and in distant processes. Biochemical approaches currently in use are insensitive to the heterogeneity of neuronal populations and the heterogeneity from soma to process to terminal specialization.

Phospholipid and membrane protein metabolism in the neuronal soma are fundamentally the same as in other cells. The enzymes used in phospholipid metabolism are formed locally on free or bound polysomes. Some lipid enzymes remain associated with and function within rough endoplasmic reticulum while others are "processed" by posttranslational modification and routing to other membrane organelles. The cellular and subcellular distribution of many of the enzymes of lipid metabolism have been determined (see Dawson, this volume). However, little information is available on how the enzymes are directed to their functional sites or how long they function at these sites. Furthermore, although many studies have demonstrated links between lipid metabolism and somal activities, that is, generation and regulation of ionic currents (see Agranoff and Fisher, this volume), studies have by and large not considered altered lipid metabolism in models in which these somal properties are altered (see Section 9.4.2).

Phospholipids, glycolipids, and cholesterol are needed for the growth and maintenance of axonal and dendritic membranes and their preterminal and terminal specialization (see Section 9.4.3). There is evidence that a continued synthesis of somal phospholipid and cholesterol is required for the delivery of membrane proteins (and presumably lipids) to distant locations in the axonal process and nerve terminals by fast axonal transport (Agranoff, 1977; Longo and Hammerschlag, 1980; Heacock et al., 1984).

Whether impairment of somal lipid metabolism can lead to axon dwindling and dying back axonopathy has yet to be established.

The central role of fast axonal transport in supplying proteins and lipids to distant processes and terminals has been extensively studied and reviewed (Grafstein and Forman, 1980; Ochs, 1983; Weiss, 1982; Ledeen, this volume). Since enzymes of lipid metabolism are present in axons and terminals (Holtzman and Mercurio, 1980; Gould et al., 1983a,b), it is feasible that process and terminal lipid metabolism at these sites contribute to their properties and function. The maintenance of axon and terminal lipid metabolism depends on a continuous supply of enzymes that are synthesized in the perikaryon and then undergo axonal transport. Whether surrounding glial cells provide metabolites, cofactors, or enzymes that participate in or regulate neuronal process and terminal metabolism is unknown. Furthermore, the influence of metabolites and other agents in cerebral spinal (in CNS) and endoneurial (in PNS) fluids on neural lipid metabolism has not been investigated. Few investigators recognize the need for and existence of pathways for getting lipid metabolic machinery to distant axons and terminals. Therefore, there have been few investigations directed at demonstrating any relationship between lipid metabolism in axons and terminals and an experimental disease (Section 9.6) (Souyri et al., 1981; DeMedio et al., 1983). The secretion-related and receptor-mediated metabolism of inositol and choline phosphoglycerides at pre- and postsynaptic sites may be an impetus for developing further research in these areas.

9.2.3   Glial Lipid Metabolism

This discussion will focus on myelin-forming oligodendroglia and Schwann cells (Pevzner, 1982; Gould et al., 1982a), since models in which the lipid-rich myelin sheaths are affected is a major part of this review (Sections 9.4 and 9.5). A major role of these cells, elaboration of myelin sheaths around large caliber axons, is a substantial part of normal nervous system development. Roughly a third of the dry weight of the total human brain is from myelin sheaths formed by oliogodendroglial cells (Norton, 1981; Gould in press). Even higher proportions of brain white matter, spinal cord, and "myelinated" peripheral nerves (e.g., trigeminal, sciatic, dorsal and ventral roots) are myelin. Furthermore, myelin is uniquely lipid-rich, containing roughly 70–80% lipid (phospholipid–cholesterol–glycolipid in molar ratios of between $4:4:2$ and $3:4:2$ (Norton, 1981; Norton and Cammer, 1984a)) compared with roughly 50% lipid for most other biological membranes. (White, 1973; Finean and Michell, 1981). The synthesis and metabolism of myelin lipids (and myelin-specific proteins) is a dominant activity of these glial cells.

Myelination is an end product in a sequence of developmental steps. Before Schwann cells and oligodendroglial processes begin to form compact multilayered myelin sheaths, they must establish defined sections (internodes) on the axons they will myelinate. Myelination depends on axon contact (Sears, 1982; Gould, in press). The "signal(s)" that axons transmit to the oligodendroglia and Schwann cells must be similar, if not identical, for oligodendroglia and Schwann cells myelinate the same axon process (e.g., motor and sensory neurons). However, there are differences in the metabolic responsiveness of Schwann cells and oligodendroglia to these signals (see Sections 9.4.1 and 9.4.5).

In addition to oligodendroglia and Schwann cells involved in myelination, there are other related glial cells that interact with neuronal perikarya, small caliber axons and terminal specializations, but do not form myelin. Furthermore, the CNS contains astroglia and microglia. Knowledge of the lipid composition and metabolic properties of these cells is for the most part limited to studies of purified cells in culture environments (Yavin, this volume). Cytochemical approaches might be used to provide a means for studying and comparing lipid metabolism of these cells *in situ* in normal animals and those with neurological impairment.

9.3   APPROACHES FOR STUDYING PHOSPHOLIPID METABOLISM IN ANIMALS

A major reason for using animal models to understand the etiology of diseases is the control that may be exercised over the experimental conditions and the history of the animals, for example, diet, housing, light–dark cycle, and the availability of tissue. The relevance of these factors will be briefly assessed with some of the animal models selected in this chapter. Obviously, consideration of these factors is an important part in developing a program based on any neurological model.

From preceding chapters, it would be relatively easy to compile a list containing many of the strategies and approaches used by lipid biochemists. In this section the applicability of some of the approaches to studies of phospholipids in neurologically affected animals will be evaluated.

The most straightforward approaches to uncover derangements in lipid metabolism would be those that measure the levels of the lipids themselves (Section 9.1.1), activities or levels of enzymes involved in their metabolism, and levels of cofactors and substrates relevant to lipid metabolism. Even though these studies are easy to perform on whole tissue samples, difficulties lie in detecting changes that affect a specific cell population of the tissue, and in establishing the relationship between measured changes and the specialized membranes of glia and/or neurons where they might occur.

The application of fractionation methods requires both a satisfactory method of purification and the stability of the components during fractionation. Furthermore, fractionation methods are generally limited to major components and are not yet available for isolating specialized minor structures, such as nodes of Ranvier or dendritic spines. If exposed proteins specific to these specializations are identified and isolated and antibodies raised, the antibodies may provide the specificity needed for developing methodology for purifying the specialized membranes and studying their properties. Fractionation is not, however, the only approach for studying abnormalities localized to specific minor membranes. Altered nodal properties, for example, might be demonstrated with biochemical studies of node-specific proteins (sodium channels or Na^+-K^+-ATPase) and morphological (e.g. freeze fracture, and special cytochemical) procedures. A possible application relevant to these approaches is discussed later (Section 9.6).

Another strategy is one in which lipids and lipid metabolism are not the main, or at least initial, focus. Experiments would be planned to determine if "membrane properties" such as transport (e.g., of ions, sugars, neurotransmitters), activities of membrane-associated enzymes, and physical and structural characteristics of the membranes are changed. Studies demonstrating that membrane-associated function(s) are compromised might be a basis for others to determine if the impairment could be a consequence of altered lipid composition and metabolism. Studies using this latter strategy are largely outside the scope of this chapter.

9.4 WALLERIAN DEGENERATION

The most widely studied model for a degenerative nervous disease is Wallerian degeneration (Waller, 1850). The popularity of this model stems from (1) the simplicity and reproducibility in causing degeneration, not only of peripheral nerves, but also of fiber tracts in the central nervous system, (2) the fact that early distal degeneration is comprised of changes specific to neuronal processes and their associated glia, and (3) that the completeness of the degeneration is a factor in subsequent regeneration, including the reestablishment of functional connectivity and the formation of myelin sheaths around the larger-caliber regenerating axons.

Damage to any part of the axon causes not only degenerative changes in the nerve distal to the site of injury, that is, classical Wallerian degeneration (Section 9.4.1), but also structural and functional changes in the cell soma, the proximal axon and dendrites (retrograde reaction, Section 9.4.2), which are relevant to successful nerve regeneration (Section 9.4.3), and myelination of the regenerating fibers (Section 9.4.4). Studies on CNS degeneration and regeneration will be covered separately (Section 9.4.5). The time course and magnitude of these changes depend on a number of factors, including (1) the nature of the injury, for example, crush, freezing, ligation, or severance; (2) the characteristics of the nerves, their length and breadth, and the caliber spectrum of component fibers, their modality, and so on; (3) the species and age of animal; and (4) the proximity of the lesion to the cell body, since this affects the volume of axoplasm and number of collaterals displaced (cf. Cragg, 1970; Watson, 1976; Grafstein and McQuarrie, 1978; Kao et al., 1983). Although these and other variables influence the pattern of degenerative and regenerative changes observed, when they are controlled, the changes are highly reproducible. Furthermore, by varying one specific parameter (e.g., age), it is possible to learn how this parameter influences the degenerative and regenerative responses of the nerve.

In considering this model in terms of criteria discussed in the previous section, Wallerian degeneration is an attractive experimental model because: (1) Crushing, cutting, or freezing the nerve initiates changes identical to those in physically traumatized human nerves. (2) Nerves of all animals, including such diverse species as lamprey eel, goldfish, mice, and monkeys, degenerate following their interruption. (3) The amounts and accessibility of tissue depend on size of the animal and on the nerve chosen; the sciatic and tibial nerves are most commonly used in peripheral nerve studies, while the optic nerve is a favorite for CNS studies. (4) The contralateral nerves are the usual controls because they exhibit identical development and nutrition. Littermates and age- and weight-matched controls are acceptable alternatives. (5) Transection, freezing, and crush will disrupt all the nerve processes, maximizing alterations in tissue metabolism. However, the time course of the changes is not uniform for all nerves but is caliber dependent, since thinner fibers degenerate faster (Lubinska, 1977). The remainder of this section will consider changes in lipids in relation to other known morphological and biochemical events in Wallerian degeneration.

Several reviews detailing lipid changes in Wallerian degeneration should be consulted for additional information (cf. Domonkos, 1972; Hallpike, 1976; Norton and Cammer, 1984b; Allt, 1976; Smith and Benjamins, 1984; Natarajan and Schmid, 1984; Yao, 1984). Few studies have focused on lipid changes in central nerve degeneration, although a growing interest in developing approaches to facilitate CNS regeneration (Kao, Bunge, and Reier, 1983) will hopefully encourage further studies in this area (Section 9.4.5).

9.4.1 The Distal Nerve

Morphological changes that occur in nerves undergoing Wallerian degeneration have been discussed in a number of papers and reviews (cf. Thomas, 1974; Schroder, 1975; Allt, 1976; Hallpike, 1976). Donat and Wisniewski (1973; see also Watson, 1976) divided the degenerating nerve into three zones based on organelle accumulation, which from the site of injury include a traumatic zone ($\sim$ 2–3 mm),[†] a peritraumatic zone (2–3 cm), [†] and the rest of the nerve. This spatial division and a temporal one (see below) are important in conceptualizing the degenerative process. Degeneration in the far distal nerve is similar to that in the peritraumatic zone, although it probably follows a protracted time course (e.g., Joseph, 1973; Lubinska, 1977; Cancalon, 1983). Few biochemical studies have focused on the far distal nerve or compared changes in the peritraumatic areas with regions further distal. In smaller animals, the extensive branching of distal nerve and the concomitant increased fasciculation could restrict biochemical studies of this nature. The focus of most biochemical studies is the peritraumatic region characterized by early, transient accumulations of axonal organelles in paranodal regions. The traumatic zones, comprised of regions on both sides of the injury, are characterized by temporal accumulations over hours to several days of axonal organelles that are both retrogradely and anterogradely transported. Biochemical studies directed toward degeneration of the traumatic zone (just distal to the injury) would be confounded by ischemia and anoxia resulting from the damaged vasculature. The axonal organelles accumulating in the distal-side traumatic region (products of retrograde transport) include lysosomes and dense bodies and are different from anterogradely accumulating organelles, that is, specialized tubulovesicular membrane systems (Holtzman and Novikoff, 1965; Tsukita and Ishikawa, 1980; Smith, 1980; Ellisman and Lindsey, 1983). It is not known how the anterogradely transported organelles are transformed into lysosomes and dense bodies prior to the return, although the transformation is likely a consequence of membrane recycling at terminals. The formation of preterminal interruptions might initiate similar organelle transformation.

† Distances come from studies of rabbit and cat sciatic nerve.

The cause of degeneration in the distal nerve is unknown, although it is probable that a reduced supply of "trophic" factors from the axon (Section 9.4.2) might "initiate" the degenerative responses, including those by associated Schwann cells (Singer and Steinberg, 1972; Schroder, 1975). Another hypothesis that a "wound" substance is taken up at the site of injury transported retrogradely to the cell bodies to influence their expression has not been disproved.

The temporal changes that occur have been divided into three stages by Rossiter (1961): stage I is characterized by axon collapse and physical destruction of myelin, stage II by cell proliferation and chemical degradation of myelin, and stage III by fibrosis or regeneration; the later occurs when axon sprouts reach and grow into the distal stump. The duration of each stage varies with different models. There is also the more subtle variation from fiber to fiber and even within each internode.

The earliest changes, which occur within minutes to hours in the peritraumatic zone, include retraction of Schwann cell processes from nodal regions and swelling adjacent to the Schmidt–Lantermann incisures primarily along intraperiod myelin. These events precede and are causally related to the breakup of myelin internodes into discreet ovoids over a 1–3-day period. The formation of ovoids is observed in smaller fibers before larger ones, and it spreads proximodistally in all size classes of fibers (Lubinska, 1977, 1982). Some of the biochemical changes that accompany and follow these morphological changes are listed in Table 9.1 (cf. Rossiter, 1961; Porcellati, 1972; Domonkos, 1972; Dewar and Moffatt, 1979; for additional information and references). There are few, if any, biochemical changes that are detected as early as morphological Schwann cell changes. Although the cause of these changes is unknown, a possible consequence of the paranodal retraction and swelling in the region of incisures might be to perturb the ionic gradients across the axolemma.

That the axon is an early target is seen in the rapid loss of the neurofilament (NF) proteins (Table 9.1). A possible cause of NF protein degradation is the rapid rise in intracellular calcium in axoplasm with concomitant activation of NF-specific calcium-activated protease (Schlaepfer, 1974a,b; Schlaepfer and Micko, 1978). The breakdown of cytoskeletal proteins could precipitate the collapse of axoplasm associated with ovoid formation. Loss of cytoskeleton accompanies shrinkage of the degenerating garfish olfactory nerve (Cancalon, 1983). There is still little information as to the loss of other axon constituents. Autoradiographic studies with Dr. Ray Sinatra showed that membrane-associated axoplasmic inositol lipid synthesis is lost from distal axons (near the traumatic zone) but not proximal axons within 3 days of injury (compare a and b in Fig. 9.1). The paucity of axonal organelles relative to Schwann

TABLE 9.1 Compositional Changes of Distal Nerve Following Injury

	Injury	Changes	Time	References
Axonal proteins	Transection (rat) sciatic nerve	Decrease in NF[a] triplet	24–48 h	Schlaepfer and Micko, 1978
	Enucleation (rabbit) optic nerve	Decrease in NF triplet	2–4 wks	Soifer et al., 1981
	Enucleation (rat) optic nerve	Decrease in NF triplet	1–2 wks	Dahl et al., 1981
	Ligation (cat, rat) sciatic nerve	Decrease in Na^+ channel (saxitoxin binding)	3–4 days	Spencer et al., 1981
	Crush (rat) optic nerve	Decrease in Na^+ channel (saxitoxin binding)	3–7 days	Politis, et al., 1983
Myelin and Schwann cell proteins	Transection (rat) sciatic nerve	Decrease in P_0 and P_1 basic protein	8 days	Wood and Dawson, 1974
	Transection (rabbit) sciatic nerve	Decrease in P_0, P_1 and P_2	14–18 days	McDermott and Wisniewski, 1977
Myelin and Schwann cell lipids	Transection (rabbit) sciatic nerve	Decrease in lipid P, fatty acid esters, fatty aldehyde	6 days–2 wks	Domonkos and Heiner, 1968a,b
	Crush (rat) sciatic nerve (and endoneurial preparation)	Decrease in cholesterol; increase in cholesterol esters and free fatty acids; increase in esterification of cholesterol	3–6 days	Wood and Dawson, 1974; Belin and Smith, 1976; Yao et al., 1980; Yao and Dyck, 1981

	Transection (rabbit) sciatic nerve	Decrease in cholesterol, phospholipid and galactolipid; relative increase in PC and decrease in PE plasmalogen	1–7 wks	Hofeig et al., 1981, 1982
	Transection (rat) sciatic nerve	Decrease in hydroxy and nonhydroxy cerebrosides and sulfatides	3–16 days	Yahara et al., 1982
	Transection (rabbit) tibial (t) and optic (o); nerves	Increase in fat free dry weight; decrease in phospholipid and cholesterol	14–100 days (t) 100–200 days (o); 19–100 days (t) 100–200 days (o)	McCaman and Robins, 1959
	Transection (rabbit) sciatic nerve	Change in ganglioside Decrease: G1 and G2; Increase: G5 and G6; No change: G3 and G4	Main change; 14–28 days	Yates and Thompson, 1978
Other metabolites	Transection (rabbit) sciatic nerve	Decrease in ATP and P creatinine; decrease in creatine; increase in glucose, lactate, and fucose	3–4 days	Stewart et al., 1965
	Crush (rabbit) sciatic nerve	Increase in 3′,5′ cAMP	1 h	Appenzeller and Partlow, 1972

[a] NF, neurofilament.

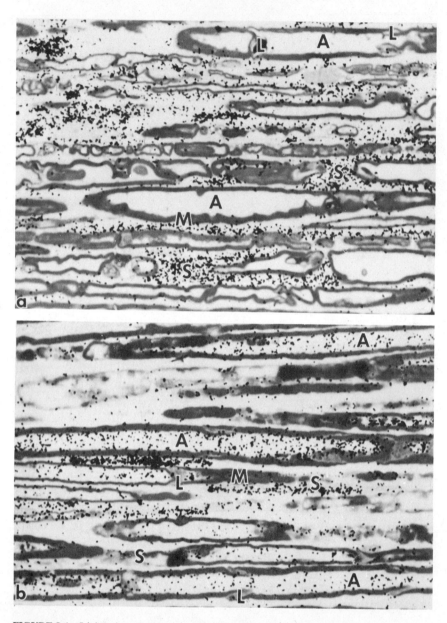

FIGURE 9.1 Light microscope autoradiographs of mouse sciatic nerve crushed for 5 s with watchmaker forceps. At times indicated following the crush, the nerves were reexposed and injected both promixally and distally with [³H]inositol (a and B) or choline (c). After 2 h the mice were anesthetized, perfused with fixative, and the tissues worked up for light microscope autoradiography as previously described (Gould and Dawson, 1976; Gould et al. 1982b). (*a*) Distal nerve injected 3 days after crush with tritiated inositol. The axons are clear and devoid of label; in contrast, (*b*) axons in the proximal nerve remain highly labeled with this precursor.

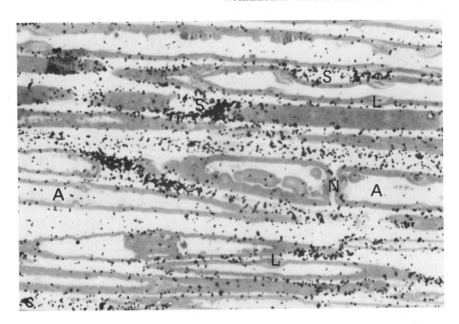

FIGURE 9.1 (*continued*)   (*c*) Choline is the precursor and, as in A, the Schwann cells are most avidly labeled, indicating that sites in the Schwann cell, not the axon, respond to the injury. Similar labeling patterns are seen proximal (not shown) as well as distal (c) to the crush. Symbols: A, axon; S, Schwann cytoplasm; L, Schmidt-Lanterman incisure; M, myelin sheath; n, node of Ranvier.

cell and myelin membranes makes it unlikely that biochemical approaches, including composition, enzyme, or metabolic precursor studies, would be useful in detecting and characterizing the degeneration and loss of axon organelles.

The metabolic and enzymic lipid changes detected in distal degenerating nerve represent predominantly those of Schwann cells and their myelin sheaths and at later times also of invading hemotogenous cells. The early morphological changes seen in Schwann cell and myelin membranes (Abrahams et al., 1980; Lassmann et al., 1978b) might relate to increased phospholipase A_1 and A_2 activities found to occur during this time period and/or that of cholesterol-esterifying enzymes (Table 9.1). It would be useful to establish that the sites where lysophospholipids and/or cholesterol esters accumulate are those in which morphological abnormalities in Schwann cell and myelin membranes are occurring. In model systems lysophospholipids and cholesterol esters destabilize bilayer structures, making these lipids plausible candidates for initiating the physical and subsequent chemical events of myelin destabilization and digestion. Superoxide radicals (and a variety of other unknown agents) may also cause myelin instability and therefore be a factor in demyelinating events (Cammer, 1980; Chia et al., 1983). It will be necessary to develop new avenues before the mechanisms underlying the destruction of axon and myelin membranes can be better understood.

A popular and potentially sensitive approach for detecting changes in lipid metabolism is to use radioactive precursors. Lipid and protein precursor studies applied to studies of distal degeneration are listed in Table 9.2. In these studies distal peritraumatic segments plus proximal segments and contralateral segments (as controls) were removed from animals and incubated with precursors, usually for incubation times in which the incorporation rates were linear. In the study of Rawlins and Smith (1971) myelin and nonmyelin fractions were separated, while in those of Koeppen et al. (1979) and Natarajan et al. (1982), homogenates of the nerve were used. The epineurium and perineurium had not been removed in most investigations, and these probably both impede the access of precursor to the Schwann cells and axons (Brown et al., 1976; Greene et al, 1979; Yao, 1984) and contribute significantly to the metabolic activity of the tissue (see Gould and Dawson, 1976). Future studies based on endoneurial preparations and homogenates of these might be informative. In this regard, Greene and his colleagues (1979) have developed a medium that appears to be quite satisfactory for maintaining endoneurial preparations during short-time (up to 2–3 h) incubations *in vitro* (see also Simmons et al., 1982, and Ganser et al., 1983).

In general, lipid and protein precursor incorporation is increased during the first 1–2 weeks of Wallerian degeneration (Table 9.2). The increased incorporation occurs prior to the breakdown of myelin lipids and protein and probably reflects primarily the proliferation of Schwann cells (reviewed in Gould et al., 1982a; Gould, in press). After 3–4 days, invading hemotogenous cells (Gibson, 1979) and activated endoneurial fibroblasts (Schubert and Friede, 1981) would begin to contribute to the increased metabolic activity. Natarajan et al. (1982) showed a rather rapid and specific increase in the formation of phosphatidylcholine (PC) by degenerating nerve. Furthermore, this increase was found to be due to enhanced enzyme activity. In unpublished studies we found that the sites of choline incorporation into lipid are largely in Schwann cells in distal degenerating nerve (Fig. 9.1). The rise in the synthetic enzyme activities might be an indirect effect of their stimulation by lysophospholipids produced in the nerve (Natarajan et al., 1982). In light of these results it is also of interest that Henry and Hodge (1983) demonstrated increased choline lipid synthesis in cultured HeLa cells during proliferation (see also Warden and Friedkin, 1984). Their autoradiographic studies localized a significant por-

TABLE 9.2 Metabolic Changes in Distal Nerve Detected with Radioactive Lipid and Protein Precursors

Precursor		Change in Incorporation	Time (days)	References
[^{32}P]phosphate	1.	Increase mainly in PC + PE	8–32	Rossiter, 1961
	2.	Increase mainly in PC	3	Natarajan et al., 1982
[^{14}C]acetate	1.	Decrease	½–32	Karnovsky and Mano, 1961
	2.	Decrease (then increase)	3–14	Rawlins and Smith, 1971
		all lipids, especially PE + Chol	28–60	
	3.	Decrease	3	Natarajan et al., 1982
	4.	Increase in PL and Chol	16–32	Rossiter, 1961
[^{14}C]choline	1.	Increase in PC	3–30	Natarajan et al., 1982
[^{14}C]glycerol	1.	Increase	16–32	Rossiter, 1961
	2.	Increase in PC and TG	3	Natarajan et al., 1982
[^{14}C]ethanolamine	1.	Increase	16–32	Rossiter, 1961
	2.	Unchanged	3	Natarajan et al., 1982
[^{14}C]serine	1.	Increase	16–32	Rossiter, 1961
[^{14}C]malonyl CoA	1.	Increase	4–20	Koeppen et al., 1979
[^{14}C]leucine	1.	Increase	1–7	Rawlins and Smith, 1971
	2.	Increase	7–15	Buse et al., 1976
	3.	Increase	2–4	Peterson et al., 1981
[^{3}H]- and [^{14}C]glycine	1.	Decrease in myelin proteins	1–5	Bell et al., 1982a

Key: The times are those at which distal degenerating (regenerating) nerves were taken and incubated with precursor. Changes are relative to noninjured controls. PC, phosphatidylcholine; PE, phosphatidylethanolamine; PL, phospholipid; TG, triacylglycerol; Chol, cholesterol.

337

tion of the labeling to the nuclear envelope. It is certainly possible that the enhanced PC synthesis in degenerating nerve might be related to increased nuclear envelope activity associated with Schwann cell proliferation. Natarajan et al. (1982) found that [^{33}P]orthophosphate and [2-^{3}H]glycerol incorporation into phosphatidylinositol (PI) was not increased in 3-day degenerating nerve; in fact, phosphate incorporation was substantially decreased. This result suggests that enhanced PI turnover is probably not a feature of these early stages of distal degeneration. It is unfortunate that no information was presented on [^{33}P]orthophosphate and [^{3}H]myo-inositol incorporation into polyphosphoinositides, as these are metabolically the most active lipids in this tissue (e.g., Sheltawy and Dawson, 1969b; White et al., 1974; Shaikh and Palmer, 1977).

A consistent finding in precursor incorporation experiments is the reduced incorporation of acetate into phospholipids and cholesterol in degenerating nerve (Table 9.2). Since fatty acid, dolichol, and cholesterol synthesis from acetate in other systems are product inhibited (e.g., Tsai and Geyer, 1977; James and Kandutsch, 1979), depression in acetate utilization might be a reflection of fatty acid and cholesterol mobilization during the early phase of myelin breakdown. Since most recently formed myelin proteins (Patsalos et al., 1980) and presumably lipids as well are broken down earliest, the mobilized cholesterol and fatty acid release might occur near sites in the Schwann cell cytoplasm (Gould et al., 1982a) where myelin lipids are being made. Furthermore, cholesterol and fatty acids at these sites might be incorporated into cholesterol esters. The accumulation of cholesterol esters could dually inhibit myelin lipid synthesis and destabilize the myelin membrane activating lipolysis of myelin lipids (see above).

In summary, there is good biochemical evidence that changes in lipid and protein composition and metabolism primarily related to Schwann cells occur during early acute stages of nerve degeneration. The importance of these changes to the degenerative and demyelination processes are as yet largely unknown. A principal limitation of the biochemical approaches that have been used is their inability to pinpoint changes to cellular and subcellular sites where the specific degenerative events are occurring. Knowledge of the compositional, metabolic, and enzymatic changes that occur might act as a framework for cytochemical (autoradiographic, immunocytochemical, and histochemical) approaches that could focus the observations to the cellular and subcellular levels.

It is likely that the rapidly advancing field of molecular biology will strengthen our understanding of nerve degeneration in terms of gene and gene product expression of Schwann cells and their involvement in the degenerative and regenerative responses. Lipid biochemists will hopefully be able to take advantage of this technology in exploring the "gene expression" of lipid-directed enzymes. The repression of those enzymes involved in myelin maintenance and the enhancement of activities required for breakdown and removal of myelin and axon debris are facets of degeneration. Unraveling the posttranslational control of biosynthetic and hydrolytic enzymes, including the influence of their activities by the physiochemical features of membranous substrates, would be another important facet for future investigations. Because the numbers of Schwann cells are increasing, knowledge of Schwann cell survival and proliferation should provide the basis for interpreting studies along these lines.

9.4.2 The Retrograde Response

While the metabolic events in the distal axon are directed toward clearing pathways for regenerating axons, the "retrograde response" [see Lieberman (1971) and Barron (1983) for reviews] encompasses both the preparation of the surviving neurons for regeneration and the degeneration of those incapable of survival. Regeneration (Section 9.4.3) includes the growth of new axon processes to appropriate targets, the establishment of functional contacts at these targets, and the myelination of the regenerating axons.

The "retrograde reaction" describes interrelated events occurring both at the site of injury (Section 9.4.3) and in the cell soma. An important question in understanding the "retrograde reaction" is: How does the cell body find out that its process is damaged? Several hypotheses on this topic have been presented (cf. Cragg, 1970; Joseph, 1973; Grafstein, 1975; Watson, 1976; Lubinska, 1977; Grafstein and McQuarrie, 1978). A clue lies in the delay between injury and regeneration, which is time for (1) retrograde transport of "chromatolytic signals" to the soma, (2) modified transcription and translation yielding proteins and lipids required for axon elongation, and (3) the rapid anterograde transport of these components to the sites where axon sprouting and growth commence.

A scenario for lipid-related events will be described, although studies of the role of lipid metabolism in relation to the retrograde reaction is largely unknown. Interruption of axons blocks both the passage of anterogradely transported organelles, causing them to either accumulate proximal to the injury or prematurely return to the cell body (Edstrom and Hanson, 1973; Bisby and Bulger, 1977; Bulger and Bisby; 1978), and the return of retrogradely transported organelles from the terminal. Accumulation of retrogradely transported material occurs directly adjacent to the site of injury and at nodes in the peritraumatic regions of the distal axons. In addition to blockage of normal anterograde and retrograde transport systems is the entry of exogenous substances, including leaked humeral solutions at the site of injury into the damaged axon tips and their transport back to the soma (Kristensson and Olson, 1974, 1975, 1976; Sparrow and Kiernan 1981). It is reasonable that one or more of these above events trigger the cell body responses required for regeneration.

As constituents of rapidly transported organelles, there is no doubt that lipids are a necessary ingredient for the retrograde reaction. Phospholipid constituents of retrogradely transported organelles originate during retrieval of plasma membrane endocytozed at natural and injury-induced terminals and afterward, through exchange with other local membranes and/or synthesis by enzymic components of the transport organelles. Studies of the source(s) of retrogradely transported lipids could be undertaken by adaptation of procedures already established to characterize retrogradely transported proteins (cf. Edstrom and Hanson, 1973; Bisby and Bulger, 1977; Sahenk and Mendell, 1981). Lipid-directed precursors would be used to tag anterogradely transported lipids, and those labeled lipids that are subsequently returned toward the soma could be collected at the distal side of a ligature and characterized (Armstrong et al., in press). Because of the possibility of precursor reutilization (dependent on enzymes in axons and terminals), the returning label would either mark the original transported lipid or another lipid into which the tagged moiety was reincorporated.

An independent approach would be to label returning lipid with a probe such as the Bolton–Hunter reagent. This reagent, used in protein transport studies (Fink and Gainer, 1980), will penetrate into the axon and tag transported amino lipids, phosphatidylethanolamine (PE), and phosphatidylserine (PS). If injected into the distal region of a nerve, the retrogradely transported PE and PS would be labeled and collected at a more proximal ligation site and characterized. However, it is possible that retrogradely transported lipids might not remain with the transport vesicles (due to lipid exchange) or be handled abnormally due to the covalent probes. Further metabolism could occur in the axon, including hydrolysis or exchange into other axonal membranes and even glial cell membranes and myelin (Ledeen, this volume). Recognition of the dynamic properties of axonal lipids is important in designing and interpreting experiments that investigate their retrograde transport in normal and degenerative circumstances.

An extension of investigations of this nature would be to determine the degree of unsaturation of the acyl chain in the classes of various transported phospholipids. This characterization would be carried out on radiolabeled lipids accumulating proximal and/or distal to a ligature by argentation thin-layer chromatography (TLC) separation (following derivatization as appropriate). These studies could demonstrate differences in acyl chain compositions within membranes of anterograde and retrograde transport vesicles.

It seems likely that the membrane proteins of the transported vesicles and/or the vesicle contents, and not the lipids, contain the "information" needed for chromatolysis. The major roles of anterogradely and retrogradely transported lipids are (1) as constituents needed for membrane growth and maintenance, that is, retrograde transport being one means of lipid recycling; (2) as "media" for transported membrane proteins; and (3) as a vehicle to restrain the "water-soluble" vesicle contents. Because of the evidence that perikaryal lipid synthesis is needed for steps in the initiation of anterograde protein transport (Longo and Hammerschlag, 1980; Heacock et al., 1984), it is possible that lipids may have additional roles.

Following nerve damage, some neurons degenerate, while others survive and regenerate. Both of these processes are part of the retrograde response, and biochemical determinations on tissue containing chromolytic neuronal soma are a reflection of the component degenerative and regenerative activities of the system. Kauffman and his colleagues have been the main group to focus on elucidating lipid changes in chromatolytic ganglia. Harkonen and Kauffman (1973, 1974) demonstrated that the lipid but not protein or RNA content of an axotomized superior cervical ganglion (SCG) increased within 3 days of injury. Ando et al. (1984), however, reported increases in wet weight and protein following either axotomy or denervation. The time points studied (1–7 days) were well before cell necrosis occurred in this system (Matthews and Raisman, 1972). This change was correlated with a selective elevation of enzymes of the pentose phosphate shunt, a pathway that provides NADPH for lipid synthesis. Furthermore, these investigators used histochemical methods to pinpoint the enzyme changes to neurons. In a follow-up study Sinicropi and Kauffman (1979) showed that the increased activity of 6-phosphogluconate dehydrogenase was due to an increased level of this protein, that is, the enhancement of the pathway was "translation" related.

Several investigations have provided evidence for a phospholipid requirement in the retrograde response. Jerkins and Kauffman (1983) showed that phospholipids were the principal macromolecules that increased in amount in 3-day axotomized ganglia. Miani (1962) found that [^{32}P]orthophosphate incorporation into lipid, mainly PE and PI, was selectively increased in axotomized spinal ganglia at 5 days, the earliest time point of this study. Similarly, Jerkins and Kauffman (1983) found that the incorporation of exogenously added glycerol, though not glucose, into lipid was increased in 3-day axotomized SCG ganglia. Contrarily,

Nagata et al. (1973) found a reduction in the rate of incorporation of [^{32}P]orthophosphate into all phospholipids, including PC, PI, PE, and phosphatidic acid (PA), in 1-week axotomized SCG. The causes of the selective alterations of lipid metabolism in axotomized neuronal tissue are unknown, as are the reasons for differences in the various studies. In general, needs for an increased lipid metabolism (see also Dombrowski and Kauffman, 1981; Heacock et al., 1984) would be similar to those suggested for enhanced protein metabolism (cf. Watson, 1974; Grafstein and Forman, 1980). However, in the studies described above, the changes showed some selectivity for lipid. The interrelated demands for lipid and proteins would be in "housekeeping" or maintenance requirements of the soma itself, including endoplasmic reticulum proliferation, the reestablishment of plasma membrane specializations to accommodate incoming boutons, the support of axon sprouting and regeneration, and finally the establishment of contact with target cells and with glia.

9.4.3   Nerve Regeneration

The growth and maintenance of axonal processes and terminals require a continual supply of perikarya-formed proteins, lipids, and other constituents to axon and terminal regions (Section 9.2.2). In nerve regeneration the demands for proteins and phospholipids as measured with radiolabeled precursors are increased. This enhanced transport of proteins and lipids would take place under circumstances in which an extensive portion of axon process and terminal arborizations has been separated from the perikaryon and is no longer a metabolic responsibility of the neuron. The demands for lipid and membrane proteins to fuel elongation and enlargement of regenerating axons is presumably far greater than that required for maintenance of established processes and terminals. The previous section reviewed the early somal and terminal changes that follow injury. In this section the topic will be the impact of the retrograde response, that is, heightened RNA and protein and lipid syntheses, on growth of the regenerating axons.

The lipid-requiring constituents of axons and terminals are the extensive plasma membrane and intracellular membrane systems. The latter include agranular reticulum, vesicular transport organelles, and mitochondria, all of which are transported down the axon at more rapid rates than the cytoskeletal and cytosolic proteins (Lorenz and Willard, 1978; Tytell et al., 1981). Although most of the current evidence suggests that the phospholipid components of the transport vesicles travel exclusively at the rapid rate (Grafstein and Forman, 1980; Guy and Bisby, 1983), they behave differently from fast-transported proteins (e.g., Grafstein et al.,

1975; Gould et al., 1982b). This behavior is due to their prolonged release from the cell body, the exchange of lipids between migrating and stationary elements within the axons, and their exchange into myelin (see Ledeen, this volume).

Regeneration causes an increase in the amount of rapidly transported protein, but not its rate of movement (e.g., Griffin et al., 1976; Cancalon and Elam, 1980). The composition of transported proteins is very similar to that in normal nerves (e.g., Hall et al., 1978; Perry and Wilson, 1981), although there are a few proteins whose levels are uniquely elevated during regeneration process before contacts with targets are reestablished (reviewed by Skene 1984). Since these proteins are membrane associated, it is not surprising that there are also increases in the quantities of transported phospholipids during regeneration (Dziegielewska et al., 1980; Alberghina et al., 1983a,b). Dziegielewska et al., (1980) found a rapid (within 10 h of the injury) increase in the transport of choline-labeled lipid along nerves, while the transport of leucine-labeled protein was unaffected. This specific increase in the transport of labeled lipid may relate to the early and selective increase in lipids in the cell soma of regenerating tissue (Jerkins and Kauffman, 1983). Certainly further work, including the use of dual-isotope procedures (choline plus amino acid), of other lipid precursors and methodology that will measure neuronal precursor pools will strengthen and clarify the notion of a selective demand for somal phospholipids during very early stages of nerve regeneration.

Another facet of regeneration that requires attention is the role of local lipid metabolism, specifically that of inositol lipids, in the growth cone region and along the neurites (Matsumoto and Gould, 1983). Interruption of the axon causes the buildup of those enzymes of lipid metabolism that are axonally transported (Kumara-Siri and Gould, 1980), and these enzymes would, if substrates were not limiting, cause enhanced metabolism of lipids in regions where axon sprouts and growth cones are formed. The relationship of local lipid synthesis to axon outgrowth is not understood. Because there is a delay of several days before axon elongation commences in rat sciatic nerve (Forman and Berenberg, 1978), but no delay in the buildup of axonally transported enzymes of lipid metabolism (Kumara-Siri and Gould, 1980), factors other than locally generated inositol lipids, such as the growth-associated proteins (GAPs) (Skene, 1984), are needed for growth cone formation, sprouting, and axon elongation.

9.4.4   Myelination of Regenerating Axons

Axon growth and reinnervation is accompanied by the reestablishment of functions, of axon impulse propagation and terminal chemical transmission or reception. Rapid saltatory conduction of the larger-caliber axons requires their myelination. Myelination during nerve regeneration is largely a recapitulation of the developmental process. However, myelin sheaths formed during regeneration are thinner relative to axon caliber (e.g., Schroder, 1972) and are in general far shorter in internodal length (Vizoso and Young, 1948) than those formed during development. The Schwann cells that form the myelin sheaths around regenerating axons are those already present in the distal stump. Schwann cell division is required, for when it is inhibited, myelination is arrested (Hall and Gregson, 1977; see also Gould et al., 1982a). Exactly why the myelin sheaths formed around regenerating axons are smaller than those around the original axons is unknown. However, because the region of contact between the Schwann cell and axon is proportionally reduced, some facet of axon–Schwann cell interaction may control myelination (Smith et al., 1982). Other parameters that may be important in the process of myelination during regeneration include the age and disposition of the glial cells and axons involved and the influence of accompanying degeneration and demyelination. Aging has been shown to contribute to reduced rates of regeneration as measured by axon elongation and axonal transport (Black and Lasek, 1979; Pestronk et al., 1980).

The two principal components for remyelination of the distal segment are regenerating neurons and proliferating Schwann cells. Studies with radiolabeled protein and lipid precursors have demonstrated that axonal transport is stimulated in nerve regeneration (Section 9.4.3). Axonally transported lipids can enter the glial cells, particularly the myelin sheaths (see Ledeen, this volume). Using autoradiographic techniques, Tessler et al. (1980) and Griffin et al. (1981) have shown that the metabolism of rapidly transported fucose-labeled proteins is restricted to the regenerating axons; that is, axonally transported proteins did not migrate into regions of compact myelin.

Although it is unlikely that axonal transport contributes structural proteins for myelin sheath formation (Gould et al., 1982a,b), it is plausible that transported proteins that become exposed on the external surface of the axolemma or others that enter adaxonal Schwann cytoplasm could influence Schwann cell differentiation, including the induction of myelin formation. A transfer of these vesicle-bound "trophic" components to adaxonal Schwann cell cytoplasm would cause membrane proteins and axonally transported lipids to enter Schwann cell plasma membrane. Via lateral diffusion, as envisioned by Gould and Dawson (1976), lipids would redistribute into and throughout the myelin sheath. The observation that axonally transported lipids and their metabolites enter myelin of normal and regenerating nerves could also be a reflection on an economic reutilization of lipids no longer needed for axon membrane maintenance.

The major contributors to nerve remyelination are the local Schwann cells and their progeny. The biochemical aspects of remyelination of the distal stump are intermingled with the prolonged degradation of myelin debris and other regenerative events occurring within the same time frame. The Wallerian degeneration model is, therefore, not a particularly useful choice for biochemical studies of nerve myelination in disease (see Section 9.5).

However, two approaches have been employed to dissociate the biochemical events of degeneration and regeneration. One approach has been to compare activities in distal nerve under conditions in which there is an active regeneration, that is, following a crush or freezing lesion, with those in which regeneration is inhibited by transection and ligation (e.g., Miani, 1962). The condition in which regeneration occurs would include not only the myelination of the regenerating axons, but also the growth and differentiation of regenerating axons as well as endoneurial and perineurial cells involved in fascicle formation. Later degeneration (including demyelination) of those axons unable to establish stable terminal contacts would also occur.

A second approach has been developed by Spencer and his colleagues (Spencer et al., 1981; Politis et al., 1982). In this model the timing of degeneration and regeneration are dissociated using two adjacent branches of the sciatic nerve. One of the branches (tibial) is transected and ligated. After a suitable time interval to allow the completion of distal degeneration, the site of transection is reexposed and the common peroneal nerve, another branch of the sciatic, cut. The proximal end of this branch is sutured to the distal tibial, allowing the peroneal fibers to grow into the already degenerated tibial nerve. With this system, biochemical events, compared with controls in which the peroneal was not so attached, will largely reflect regeneration and myelination. Politis et al. (1982) used this system to demonstrate that the influx of regenerating axons stimulated the synthesis of myelin proteins. Furthermore, they found that the synthesis of myelin-specific proteins, P_0 and the basic proteins, was not synchronous; they detected radioactive basic protein prior to that of P_0. Studies along these lines with phospholipid and glycolipid precursors would be of interest in determining the influence of axon regeneration on the timing of the formation of lipids (in relation to myelin proteins) characteristic of PNS myelin (see also Section 9.5).

9.4.5 Degeneration of the CNS

The CNS has been less frequently used for studies of Wallerian degeneration. The paucity of studies is probably due to the facts that CNS tracts are less accessible than those of the PNS and that regeneration normally does not occur. An exception is the optic nerve of nonmammalian in-vertebrates (cf. Agranoff, 1977; Grafstein and McQuarrie, 1978). The optic nerve has been the focus of most studies on CNS degeneration, probably for reasons of its accessibility (enucleation is an easy operation) and the natural isolation of this pathway from the rest of the CNS. Recent studies have favored nerve section and removal of the retina over enucleation as these procedures would minimize edema, hemorrhage, and macrophage infiltration (cf. Lassmann et al., 1978a; Reigner et al., 1981). Studies with this system and others have shown that the degenerative changes in CNS tissue are qualitatively similar but far slower than those with PNS. For example, McCaman and Robins (1959) found that the maximum loss of lipid constituents of degenerating PNS (tibial nerve) occurred about 14 days after nerve transection, while with CNS (optic nerve) lipid levels declined for 100 days.

To understand why degeneration is so sluggish in the CNS compared with peripheral nerve, one must consider the respective glial cells, oli-godendroglial cells plus astrocytes in the CNS and Schwann cells in the PNS. The intimate relationship between myelin-forming Schwann cells with their single internode of axon (see Caley and Butler, 1974) would favor their ability to initiate axon and myelin sheath destruction. CNS glial cells, on the other hand, have their perikarya separated from the axons they myelinate by long and tortuous processes. The lack of "re-sponsiveness" to axon damage may be due to this physical separation of sites where degradative enzymes would be made from their target inter-nodes. Furthermore, there is still controversy over the respective roles of astrocytes, oligodendroglia, and multipotential glial cells in initiating the degenerative responses (cf. Vaughn and Peters, 1968; Cook and Wis-niewski, 1973; Lassmann et al., 1978a; Wender et al., 1981). This con-troversy stems from studies in which the identification of the cells is based on morphological grounds. Since all of the candidates are probably de-rived from a common precursor (cf. Privat et al., 1981; Raff et al., 1983), it is probably unwise to place too much emphasis on the specific cells that initiate CNS degeneration. Dedifferentiation and/or the recruitment of nondifferentiated precursor cells are the most likely basis of the CNS glial response, and these cells may show properties common both to as-trocytes and oligodendroglia. Whether the degenerative change is caused largely by dedifferentiated CNS glia or whether invading macrophages participate might depend on the tissue selected, the type of injury, and the times studied.

McCaman and Robins (1959) found that it took between 45 and 100 days to detect substantial losses of lipids in degenerating optic nerve, compared with 8–14 days with tibial nerve. They concluded that the different time scales reflected different rates of myelin loss in CNS and PNS tissues. The same time frame of CNS myelin breakdown was found by Reigner et al. (1981) based on yield of myelin in subcellular fractionation. These investigators further showed that the myelin isolated at different stages of degeneration had differing protein composition and fractionation characteristics. These results support the view of Lassmann et al. (1978a) that structural changes in myelin generation reflect differing stabilities of the components of myelin during degeneration. Both Reigner et al. (1981) and Wender et al. (1981) noted increased levels of cholesterol esters by 8 days and suggested their involvement in myelin breakdown.

Enzyme and metabolic changes associated with CNS degeneration have been considered in a few instances. Karnovsky and Majno (1961) found, using isolated tracts from degenerating rat spinal cord, that oxygen uptake is rapidly and persistently depressed in degenerating white matter. In contrast, oxygen consumption by transected sciatic nerve increased following a brief decline. Radioactive acetate incorporation into lipids was found to decline in both CNS and PNS preparations. However, the incorporation of this precursor into lipid increased and actually exceeded controls (two- to threefold) in peripheral nerve preparations examined after 10 days; it remained low in CNS. These studies support the view that the metabolic response of CNS glia is different from that of Schwann cells in the PNS. Like peripheral nerve, activities related to CNS myelin maintenance decline, namely, oxygen uptake, lipid synthesis (reflected by acetate utilization), and myelin enzyme activities (cyclic nucleotide phosphohydrolase and cerebroside sulfotransferase; Reigner et al., 1981). These changes are consistent with morphological observations of Privat et al. (1981) and Skoff (1981), who demonstrated in developing optic nerve that the loss of axon "signals" retard glial cell development and differentiation. Axon stability is apparently needed for differentiated oligodendroglia to retain metabolic properties needed for myelin maintenance. The local CNS glia appear to be less able than Schwann cells to develop autophagic and phagocytic responses needed for demyelination and degeneration.

Studies of CNS degeneration have generally not included phospholipid metabolism as a parameter. In addition to the earlier studies of McCaman and Robins (1959), Horrocks et al. (1973) demonstrated a rather rapid (30 min to 2 h) and selective, though not persistent, loss of PE plasmalogen in lipids from myelin isolated from traumatized monkey spinal cord. Since the loss of CNS myelin lipids occurs over an extended time course, changes in phospholipase activity, [^{32}P]orthophosphate incorporation, and that of other precursors, would be expected to be less dramatic than in degenerating peripheral nerve.

A major reason for understanding the process of CNS degeneration is as background for developing strategies that will promote CNS regeneration. There is the need to clear "the scar" tissue so that CNS axons will have room to grow and also be able to sense chemotrophic signals from distant targets. In this regard, lipolytic enzymes, lysolipids, and/or even Schwann cells or macrophages might act as potential stimulators of the degenerative and regenerative processes. Another facet of this story is the role of CNS glia in the successful degeneration and regeneration occurring in infra-mammalian systems (see chapters of Stensaas, Simpson, and Reier et al. in Kao et al., 1983). For example, little is known as to how astrocytes and oligodendroglia function in the regeneration and myelination that occur in systems such as the goldfish optic pathway.

9.5 MODELS FOR DEMYELINATION AND HYPOMYELINATION

There is a broad variety of animal models in which demyelination occurs. In addition to those in which mature myelin sheaths are disrupted and lost, either as a primary event or occurring secondarily to axonal degeneration (see previous section), there are models in which the process of myelin formation is impaired (hypomyelination). Recent books and reviews by Dyck et al. (1975, 1984), Waxman (1978), Morell (1984), Waxman and Ritchie (1981), and Morell et al. (1981) should be consulted for additional information on this subject. In the sections that follow several demyelination and hypomyelination models will be presented and then some studies demonstrating and/or implicating phospholipids will be considered.

9.5.1 Models of Demyelination

Demyelination is commonly caused by agents that "attack" the myelin sheaths directly and/or impair the maintenance functions of the myelin-forming Schwann cells and oligodendroglia. The causes of hypomyelination (Section 9.5.2) are usually genetic and/or hormonal in origin. The primary focus of these later defects is in the development and deployment of myelin-forming glial cells or in their transformation to specialized cells that will ensheath axon segments and form myelin sheaths. Primary demyelination models are defined as those in which the underlying axons are initially "spared." However, demyelination is not without consequences to axon structure and function. Altered axolemmal morphology has been detected with staining and freeze-fracture methods (cf. Foster et al., 1980; Rosenbluth, 1981). Impaired nerve impulse propagation is a characteristic feature (e.g., Smith and Hall, 1980; Brismar, 1981a,b; Sumner et al., 1982). Axon caliber is usually reduced (e.g., Aguayo et al., 1979a) and there is evidence that fast, but not slow, waves of axon transport, through regions where myelin has been removed, are depressed (Kidman et al., 1978, 1979). Models of PNS demyelination are attractive in that they could shed light on the etiology and consequences of a variety of human conditions characterized by segmental demyelination [see Dyck et al. (1975, 1984) and Spencer and Schaumberg (1980) for reviews]. Primary demyelination, unlike degeneration, occurs in spite of continuing axonal "signals" that would normally cause the Schwann cells to maintain their myelin sheaths. Degeneration, on the other hand, is often a consequence of the loss of these signals. Whether demyelinating agents modify or negate axon signals or simply distract or overpower the Schwann cells' myelin-forming activities is probably dependent on how the demyelination is caused. In this section two models of segmental demyelination, lysolecithin- (and phospholipase A-) induced demyelination and immune-mediated demyelination, will be considered. It is hoped that the concepts generated in the discussion of these models will be viewed in the light of the many other models currently being researched (Ludwin, 1981; Smith and Benjamins, 1984; Morell et al., 1981). In establishing a model of demyelination, it is important to demonstrate that the experimental manipulation, such as the injection of a demyelinating agent (e.g., lysoPC, immune serum, or diphtheria toxin), does not cause substantial nerve degeneration, as this will compound results and their interpretation. In most models degeneration can be readily assessed by examination of the morphology, biochemistry (e.g., axon and terminal markers, transmitters or transmitter enzymes), and/or electrophysiological properties of nerve distal to the zone where demyelination is produced.

Both lysoPC and phospholipase A cause segmental demyelination when they are injected either into sciatic nerves of mice and rats (Hall and Gregson, 1971; Gregson and Hall, 1973; Smith et al., 1983) or into central tracts (spinal cord dorsal columns and corpus callosum; Hall, 1972; Blakemore et al., 1977; Foster et al., 1980). Like the Wallerian degeneration model, the changes occur in a well-characterized temporal fashion following application of the agent. The effectiveness of both agents (phospholipase A is far less commonly used) in causing focal demyelination is likely related to the interactions between lysolipids and the myelin membranes. In a previous section (9.4.1) the potential involvement of lysolipids in demyelination associated with nerve degeneration was discussed. A reason put forward as to why Schwann cells (and presumably CNS glia) and their axons are not compromised by lysophospholipid is that the plasma membranes of these cells, unlike myelin, will neutralize the ly-solipids by acylating them. However, evidence that acylating enzymes are present in glial and axonal plasma membranes and not in myelin is equivocal (e.g., Benes et al., 1973; Fisher and Rowe, 1980). Large local concentrations of lysophospholipid presumably permeabilize and desta-bilize plasma membranes (e.g., Blakemore et al., 1977; Foster et al., 1980) of some of these cells, leading to variable nerve degeneration as well as demyelination in this model.

The reasons why Schwann cells and possibly CNS glia are activated to remove their myelin sheaths are unknown. Of possible relevance is the finding that myelin fragments prepared by subfractionation stimulate Schwann cell proliferation in tissue culture (DeVries et al., 1980). This responsiveness of Schwann cell to myelin debris (or in this case lysoPC-dispersed myelin fragments) may cause these cells to initiate activities involved in myelin sheath removal and digestion.

Another feature of the PNS demyelination model is that once the myelin debris is cleared, usually at about 14 days, the Schwann cells will ensheath the bared axons and remyelinate them. The Schwann cells that perform the remyelination are the progeny of those involved in demyelination (Hall and Gregson, 1975, 1978). Antimitotic drugs injected into the nerve in conjunction with the lysoPC treatment prevented Schwann cell prolif-eration and remyelination did not occur. The Schwann cells thus need to divide and dedifferentiate before they can ensheath axons and form myelin (Hall, 1978). Furthermore, without proliferation the myelin debris is not completely removed, and cell division may be needed to help dilute myelin debris so the catabolic machinery of the Schwann cells can effectively digest it. Antimitotic agents should be effective in blocking the biochem-ical activities associated with remyelination and, therefore, might prove useful in helping to dissociate some of the biochemical events involved in demyelination and remyelination (see Section 9.5.4).

LysoPC- and phospholipase A–induced demyelination models have attracted little attention from the neurochemist. A recent study of Smith et al. (1983; see also Smith and Benjamins, 1984) provides information on how models of this nature could be used in biochemical studies. Their approach was to temporally (1–30 days) determine the effects of lysoPC injection on the incorporation of amino acids and fucose into myelin pro-teins. To minimize the variability introduced by the intraneural injection procedure, minces of four pooled nerves were used for each incubation with a mixture of ^{14}C-labeled amino acids and [^{3}H]-fucose. At all time points the recoveries of labeled proteins in an isolated myelin fraction were higher in lysoPC-treated nerve samples than in the controls. Sep-aration of the proteins on gels and autoradiography revealed shifts in incorporation pattern. Amino acids entered high-molecular-weight proteins at times from 1 to 7 days, while prior to the treatment and at later times their incorporation was mainly in the low-molecular-weight structural proteins of myelin, namely the P_0 glycoprotein and myelin basic proteins (MBPs). These results are consistent with the morphological data, which show that at times prior to remyelination, the Schwann cell involvement is with cellular functions other than myelin formation and maintenance. Presumably the high-molecular-weight proteins isolated with myelin are synthesized in this time frame to function in activities such as axonolysis and myelin debris removal. Poduslo (1984) recently reported that Schwann cells continue to synthesize and maintain a form of P_0 protein for long periods of nerve degeneration. The incorporation patterns at later times reflect myelination. A possible extension of these studies would be to see if mitomycin C treatment (Hall and Gregson, 1975) prevents the shift in incorporation toward low-molecular-weight myelin proteins at these later times.

Another demyelinating agent, diphtheria toxin (DT), produces focal segmental demyelination when injected into peripheral nerves (Allt and Cavanaugh, 1969; Brismar, 1981a,b) and spinal cord (McDonald and Sears, 1970). Pleasure and his colleagues (1973) used a totally *in vitro* approach to study the effects of this agent on peripheral nerve metabolism. They showed that DT, added to media containing sciatic nerves, reduced the incorporation of labeled amino acid and sulfate into the myelin structural proteins and sulfolipids, respectively, in a time- and concentration-dependent manner. In contrast, they found that the turnover of prelabeled proteins and sulfolipids present in the nerves was unaffected by DT. This study, like that of Smith et al. (1983), indicates that one aspect of demyelination is a selective depression in the synthesis of myelin-specific constituents, presumably representing initial dedifferentiation of the myelin-forming Schwann cells.

Studies using the approaches of Pleasure and Smith could quite naturally be extended to include radiolabeled phospholipid precursors as probes. The aim of such studies could either be to determine if lipid precursor incorporation patterns (e.g., ethanolamine to plasmalogens, or choline to lysoPC) are modified during demyelination and remyelination induced *in vivo* (Smith approach) or by the demyelinating agents directly (Pleasure approach). In choosing precursors for such studies, one might consider acetate, ethanolamine, choline, phosphate, and glycerol, as these precursors have already proven useful in uncovering changes during nerve degeneration (Table 9.2). It might be instructive in proposed studies of this nature to compare changes with lipid and protein precursors, either as dual isotopes or with precursors such as serine, sulfate, methionine, and galactose that label both lipids and proteins. These studies should reveal if changes in the incorporation rates into various lipids and proteins are similarly and possibly interdependently related during the course of demyelination and remyelination by the action of agents that cause demyelination. Since demyelination involves the hydrolysis of myelin lipids and proteins, their breakdown products will likely alter the precursor pool of the local axons and glia. In metabolic studies with exogenously labeled precursors, one should consider possible changes in precursor pools in the interpretation of results.

It would be wise to extend findings from precursor incorporation studies to others based on tissue homogenates to determine whether enzymic reactions, substrate, and/or cofactor levels were changed. Amounts of cholesterol esters, other lysolipids, and ethanolamine plasmalogen have not been measured in these demyelinating models. Horrocks and his colleagues (1980) have reported that plasmalogenase activity was increased in a variety of demyelinating disease models and may be a sensitive marker of demyelinating diseases. If reproducible and profound changes associated with demyelination and/or remyelination are identified, they would serve as a basis for formulating mechanisms by which these processes occur. Furthermore, it might be possible to use various inhibitors, such as mitomycin C, to further elucidate requirements for processes of demyelination.

The myelin-forming oligodendroglia and Schwann cells and their respective myelin sheaths are potential targets of autoimmune attack by both humoral (complement-mediated) and cell-mediated mechanisms. In studying animal models with immune involvement, one is faced with complex and multifaceted demyelination processes. Variation in the initiation and time course of the demyelination in different regions of the tissue in different animals and in the mechanism involved make it difficult to develop a rational strategy with biochemical methods as the basis.

Immunological attack(s) on the myelin machinery can be immune-mediated disorders directed either toward myelin components or other glial cell constituents or toward viral proteins that become expressed on surfaces of infected myelin-forming cells. It is also possible that viral infection might cause abnormalities in the formation or subsequent metabolism of myelin components, rendering the system susceptible to immune attack (Dal Canto and Rabinowitz, 1982). Although there are a wide variety of models in which immune-mediated demyelination occurs (see Ludwin, 1981; Morell, 1984; Morell et al., 1981; Alvord et al., 1984; Waksman and Reynolds, 1984; for reviews), only experimental allergic encephalomyelitis (EAE) and experimental allergic neuritis (EAN) will be considered here. The former is directed toward antigens of the CNS and has been long considered a model of multiple sclerosis, while the latter is directed toward the PNS and is a model of Landry–Guillain–Barre syndrome. This relevance has given them a popularity that has created an extensive literature.

There are two general forms of EAE, an acute monophasic form and a chronic relapsing one. Demyelination is far more prevalent in the latter, which is currently felt to be a more appropriate model for multiple sclerosis (Waksman and Reynolds, 1984; Alvord et al., 1984; Wisniewski et al., 1980a). The limited demyelination that occurs during acute EAE is believed to result from nonspecific reactions associated with local inflammation and edema (Wisniewski et al., 1980b). The demyelinating lesions are usually focused in perivascular cuffs. The acute form has been more widely used in biochemical studies, in part because of its induction by highly purified antigens, including MBP and peptide fragments derived from this protein, and in part because of its ease of generation. Both the chronic-relapsing and acute forms are produced by injection of antigens (e.g., MBP, spinal cord, brain white matter, or purified myelin homogenates) suspended in complete Freunds adjuvant containing *Mycobacterium tuberculosis* into the dorsum of the hind feet. The type of the disease depends largely on the antigen and the species and age of the animal used. The chronic-relapsing form is usually produced in juveniles, with large doses of complex (myelin-containing) antigen. Acute and chronic forms of EAN have been produced using peripheral nerve, PNS myelin, and purified P2 protein mixed with lipid (reviewed in *Annals of Neurology*, Vol. 9, supplement 1981). The several lipid-related aspects of this class of diseases that will be considered here are (1) the antigenicity of lipids, (2) the removal and destruction of myelin lipids, and (3) the changes in lipid metabolism that accompany the demyelination process.

The chronic-relapsing forms of EAE and EAN are only produced with lipid-containing antigens. Experiments have been carried out in which pure lipids and lipid mixtures are added to the MBP protein or are depleted from an antigen as myelin by organic solvent extraction (e.g., Ishaque et al., 1981; Madrid, et al., 1981; Maggio et al., 1981). These variations have been shown to affect the resulting disease as judged by clinical assessment and morphological and/or biochemical criteria. There are at least two reasons why lipids might affect antigenicity: either they are antigenic themselves or they influence antigenicity of proteins by altering their conformation. Of potential interest are the recent observations that the most actively metabolized phospholipids in myelin, the polyphosphoinositides, are antigenic (Richards et al., 1983). It would be of interest to see if antibodies to these lipids are formed in those models where active demyelination occurs. Furthermore, the autoantigenicity of these antibodies could be tested (see below).

In studies of lipid changes in brains from animals sensitized with different antigens, Maggio and his colleagues (1981) showed that lipid loss was correlated with the protein antigens involved in the autoimmune response. Acidic sulfatides were preferentially lost when myelin basic protein was the antigen, while cholesterol was lost when the Folch–Lees proteolipid protein (also called lipophilin) was the antigen. The evidence for the interactions of sulfate with MBP and cholesterol with proteolipid protein is from model system studies [viz. reviews by Rumsby and Crang (1977) and Boggs and Moscarello (1978)]. Recent work of Tennekoon et al. (1983) is of importance in demonstrating that sulfatides are probably not the acidic lipids with which MBPs interact. Since these are formed at the lumenal side of the Golgi apparatus, their path to and insertion into the external face of the myelin membrane would not expose them to cytosolic MBP. Another relevant point considered by Mithen et al. (1982), among others, is the difficulty in generating autoimmune-mediated demyelination with a protein (MBP) normally expressed on the internal, nonexposed surfaces of myelin and glial cell plasma membranes. The mechanisms involved in exposing MBP (or its antigenic fragments) to sites where it could initiate demyelination have not been clarified. The role of membrane asymmetry of myelin in demyelinating diseases will be considered in the discussion of mutant mice (Section 9.5.2).

Important, though difficult, questions in autoimmune demyelination are: how are the myelin-maintaining (-forming) glia affected by the immune reactions and how are myelin sheaths destroyed? Biochemical studies of this nature have to date been largely conducted with acute EAE models (Smith and Benjamins, 1984) where demyelination is limited. The main biochemical alteration found in nervous tissue from acute EAE include (1) reduction in the tricarboxylic acid cycle seen as increased lactic acid accumulation and decreased production of $^{14}CO_2$ from glucose (Smith, 1969); (2) increased incorporation of amino acids into proteins, including those of myelin (Wender et al., 1971; Smith and Rauch, 1974; Babitch et al., 1975); (3) increased proteolytic activity (see reviews); (4) decreased incorporation of acetate and glucose into lipid (Smith, 1969; Smith and Rauch, 1974); and (5) increased phospholipase A_1 and A_2 activities (Woelk and Kanig, 1974; Woelk et al., 1974). These diverse changes have provided little insight toward understanding the relationship between humoral and cell-mediated reactions and ensuing paralysis and death of the experimental animal. The above results, however, do provide parameters for assessing autoimmune demyelination in chronic-relapsing models.

⟩ Although it is possible to develop experimental protocols for studying tissue changes (such as those listed above) in these models, the inevitable problem will be to relate these changes to myelin-maintaining glia, invading macrophages, endothelial cells, and other cells damaged and malfunctioning as a result of the complicated sequences of events occurring focally in selected regions of the tissue. For example, does the increase in lipolytic enzyme activities in EAE tissue versus control (Woelk and Kanig, 1974; Woelk et al., 1974) reflect activity of the invading cells or is it due to an activation of machinery present in indigenous cells? Furthermore, how will it be possible to place the activation of lipolytic enzymes in the framework of a model for chronic EAE without knowing the nature of cells from which the enzymes are derived or their sites of action in relation to ongoing cellular destruction?

It might be reasonable to develop alternative strategies to study EAE and EAN based on simpler model systems, such as tissue culture (e.g., Fry et al., 1972, 1974), isolated macrophages (Trotter and Smith, 1984), and sciatic nerve injected with EAE or EAN serum (Saida et al., 1978, 1979a; Harrison et al., 1984). Studies with these systems have the advantage that the demyelination is spatially and temporally regulated. In the case of models where agents are directed into the nerve, biochemical approaches discussed in Sections 9.4.1 and with the lysolecithin model above could be applied directly. Even with these simpler systems, the problem of defining the alteration to a specific cell type or interactive event (e.g., stripping of myelin by invading cells) must also be approached with cytochemical methods.

9.5.2 Mutants and Hypomyelination

Deficiency in the formation of myelin sheaths is a characteristic of a number of animal mutants. These hypomyelination mutants have been the focus of numerous morphological and biochemical investigations (Baumann, 1980; Baumann and Lachapelle, 1982; Hogan and Greenfield, 1984). The principal aims of the later studies have been to elucidate the genetic defect and determine its role in preventing myelination. Approaches to characterize the defective gene product have included analysis of the chemical (lipid and protein) composition of brains and isolated myelin, measurements of enzyme activities [both those copurifying with myelin, e.g., cyclic nucleotide phosphohydrolase (Norton, 1980) and others involved in myelin lipid metabolism], and the determination of incorporation of labeled precursors into myelin proteins and lipids. Through these approaches, two MBP-deficient mutants, shiverer and *mld*, as well as the twitcher mouse, a mutant that lacks galactocerebrosidase, an enzyme required for cerebroside catabolism, have been characterized. Studies along these same lines have failed to demonstrate specific genetic abnormalities in other commonly studied mutants, including quaking, jimpy, dystrophic, and trembler mice and myelin-deficient rats. It is plausible that the genetic defects in these mutants are not "myelin"-specific components per se; they may be minor-occurring regulatory components of the myelination process or they could be essential for earlier stages of gliogenesis, including cell proliferation, migration, or the "premyelin" events of establishing contact with axons and initiating the ensheathment. Another possibility would be abnormal synthesis, transport, or transfer of axon (neuron-derived) signals for myelination. This possibility can be tested by a grafting paradigm, which has been developed and used by Aguayo and his colleagues (1979a,b) to show that the trembler, quaking, and dystrophic abnormalities were not caused by aberrant axonal signals. The defects were of Schwann cell (glial) origin. It is unlikely that the genetic defect in these above mutants will be imminently forthcoming or that it will be due to an abnormality in formation of a specific lipid. The focus of this section will be on considering how myelin arrest occurs in shiverer and twitcher mutants. It is hoped that these discussions will be of value in developing additional approaches for other hypomyelinating mutants.

Shiverer and *mld* mutant mice are allelic (Lachapelle et al., 1980). They are characterized biochemically by the complete absence of MBPs and morphologically by a limited and abnormal myelination in the CNS (Jacque et al., 1983; Privat et al., 1979; Dupouey et al., 1979; Rosenbluth, 1980a; Ginalski-Winkelmann et al., 1983; Barbarese et al., 1983; Roach et al., 1983; Campagnoni et al., 1984). Absence of the major dense line in central myelin sheaths of these mutants has been considered evidence for the localization of MBPs to the apposed cytoplasmic surfaces of myelin. It might follow that the function of MBP is in the compaction (extrusion of the cytoplasm) during CNS myelin sheath formation and it is their absence that limits this compaction and consequently limits myelination. The PNS of these mutants is ultrastructurally normal although MBPs are lacking (Kirschner and Ganser, 1980; Rosenbluth, 1980b; Peterson and Marler, 1983). Evidently, MBP is not needed for PNS myelination, possibly because other proteins of PNS myelin, such as the P_0 glycoprotein, can function in this compaction role at cytoplasmic surfaces.

Since the "turning on" of genes for myelin sheath (protein) formation is a late event in gliogenesis, it would follow that the developmentally earlier events would occur normally. These would include the proliferation of glia, their deployment to areas where the myelin sheaths are needed, and the extension of processes to axons and internodal ensheathment. It might be possible to find out if these events had indeed proceeded normally by morphometric or cytomorphometric analyses. It would follow that the defect in MBP synthesis would only become important when the machinery for making compact myelin sheaths is activated. Precisely how the lack of basic protein synthesis affects other events of the myelination process is not known. A worthwhile aim for studies of myelination with the shiverer and *mld* mutants would be to learn how the inability of myelin-forming glial cells to make MBP would affect other aspects of the myelination process.

Using molecular biology technology (with cloned DNA sequences to MBP), Roach et al. (1983) have demonstrated that mRNAs for the basic proteins are absent in shiverer brains and that segments of the DNA genome coding for these proteins are also missing. The mRNA deficit has also been revealed in studies with shiverer and *mld* cell-free protein-synthesizing systems. These brain-derived systems do not make the four MBPs of 21,000, 18,500, 17,000, and 14,000 molecular weight found in normal rodent brains (Barbarese et al., 1983; Ginalski-Winkelmann et al., 1983; Campagnoni et al., 1984). With heterozygous *mld/+* and *shi/+* mutants, synthesis of these four proteins proceeded at roughly half the rate of normal mice. Whether this result has meaning in terms of the numbers of normal oligodendroglia present in the heterozygote or whether the synthetic capacity of individual oligodendroglia is limited has not been addressed by morphological study or with other biochemical criteria. Campagnoni (personal communication) is studying proteolipid protein synthesis in the heterozygous mutant; it will be of interest to see if levels of this protein are also halved.

In spite of the reduction in CNS myelin in homozygous mutants, levels of myelin-associated enzymes, 5'-nucleotidase, cyclic nucleotide phosphohydrolase, and carbonic anhydrase are not reduced. Not surprisingly, they fractionate differently from enzymes in preparations from normal mouse brain (Mikoshiba et al., 1980; Cammer and Zimmerman, 1983). These findings indicate that these enzymes are not constituents of compact myelin and/or that their synthesis occurs independently and is independently regulated from that of MBP and the formation of myelin sheaths. Immunocytochemical approaches based on antibodies to these enzymes and/or histochemical approaches might provide a means of characterizing the distribution of myelin-forming glial cells in the mutants (homozygous and heterozygous) and sites within these cells where the enzymes are accumulating. Additionally, the staining patterns could be compared with those of other myelin constituents, such as proteolipid protein, myelin-associated glycoprotein, galactocereberoside, and sulfatide, to see if the enzymes accumulate in the same regions of oligoden-droglia as these other myelin constituents.

As might be expected, other components of compact myelin are re-duced in shiverer brain. Bird et al. (1978) demonstrated that cerebral lipid levels were altered in both young and adult mutants. These gross changes, including reduced amounts of cerebroside, sulfatide and cholesterol rel-ative to phospholipid, surely reflect the lack of formation of normal myelin membrane. An increased cholesterol ester content in the mutant brain may correlate with ultrastructural observations of myelin breakdown in the mutant CNS (Rosenbluth, 1980a). The other major CNS myelin pro-tein, the proteolipid protein, is likewise reduced (Matthieu et al., 1981), in accordance with the reduction of compact myelin.

What direction might future studies take to clarify abnormal myeli-nation in these mutants? One might consider the premise that MBPs are involved in compaction of cytoplasmic leaflets of the glial plasma mem-branes. These MBP-deficient mutants might be ideal candidates to use in characterization of the acidic lipids present at those sites with which MBP would interact. It would therefore appear reasonable to determine whether the composition and metabolism of specific acidic lipids are al-tered during early periods of both CNS and PNS myelination. Plausible candidates are polyphosphoinositides, as these lipids interact with basic protein in model systems (Palmer and Dawson, 1969) and they probably reside on the cytoplasmic leaflet of the plasma membrane where (in crude brain preparations) their rapid metabolism is controlled by cytoplasmic kinases and phosphomonoesterases (Fisher et al., 1984). The acidic gly-colipids, sulfatide and ganglioside, which also interact with basic protein in model membrane systems, would probably never encounter MBP dur-ing their formation and migration to the external side of the myelin sheath (see Section 9.5.1). In addition to compositional and metabolic avenues for these studies, it might be possible to use specific antibodies to po-lyphosphoinositides to determine if they are lacking or abnormally dis-posed in CNS and PNS myelin.

The twitcher mutant is an attractive new model of a lipid storage dis-ease, since the enzyme defect, galactosylcerebrosidase plus lactosylcer-amidase I activities, is the same as found in human globoid cell leuko-dystrophy or Krabbe's disease (Duchen et al., 1980; Kobayashi et al., 1980). The disorder in both the PNS and CNS has been characterized in recent morphological studies (Duchen et al., 1980; Jacobs et al., 1982; Nagara et al., 1982; Takahashi et al., 1983a,b; Takahashi and Suzuki, 1984). Jacobs and her colleagues showed that sciatic nerve myelination proceeds normally until the 10th to 11th day at which time demyelination is first observed. Krabbe-type inclusions are present in both Schwann cells and macrophages (globoid cells) a few days later. From then on extensive demyelination and remyelination occur and the axons, which are spared, are of somewhat smaller caliber than those from controls. These results are in line with the arguments that events of PNS gliogenesis, including proliferation and migration of Schwann cells, ensheathment of axons, and early myelination, all proceed normally. Studies in the CNS, mainly the spinal cord, by Suzuki and his colleagues have demonstrated that, there also, gliogenesis and initial myelination occur normally. With time the process is slowed and myelin degradation becomes more prevalent. As in the shiverer and *mld* mutations the defect, being developmentally late, allows many earlier stages of gliogenesis to occur.

The defect is presumably first manifested when galactocerebroside, the substrate of the missing enzyme, has accumulated. The resulting pathology is presumably due, at least in part, to the formation of abnormal galactocerebroside-rich inclusions in the myelin-forming (and metabolizing) glial cells and to the subsequent recruitment of globoid cells (presumably of macrophage origin) that participate in absorbing these inclusions and precipitating the demyelination process. It might be of importance that both galactocerebroside and antibodies can effect autoimmune demyelination (Saida et al., 1979b, 1981; Sumner et al., 1982; and Section 9.5.1).

An advantage of this mutation is its early detectability, before clinical signs develop, by means of enzyme assays on clipped tail (Kobayashi et al., 1982). That the defect is of glial and not neuronal origin was shown by Scaravilli and Jabobs (1981) with the nerve-grafting paradigm developed by Aguayo et al. (1977, 1979b). In further grafting studies Scaravilli and Jacobs (1982) and Scaravilli and Suzuki (1983) showed that twitcher grafted into trembler and normal hosts are able to form normal myelin sheaths. Presumably, an enzyme-replacement mechanism operates in which the Schwann cells in the graft are able to obtain circulating enzyme from the host animal.

Studies of lipids and lipid metabolism in CNS by Igisu et al. (1983) have shown that (1) alterations in amounts of total brain lipid decreased only in the later stages (37–42 days) of the disease; (2) levels of galactolipid, both cerebroside and sulfatide, were altered [both are increased or normal at early times (1–15 days) and decreased at later times]; and (3) phospholipids and cholesterol levels remain very close to normal throughout the disease. Studies have not been conducted on lipid changes in peripheral nerve.

In considering directions for future studies with twitcher, one might consider it in the framework of shiverer. With this mutant, however, the defect concerns an outwardly oriented myelin component. In an analogous fashion to the discussion of the MBP-deficient mutants, studies of the metabolism of externally disposed proteolipid protein in the CNS and P_0 in the PNS would be appealing, as it would be these proteins with which cerebroside would most likely interact. Furthermore, it would be of interest to learn how cerebroside catabolism is related to sulfatide metabolism as well as that of myelin gangliosides. It might also be worthwhile to consider the changes in light of those observed in Wallerian degeneration. For example, the metabolic properties of twitcher Schwann cells containing lipid-rich inclusions may be similar to distal Schwann cells in nerve degeneration, whose metabolism is altered by accumulations of myelin debris (Section 9.4.1).

One reason for developing morphological and cytochemical approaches in studying this model is that compositional and metabolic changes will reflect both malfunctioning glial cells and that of invading globoid cells. The grafting model of Scaravilli and Suzuki (1983) is of potential interest in biochemical studies, since twitcher Schwann cells in the graft are morphologically normal. Metabolic studies of the graft could be carried out to see if biochemical abnormalities in the mutant are fully corrected.

Two other lines of study related to this mutation will be discussed briefly. The first would be based on the finding of Igisu and Suzuki (1984) that galactosylsphingosine (psychosine) accumulates in brains of twitcher mice. These authors discuss the possible effects of psychosine deposition (see also Suzuki and Suzuki, 1983), including the evidence that the compound is toxic to cells in which it accumulates. The basis of psychosine toxicity is largely unknown and it might be fruitful to carry out experiments to determine if psychosine and/or exogenous cerebroside alter the activities (K_m or V_{max} values) of lipid enzymes present in myelin (Norton, 1980; Ledeen, this volume) or with other enzymic activities involved in myelination (both anabolic and catabolic activities).

The second line involves the use of cyclic amino acids as potential inhibitors of myelination. These studies are of potential relevance to the twitcher model because cycloserine has been reported to block cerebroside synthesis (Sundaram and Lev, 1984), and it may be possible to use this drug in studies to alleviate twitcher pathology through blocking the buildup of cerebroside and possibly psychosine as well.

Another use of cycloserine is based on studies with another cyclic amino acid, cycloleucine. This drug has been shown to produce spongiform demyelination (Jacobson et al., 1973; Gandy et al., 1973; Nixon, 1976; Nixon et al., 1976; Greco et al., 1980), and the defect has been ascribed to competition with natural amino acids in transport and inhibition of various methylation reactions. It would also be of interest to see if these agents cause demyelination when either injected into peripheral nerve (Section 9.5.1) or introduced into myelinating tissue cultures. If reproducible demyelination occurred in these systems, studies along the lines considered for nerve degeneration and lysolecithin-induced demyelination could be carried out.

9.6 EXPERIMENTAL DIABETIC NEUROPATHY

The experimental models of diabetes have attracted many investigators interested in contributing to our understanding of the disease. The animal models develop the same complications expressed in human diabetes, namely neuropathy, retinopathy, and nephropathy. The background of most available models can be found in the reviews of Renold (1968), Rerup (1970), Bray and York (1971), and Seemayer et al. (1980). In addition, related galactosemic (Gabbay and Snider, 1970, 1972) and *myo*-inositol-induced uremic (DeJesus et al., 1974; Liveson et al., 1984) models have many of the characteristics of experimentally diabetic animals. The elucidation of the etiology of these neuropathies might also prove relevant to mental retardation (galactosemia) and complications of renal disease.

The principal characteristics of the experimental diabetic models that correlate with the human condition are (1) hyperglycemia, (2) insulinemia, (3) elevated fructose and sorbitol levels in plasma and selected tissues including lens and peripheral nerve, (4) depressed *myo*-inositol levels in plasma and selected tissues, and (5) lowered nerve conduction velocities as measured from the velocities of the largest-caliber fibers. This section will cover only a limited number of morphological and biochemical studies carried out with diabetic rats. Several recent reviews (Prockop and Pleasure, 1977; Clements, 1979; Anderson, 1976; Brownlee and Cerami, 1981; Thomas and Eliasson, 1984) provide a broader picture of this complication of diabetes and should be consulted for further references and information.

All classes of diabetic animal models, including those caused by pancreatectomy or by drug (alloxan or streptozotocin) administration as well as genetic mutants, have been shown to reproduce diabetic neuropathy. The characteristic features of the experimental neuropathy are altered nerve sugar and polyol levels, reduced nerve (commonly sciatic or tail) conduction velocities, and limited ultrastructural pathology. Similarly, galactosemic and uremic models caused by feeding diets containing high (35–40%) amounts of galactose or *myo*-inositol, respectively, change nerve polyol levels and reduce nerve conduction velocity. In choosing a specific model, the streptozotocin rat is advantageous in that it is relatively easy to produce diabetes with this drug and the rats are quite easy to maintain. In long-term studies it may be important to keep the animals in smooth-floored cages, as wire bottoms (though easier to clean) cause pressure-induced distal neuropathy, which is unrelated to the diabetes (Peter Spencer, personal communication). Another advantage of a chemical model versus the genetic models is that the time course of diabetes commences within a few days of injection of the drug. The major drawback of chemically induced models is the possible neurotoxic side effects of the drug, that is, neural changes produced independent of the diabetes. An apparently important factor is the age of the animal. Jefferys et al. (1978), using older and larger rats than Greene et al. (1975), were unable to reproduce reversal of the neuropathy with *myo*-inositol feeding. However, with younger rats (where 1% *myo*-inositol in the feed reverses the neuropathy) there is a question as to whether the effects of the diabetes are due solely to hyperglycemia or also to the arrest of nerve growth. In this regard, it would be useful to consider as controls diabetic rats in which the neuropathy was treated. Insulin (Greene et al., 1975), *myo*-inositol feeding (Greene et al., 1975; Greene and Lattimer, 1983), and aldose reductase inhibitor treatment (Finegold et al., 1983; Gillon and Hawthorne, 1983) will reverse experimental diabetic neuropathy.

The available genetic models include the *db/db* mice, the Chinese hamster, and the BB Wistar rat. Far less biochemical, physiological, and morphological experimentation has been carried out with these models. The db/db mice are easy to maintain, while the BB Wistar rats are notoriously difficult (Seemayer et al., 1980; Mendell et al., 1981). As these models more closely approximate juvenile diabetes, it would be worthwhile to use them to validate and support results obtained with chemical models. Galactosemic and uremic models would provide additional testing grounds for new findings.

Diabetic neuropathy in animals and humans develops in relation to the duration and control of the disease. The development can be longitudinally assessed by electrophysiological means; the method described by Goto and Peters (1974) for measuring motor conduction velocity in rat tail is the most straightforward as it can be carried out with limited perturbation of the animal. Whether the causes of decreased nerve conduction observed in acute versus chronic stages of the disease are the same or not is unknown (Anderson, 1976; Clements, 1979). Likewise, the relative contributions of axonal and/or glial malfunction in the early and later developing stages of the neuropathy are obscure. Morphological studies have demonstrated both axon dwindling and nodal abnormalities on the one hand and segmental demyelination and myelin structural changes on the other. These findings might indicate that both partners (axons and

Schwann cells) of the peripheral nerve are "targets" of the diabetic condition.

The chemical basis for the neuropathy (acute and chronic phases will not be distinguished here) is likely to be tied in some way to persistent hyperglycemia and altered polyol content, for when hyperglycemia is controlled, polyol levels return to normal and nerve conduction deficits are restored (Greene et al., 1975). Furthermore, Greene et al. (1975) showed that *myo*-inositol feeding (at 1%, but not 3%) restores nerve *myo*-inositol levels and nerve conduction in streptozotocin rats. No satisfactory explanation for the failure to reverse the neuropathy with the richer inositol diet has been found. Since the distribution of polyols and sugars within the nerve (axon vs. glia) is not known, and since *myo*-inositol lipid metabolism occurs in both axons and Schwann cells (Gould, 1976), it is not known which cell type, neuron or glia, is primarily susceptible to *myo*-inositol depletion (and/or excess uremia). Ludvigson and Sorenson (1980) generated antibodies to aldose reductase and used immunocytochemistry to demonstrate that this key enzyme in sorbitol and fructose formation was concentrated in Schwann cell cytoplasm and not in the axon. It would follow that the increased sorbitol and fructose could, therefore, interfere with *myo*-inositol movements in the Schwann cells. However, since tritiated *myo*-inositol injected into the endoneurial space passes rapidly through the Schwann cells into the axons of myelinated fibers to be rapidly incorporated into lipid (Gould, 1976), it is likely that fructose and sorbitol accumulation in Schwann cell cytoplasm could deplete pools of *myo*-inositol in both Schwann cells and axoplasm.

Since the major role of *myo*-inositol is as precursor for phospholipids (Hawthorne and Pickard, 1979), the remaining discussion will focus on relationships between inositol lipid metabolism and diabetic neuropathy. An inherent problem is our lack of knowledge concerning the role of inositol lipids in the nerve conduction process. Although a variety of studies have shown that electrical stimulation of nerve causes changes in the metabolism of inositol lipids (Larrabee and Brinley, 1968; Birnberger et al., 1971; Hughes and Salway, 1973; White et al., 1974; Kilian and Schacht, 1980; Goswami and Gould, in press), these do not indicate where within the nerve the changes occur or how the changes relate to propagation of the action potential.

The biochemical evidence for a relationship between inositol lipids and diabetic neuropathy comes largely from studies of streptozotocin rat sciatic nerve. Reduction in inositol lipid levels in nerve and brain of chronically streptozotocin diabetic rats has been reported (Palmano et al., 1977; Natarajan et al., 1981). In these studies polyphosphoinositides were not measured. Clements and Stockard (1980) did show, using inositol labeling, that the proportion of radioactivity in phosphatidylinositol-4,5-bisphosphate (PIP$_2$) was slightly reduced compared with phosphatidylinositol phosphate (PIP) and PI. That the compositional studies revealed changes in peripheral nerve PI, especially that of Palmano et al. (1977), who also found changes after 72 h of diabetes, is somewhat surprising. It is well established that most of the lipids of rat sciatic nerve are present in the multilayered myelin sheaths and that the lipids (and proteins) of the sheaths, particularly in larger-caliber structures, are relatively stable compared with other membranes (Gould et al., 1982a). Hence it is unlikely that compositional changes in less dominant, metabolically more active membranes would be detected with these studies.

The metabolic studies performed by Hothersall and McLean (1979), Clements and Stockard (1980), Natarajan et al. (1981), and Bell et al (1982b) detected and characterized alterations of inositol lipid metabolism in diabetic nerves. Hothersall and McLean found that streptozotocin diabetes depressed the incorporation of [^{3}H]inositol, but not other lipid precursors, into phospholipids by intact nerve preparations. This effect was not reproduced when the incubations were carried out with nerve homogenates, and the investigators suggested that the alteration was a reflection of inositol transport into the preparation, since inositol incorporation by nerve homogenates far exceeded that of intact nerve preparations. The recent finding of Gillon and Hawthorne (1983) that *myo*-inositol uptake into endoneurial preparations of diabetic nerve was reduced 40% relative to controls is in line with this hypothesis; that is, the effect is primarily related to inositol transport (see also Clements and Stockard, 1980) and not lipid synthesis. Clements and Stockard studied the metabolism of intraperitoneally injected [^{3}H]inositol in 2-week streptozotocin diabetic, insulin-treated diabetic, and control animals. The metabolic changes in inositol uptake and incorporation found in diabetic animals were not corrected by insulin treatment, although the activity of CDP-diacylglycerol: *myo*-inositol phosphatidyltransferase (inositol transferase), which was depressed in diabetic nerve, was restored with this treatment (see below).

The study of Natarajan and his colleagues showed that [^{33}P]orthophosphate incorporation into phosphoinositides was altered in chronic (20-week) diabetic versus control nerves such that labeling of PI and PIP$_2$ were depressed while that of PIP was increased. In contrast, acutely (5-day) diabetic rats showed little change in the incorporation of ^{33}P into inositides. In similarly designed experiments Bell and her colleagues found that incorporation of [^{32}P]phosphate by the nerve preparations from 10–20-week diabetic rats into PIP$_2$ was increased, whereas uptake into PI and PIP was unchanged. The differences between the results of these two studies may reflect the incubation conditions chosen, the manner of preparation of the nerves, or the concentrations of phosphate presented to the nerve preparations.

Further evidence that inositol lipid metabolism is affected in diabetic nerve comes from studies of relevant enzyme activities in homogenates of control and diabetic nerve. In published studies from two laboratories (Whiting et al., 1979; Clements and Stockard, 1980) and in our unpublished work carried out with M. H. Kumara-Siri, the levels of inositol transferase were substantially decreased in diabetic nerves. Since this enzyme is present in axons (Gould, 1976; Gould et al., 1983a,b) and is axonally transported (Kumara-Siri and Gould, 1980) and has a K_m in the millimolar range, there is a strong possibility that the loss of its activity, coupled with the decreased availability of inositol substrate, may reduce the metabolism of axonal PI and, consequently, also depress the metabolism of axonal PIP and PIP_2. Since the transport rates of other components are reduced in diabetic nerves (e.g., Meiri and McLean, 1982; Vitadello et al., 1983), the loss of inositol transferase activity might be due to its depressed axonal transport. However, in preliminary studies with M. H. Kumara-Siri, we were unable to demonstrate any reduction in the rate of accumulation of this enzyme activity proximal to a ligature. Another explanation for the reduced activity of inositol transferase in nerve might be its glycosylation at or near the active site, since myo-inositol and glucose are structurally similar and nonenzymatic glycosylation occurs in diabetic nerve (Vlassara et al., 1981).

A possible relationship between inositol lipid metabolism and nerve conduction changes may be deduced from the recent findings of Greene and Lattimer (1983) who showed that the activities of the ouabain-sensitive sodium-potassium ATPase (but not other nerve ATPase activity) was reduced in diabetic versus control nerve homogenates. Furthermore, the reduction in activity of this enzyme was prevented in diabetic rats fed 1% myo-inositol to reverse the neuropathy. This enzyme has been localized to nodal and/or paranodal neural membranes in immunocytochemical (Wood et al., 1977; Schwartz et al., 1981) and histochemical (Vorbrodt et al., 1982) studies. Greene and Lattimer suggested that the reduced activity of this enzyme in homogenates of diabetic nerve might be related to a specific requirement of PI (PIP and/or PIP_2 are also potential activators) by this lipid-requiring enzyme (Roelofson, 1981). In support of this "ATPase hypothesis" (though not inositol lipid involvement) is the work of Brismar and Sima (1981) who used single-node, voltage clamp studies to demonstrate increased Na^+ accumulation in diabetic nerves and attributed this change to a defective Na^+-K^+-ATPase pump.

A plausible avenue to examine the relationship between Na^+-K^+-ATP-ase and inositol lipids would be to see if enzyme properties (K_m and/or V_{max}) are changed when concentrations of inositol lipid are altered. The concentrations of PI in the homogenates (or an ATPase-enriched membrane preparation) could be depleted by incubations with PC liposomes and a purified bovine brain exchange protein (see Steele et al., 1982). Conversely, incubating the tissue in liposomes enriched in PI (PC–PI, 2 : 1, mol/mol) would elevate PI in the membrane. In this way it would be possible to determine both the effects of increased and decreased PI levels on Na^+-K^+-ATPase activity. Experiments of this nature using diabetic nerve would indicate whether the reduced ATPase activity could be restored with increased membrane PI. It might also be possible to alter the concentrations of polyphosphoinositides in the membrane by preincubating the ATPase-enriched membrane with preparations of enzymes that form or degrade these compounds. If peripheral nerve Na^+-K^+-ATPase activity is shown to be sensitive to membrane phosphoinositide levels, then it would seem feasible that reduced axonal *myo*-inositol could influence ionic gradients in nerve, causing a depression in nerve conduction.

Altered ionic gradients of sodium, potassium, and calcium as well as counterions in turn could affect axon and axolemma functions and metabolism, especially ATP levels and the regulation of protein and phospholipid phosphorylation.

Diabetic neuropathy is a complex experimental problem in which a cascade of underlying perturbations, including the metabolism of inositol-containing lipids, presumably have importance. It is likely that future studies will provide insight into the etiology of this clinically significant disorder and furnish understanding of the role(s) for inositol lipids in the excitable properties of neural membranes.

9.7   CONCLUSIONS

This chapter includes discussion of far fewer neurological models than originally planned and omits mention of much outstanding work. It is my feeling, however, that the wider-ranging discussion of selected models will help the reader in developing experimental strategies based on the properties of neurons and glial cells that make up nervous tissue.

The progression in the presentation from the simpler and extensively studied process of Wallerian degeneration to more difficult and complex models such as shiverer and twitcher mutant mice and diabetic rat had purpose. I chose to paint a detailed picture of Wallerian degeneration and the utility of lipid-related techniques in studying it so that these will act as guidelines in considering other animal models. My focus on the peripheral nerve stems from my long-standing acquaintance with this tissue and my intuitive feeling that studies with the PNS are simpler to interpret and will provide background for carrying out studies of CNS disorders.

Disorders of the nervous system, by the very nature of the component cells and the involved interactions between them, are complicated, and neither morphological, biochemical, or physiological approaches used in isolation will greatly clarify the origins and nature of the disorder. The neuroscientist who attempts to understand facets of specific neurological diseases must be as broad as possible in outlook. In writing this chapter, I tried to think broadly about the models and to suggest new directions for research.

ACKNOWLEDGMENTS

I would like to thank Lee Antonucci and Helen LaMantia for their continued help in typing and retyping the many drafts of this chapter. Warren Spivack provided invaluable help in critically reading the manuscript and reorganizing the references. Drs. Marion Smith, Bob Ledeen, Jeffrey Yao, Visvanathan Natarajan, Firoze Jungalwala, Kuni Suzuki, Tony Campagnoni, Regina Armstrong, and Stephen Fisher willingly sent me preprints of chapters for this and other books, which proved useful in defining the scope of this work and in finding important source material. Joe Eichberg's guidance and tremendous patience was gratefully appreciated. Finally, thanks are due to my wife and children for the time away from them required for the preparation of this manuscript.

REFERENCES

Abrahams, P.H., Day, A., and Allt, G., *Acta Neuropathol. (Berlin)*, *50*, 85–90 (1980).

Agranoff, B.W., *Adv. Exp. Med. Biol.*, *83*, 191–201 (1977).

Aguayo, A.J., Attiwell, M., Trecarten, J., Perkins, S., and Bray, G.M., *Nature*, *265*, 73–75 (1977).

Aguayo, A.J., Bray, G.M., and Perkins, S.C., *Annu. N.Y. Acad. Sci.*, *317*, 512–531 (1979a).

Aguayo, A.J., Bray, G.M., Perkins, C.S., and Duncan, I.D., *Soc. Neurosci. Symp.*, *4*, 361–383 (1979b).

Alberghina, M., Viola, M., and Giuffrida, A.M., *J. Neurochem.*, *40*, 25–31 (1983a).

Alberghina, M., Moschella, F., Viola, M., Brancati, V., Micali, G., and Giuffrida, A.M., *J. Neurochem.*, *40*, 32–38 (1983b).

Allt, G., in D.N. Landon, Ed., *The Peripheral Nerve*, Chapman and Hall, London, 1976, pp. 666–739.

Allt, G., and Cavanaugh, J.B., *Brain Res., 92*, 459–468 (1969).

Alvord, E.C., Jr., Kies, M.W., and Suckling, A.J., Eds., Alan R. Liss, Inc., New York, 1984.

Anderson, J.W., *Amer. J. Clin. Nutr., 29*, 402–408 (1976).

Ando, M., Miwa, M., Kato, K., and Nagata, T., *J. Neurochem., 42*, 94–100 (1984).

Appenzeller, O., and Partlow, L.M., *Brain Res., 42*, 521–524 (1972).

Armstrong, R., Toews, A., Ray, R., and Morell, P., *J. Neurosci.* (in press).

Babitch, J.A., Blomstrand, C., and Hamberger, A., *Acta Neurol. Scand., 51*, 211–224 (1975).

Barbarese, E., Nielson, M.L., and Carson, J.H., *J. Neurochem., 40*, 1680–1686 (1983).

Barron, K.D., in C.C. Kao, R.P. Bunge, and P.J. Reier, Eds., *Spinal Cord Reconstruction*, Raven Press, New York, 1983, pp. 7–40.

Baumann, N.A., Ed., *Neurological Mutations Affecting Myelination*, Elsevier/North Holland Biomedical Press, Amsterdam, 1980.

Baumann, N., and Lachapelle, F., in A. Lajtha, Ed., *Handbook of Neurochemistry*, 2nd Ed.,Vol. 2, Plenum Press, New York, 1982, pp. 253–279.

Belin, J., and Smith, A.D., *J. Neurochem., 27*, 969–970 (1976).

Bell, M.E., Peterson, R.G., and Wiggins, R.C., *Neurochem. Res., 7*, 99–114 (1982a).

Bell, M.E., Peterson, R.G., and Eichberg, J., *J. Neurochem., 39*, 192–200 (1982b).

Benes, F., Higgins, J.A., and Barnett, R.J., *J. Cell Biol., 57*, 613–629 (1973).

Bird, T.D., Farrell, D.F., and Sumi, S.M. *J. Neurochem., 31*, 387–391 (1978).

Birnberger, A.C., Birnberger, K.L., Eliasson, S.G., and Simpson, P.C., *J. Neurochem., 18*, 1291–1298 (1971).

Bisby, M.A., and Bulger, V.T., *J. Neurochem., 29*, 313–320 (1977).

Black, M.M., and Lasek, R.J., *Expl. Neurol., 63*, 108–119 (1979).

Blakemore, W.F., Eames, R.A., Smith, K.J., and McDonald, N.I., *J. Neurol. Sci., 33*, 31–43 (1977).

Boggs, J.M., and Moscarello, M.A., *Biochim. Biophys. Acta, 515*, 1–21 (1978).

Bonnaud-Toulze, E.N., and Raine, C.S., *Neuropathol. Appl. Neurobiol., 6*, 279–290 (1980).

Borst, P., *Trends Biochem. Sci., 8*, 269–272 (1983).

Bradbury, M., Ed., *The Concept of a Blood Brain Barrier*, Wiley, New York, 1979.

Brady, R.O., in G.J. Siegel, R.W. Albers, B.W. Agranoff, and R. Katzman, Eds., *Basic Neurochemistry*, 3rd ed., Little Brown and Co., Boston, 1981, pp. 615–626.

Brady, R.O., in J.B. Stanbury, J.B. Wyngaarden, D.S. Frederickson, J.L. Goldstein, and M.S. Brown, Eds., *The Metabolic Basic of Inherited Disease*, McGraw-Hill Book Co., New York, 1983, pp. 831–841.

Bray, G.A., and York, D.A., *Physiol. Rev., 51*, 598–646 (1971).

Brismar, T., *Acta Physiol. Scand., 113*, 161–166 (1981a).

Brismar, T., *Acta Physiol. Scand., 113*, 167–176 (1981b).

Brismar, T., and Sima, A.A.F., *Acta Physiol. Scand., 113*, 499–506 (1981).

Brown, M.J., Pleasure, D.E., and Asbury, A.K., *J. Neurol. Sci., 29*, 361–369 (1976).

Brownlee, M., and Cerami, A., *Ann. Rev. Biochem., 50*, 385–432 (1981).

Bulger, V.T., and Bisby, M.A., *J. Neurochem., 31*, 1411–1418 (1978).

Buse, M.G., Herlong, H.F., Weigand, D.A., and Spicer, S.S., *J. Neurochem., 27,* 1339–1345 (1976).

Caley, D.W., and Butler, A.B., *Amer. J. Anat., 140,* 339–348 (1974).

Cammer, W., in P.S. Spencer and H.H. Schaumberg, Eds., *Experimental and Clinical Neurotoxicology,* Williams and Wilkens Publ., Baltimore, 1980, pp. 239–256.

Cammer, W., and Zimmerman, T.R., Jr., *Brain Res., 265,* 73–80 (1983).

Campagnoni, A.T., Campagnoni, C.W., Bourre, J.-M., Jacque, C., and Baumann, N., *J. Neurochem., 42,* 733–739 (1984).

Cancalon, P., *J. Cell Biol.,* 97, 6–14 (1983).

Cancalon, P., and Elam, J.S., *J. Neurochem., 35,* 889–897 (1980).

Chia, L.S., Thompson, J.E., and Moscarello, M.A., *Biochem. Biophys. Res. Commun., 117,* 141–146 (1983).

Clements, R.S., Jr., *Diabetes, 28,* 609–611 (1979).

Clements, R.S., and Stockard, C.R., *Diabetes, 29,* 227–235 (1980).

Cook, R.D., and Wisniewski, H.M., *Brain Res., 81,* 191–206 (1973).

Cragg, B.G., *Brain Res., 23,* 1–21 (1970).

Dahl, D., Crosby, C.J., and Bignami, A., *Exp. Neurol., 71,* 421–430 (1981).

Dal Canto, M.C., and Rabinowitz, S.G., *Annu. Neurol., 11,* 109–127 (1982).

DeJesus, P.V., Clements, R.S., and Winegrad, A.I., *J. Neurol. Sci., 21,* 237–249 (1974).

De Medio, G.E., Brunetti, M., Dorman, R.V., Droz, B., Horrocks, L.A., Porcellati, G., Souyri, F., and Trovarelli, G., *Birth Defects, 19,* 175–187 (1983).

DeVries, G.H., Salzer, J.L., and Bunge, R.P., *Trans. Amer. Soc. Neurochem, 11,* 111 (1980).

Dewar, A.J., and Moffett, B.J., *Pharm. Ther., 5,* 545–562 (1979).

Dombrowski, A.M., and Kauffman, F.C., *Brain Res., 219,* 407–421 (1981).

Domonkos, J., in A. Lajtha, Ed., *Handbook of Neurochemistry, Vol. 7,* Plenum Press, New York, 1972, pp. 93–106.

Domonkos, J., and Heiner, L., *J. Neurochem., 15,* 87–91 (1968a).

Domonkos, J., and Heiner, L., *J. Neurochem., 15,* 93–98 (1968b)

Donat, J.R., and Wisniewski, H.M., *Brain Res., 53,* 41–53 (1973).

Duchen, L.W., Eicher, E.M., Jacobs, J.M., Scaravilli, J.M., and Teixeira, F., *Brain, 103,* 695–710 (1980).

Dupouey, P., Jacque, C., Bourre, J.M., Cesselin, F., Privat, A., and Baumann, N., *Neurosci. Lett., 12,* 113–118 (1979).

Dyck, P.J., Thomas, P.K., and Lambert, E.H., Eds., *Peripheral Neuropathy,* Vols. I and II, W.B. Saunders Co., Philadelphia, 1975.

Dyck, P.J., Thomas, P.K., Lambert, E.H., and Bunge, R., Eds., *Peripheral Neuropathy,* 2nd Ed., Vols. I and II, W.B. Saunders Co., Philadelphia, 1984.

Dziegielewska, K.M., Evans, C.A.N., and Saunders, N.R., *J. Physiol., 304,* 83–98 (1980).

Edstrom, A., and Hanson, M., *Brain Res., 61,* 311–320 (1973).

Ellisman, M.H., and Lindsey, J.D., *J. Neurocytol., 12,* 393–411 (1983).

Finean, J.B., and Michell, R.H., Eds., in *Membrane Structure,* North Holland Biomedical Press, Amsterdam, 1981, pp. 1–36.

Finegold, D., Lattimer, S.A., Nolle, S., Bernstein, M., and Greene, D.A., *Diabetes, 32,* 988–992 (1983).

Fink, D.J., and Gainer, H., *J. Cell Biol.*, *85*, 175–186 (1980).

Fisher, S.K., and Rowe, C.E., *Biochim. Biophys. Acta*, *618*, 231–241 (1980).

Fisher, S.K., van Rooijen, L.A.A., and Agranoff, B.W., *Trends Biol. Sci.*, *9*, 53–56 (1984).

Forman, D.S., and Berenberg, R.A., *Brain Res.*, *156*, 213–225 (1978).

Foster, R.E., Kocsis, J.D., Malenka, R.C., and Waxman, S.G., *J. Neurol. Sci.*, *48*, 221–231 (1980).

Fry, J.M., Lehrer, G.M., and Bornstein, M.B., *Science*, *175*, 192–194 (1972).

Fry, J.M., Weissbarth, S., Lehrer, G.M., and Bornstein, M.B., *Science*, *183*, 540–542 (1974).

Gabbay, K.H., and Snider, J.J., *Diabetes*, *19*, 357–358 (1970).

Gabbay, K.H., and Snider, J.J., *Diabetes*, *21*, 295–300 (1972).

Gandy, G., Jacobson, W., and Sidman, R., *J. Physiol. (Lond.)*, *233*, 1P–3P (1973).

Ganser, A.L., Kirschner, D.A., and Willinger, M., *J. Neurocytol.*, *12*, 921–938 (1983).

Gibson, J.D., *J. Anat.*, *129*, 1–19 (1979).

Gillon, K.R.W., Hawthorne, J.N., *Biochem. J.*, *210*, 775–781 (1983).

Ginalski-Winkelmann, H., Almazan, G., and Matthieu, J.-M., *Brain Res.*, *277*, 386–388 (1983).

Goswami, S.K., and Gould, R.M., *J. Neurochem.* (in press).

Goto, I., and Peters, H.A., *J. Neurol. Sci.*, *22*, 177–182 (1974).

Gould, R.M., *Brain Res.*, *117*, 169–174 (1976).

Gould, R.M., in S.J. Enna, D.W. McCandless, and R.C. Wiggins, Eds., *Developmental Neurochemistry*, University of Texas Press (in press).

Gould, R.M., and Dawson, R.M.G., *J. Cell Biol.*, *68*, 480–496 (1976).

Gould, R.M., Matsumoto, D., and Mattingly, G., in A. Lajtha, Ed., *Handbook of Neurochemistry*, 2nd Ed., Vol. 1, Plenum Press, New York, 1982a, pp. 397–414.

Gould, R.M., Spivack, W.D., Sinatra, R.S. Lindquist, T.D., and Ingoglia, N.A., *J. Neurochem.*, *39*, 1569–1578 (1982b).

Gould, R.M., Pant, H., Gainer, H., and Tytell, M., *J. Neurochem.*, *40*, 1293–1299 (1983a).

Gould, R.M., Spivack, W.D., Robertson, D., and Poznansky, M.J., *J. Neurochem.*, *40*, 1300–1306 (1983b).

Gould, R.P., and Holt, S.J., in *Cytology of Nervous Tissue*, Proc. Anat. Soc. Lond., 1961, pp. 45–48.

Grafstein, B., *Exp. Neurol.*, *48*, 32–51 (1975).

Grafstein, B., and Forman, D.S., *Physiol. Rev.*, *60*, 1167–1283 (1980).

Grafstein, B., and McQuarrie, I.G., in C.W. Cotman, Ed., *Neuronal Plasticity*, Raven Press, New York, 1978, pp. 155–195.

Grafstein, B., Miller, J.A., Ledeen, R.W., Haley, J., and Specht, S.C., *Exp. Neurol.*, *46*, 261–281 (1975).

Greco, C.M., Powell, H.C., Garett, R.S., and Lampert, P.W., *Neuropathol. Appl. Neurobiol.*, *6*, 349–360 (1980).

Greene, D.A., and Lattimer, S.A., *J. Clin. Invest.*, *72*, 1058–1063 (1983).

Greene, D.A., DeJesus, P.V., and Winegrad, A.I., *J. Clin. Invest.*, *55*, 1326–1336 (1975).

Greene, D.A., Winegrad, A.I., Carpentier, J.-L., Brown, M.J., Fukuma, M.J., and Orci, C., *J. Neurochem.*, *33*, 1007–1018 (1979).

Gregson, N.A., and Hall, S.M., *J. Cell Sci.*, *13*, 257–277 (1973).

Griffin, J.W., Drachman, D.B., and Price, D.L., *J. Neurobiol., 7,* 355–370 (1976).

Griffin, J.W., Price, D.L., Drachman, D.B., and Morris, J., *J. Cell Biol., 88,* 205–214 (1981).

Guy, J.R., and Bisby, M.A., *Exp. Neurol., 82,* 706–710 (1983).

Hajra, A.K., and Bishop, J.E., *Ann. NY Acad. Sci., 386,* 170–182 (1982).

Hall, M.E., Wilson, D.L., and Stone, G.C., *J. Neurobiol., 9,* 353–366 (1978).

Hall, S.M., *J. Cell Sci., 10,* 535–546 (1972).

Hall, S.M., *Neuropathol. Appl. Neurobiol., 4,* 165–176 (1978).

Hall, S.M., and Gregson, N.A., *J. Cell Sci., 9,* 769–789 (1971).

Hall, S.M., and Gregson, N.A., *Neuropathol. Appl. Neurobiol., 1,* 149–170 (1975).

Hall, S.M., and Gregson, N.A., *Neuropathol. Appl. Neurobiol., 3,* 65–78 (1977).

Hall, S.M., and Gregson, N.A., *Neuropathol. Appl. Neurobiol., 4,* 117–127 (1978).

Hallpike, J.F. in D.N. Landon, Ed., *The Peripheral Nerve,* Chapman and Hall, London, 1976, pp. 605–665.

Harkonen, M.H.A., and Kauffman, F.C., *Brain Res., 65,* 127–139 (1973).

Harkonen, M.H.A., and Kauffman, F.C., *Brain Res., 65,* 141–157 (1974).

Harrison, B.M., Hansen, L.A., Pollard, J.D., and McLeod, J.G., *Annu. Neurol., 15,* 163–170 (1984).

Hawthorne, J.N., and Pickard, M.R., *J. Neurochem., 32,* 5–14 (1979).

Heacock, A.M., Klinger, P.D., Seguin, E.B., and Agranoff, B.W., *J. Neurochem., 42,* 987–993 (1984).

Henry, S.M., and Hodge, L.D., *J. Cell Biol., 97,* 166–172 (1983).

Heymans, H.S.A., Schutgens, R.B.H., Tan, R., van den Bosch, H., and Borst, P., *Nature, 306,* 69–70 (1983).

Hofteig, J.H., Vo, P.N., and Yates, A.J., *Acta Neuropathol. (Berl.) 55,* 151–156 (1981).

Hofteig, J.H., Vo, P.N., Yates, A.J., and Leon, K.S., *J. Neurochem., 39,* 401–408 (1982).

Hogan, E.L., and Greenfield, S. in P. Morell, Ed., *Myelin,* 2nd Ed., Plenum Press, New York, 1984, pp. 489–534.

Holtzman, E., and Mercurio, A.M., *Int. Rev. Cytol., 67,* 1–67 (1980).

Holtzman, E., and Novikoff, A.B., *J. Cell Biol., 27,* 651–669 (1965).

Horrocks, L.A., Toews, A., Yashon, D., and Locke, G.E., *Neurobiol., 3,* 256–263 (1973).

Horrocks, L.A., Spanner, S., Mozzi, R., Fu, S.C., D'Amato, R.A., and Krakowska, S., *Adv. Exp. Med. Biol., 100,* 423–438 (1980).

Hostetler, K.Y., in J.N. Hawthorne and G.B. Ansell, Eds., *Phospholipids,* Elsevier Biomedical Press, Amsterdam, 1982, pp. 215–261.

Hothersall, J.S., and McLean, P., *Biochem. Biophys. Res. Commun., 88,* 477–484 (1979).

Hughes, I.E., and Salway, J.G., *J. Pharm. Pharmac., 25,* 745–747 (1973).

Igisu, H., and Suzuki, K., *Science, 224,* 753–755 (1984).

Igisu, H., Shimomura, K., Kishimoto, Y., and Suzuki, K., *Brain, 106,* 405–417 (1983).

Ishaque, A., Szymanska, I., Ramwami, J., and Eylar, E.H., *Biochim. Biophys. Acta., 669,* 28–32 (1981).

Jacobs, J.M., Scaravilli, F., and De Aranda, F.T., *J. Neurol. Sci., 55,* 285–304 (1982).

Jacobson, W., Gandy, G., and Sidman, R.L., *J. Pathol., 109,* XIII (1973).

Jacque, C., Delassalle, A., Raoul, M., and Baumann, N., *J. Neurochem., 41,* 1335–1340 (1983).

James, M.J., and Kandutsch, A.A., *J. Biol. Chem., 259,* 8442–8446 (1979).

Jefferys, S.G.R., Palmano, K.P., Sharma, A.K., and Thomas, P.K., *J. Neurol. Neurosurg. Psychiat., 41,* 333–339 (1978).

Jerkins, A., and Kauffman, F.C., *Exp. Neurol., 79,* 347–359 (1983).

Joseph, B.S., *Brain Res., 59,* 1–18 (1973).

Kao, C.C., Bunge, R.P., and Reier, P.J., Eds., *Spinal Cord Reconstruction,* Raven Press, New York, (1983).

Karnovsky, M.L., and Majno, G., in J. Folch-Pi, Ed., *Chemical Pathology of the Nervous System,* Pergamon Press, New York, 1961, pp. 261–267.

Katzman, R., in G.J. Siegel, R.W. Albers, B.W. Agranoff, and R. Katzman, Eds., *Basic Neurochemistry,* 3rd Ed., Little, Brown and Co., Boston, 1981, pp. 497–510.

Kidman, A., Hanwell, M., and Cooper, N., *J. Neurochem., 33,* 357–359 (1979).

Kidman, A.D., Dolan, L., and Sippe, H.T., *J. Neurochem., 30,* 57–61 (1978).

Kilian, P.L., and Schacht, J., *J. Neurochem., 34,* 709–712 (1980).

Kirschner, D.A., and Ganser, A.L., *Nature, 283,* 207–210 (1980).

Kobayashi, T., Yamanaka, T., Jacobs, J.M., Teixeira, F., and Suzuki, K., *Brain Res., 202,* 479–483 (1980).

Kobayashi, T., Nagara, H., and Suzuki, K., *Biochem. Med., 27,* 8–14 (1982).

Koeppen, A.H., Papandrea, S.D., and Mitzen, E.J., *Muscle & Nerve, 2,* 369–375 (1979).

Kristensson, K., and Olsson, Y., *Brain Res., 79,* 101–109 (1974).

Kristensson, K., and Olsson, Y., *J. Neurocytol., 4,* 653–661 (1975).

Kristensson, K., and Olsson, Y., *Brain Res., 115,* 201–213 (1976).

Kumara-Siri, M.H., and Gould, R.M., *Brain Res., 186,* 315–330 (1980).

Lachapelle, F., De Baecque, C., Jacque, C., Bourre, J.M., Delassalle, A., Doolittle, D.G., Hauw, J.J., and Baumann, N., in N. Baumann, Ed., *Neurological Mutations Affecting Myelination,* Elsevier/North Holland Biomedical Press, Amsterdam, 1980, pp. 27–32.

Lajtha, A., Ed., *Handbook of Neurochemistry,* Plenum Press, New York, 10 vols., 1982–1985.

Larrabee, M.G., and Brinley, F.J., Jr., *J. Neurochem., 15,* 533–545 (1968).

Lasek, R.J., and Brady, S.T., *Cold Spring Harbor Symp. Quant. Biol., 46,* 113–124 (1982).

Lassmann, H., Ammerer, H.P., and Kulnig, W., *Acta Neuropathol. (Berl.), 44,* 91–102 (1978a).

Lassmann, H., Ammerer, H.P., Jurecker, W., and Kulnig, W., *Acta Neuropathol. (Berl.), 44,* 103–109 (1978b).

Lieberman, A.R., *Int. Rev. Neurobiol., 14,* 49–124 (1971).

Liveson, J.A., Gardner, J., and Bornstein, M.B., *Einstein Quarterly J. Biol. Med., 2,* 41–45 (1984).

Longo, F.M., and Hammerschlag, R., *Brain Res., 193,* 471–485 (1980).

Lorenz, T., and Willard, M., *Proc. Natl. Acad. Sci. USA, 75,* 505–509 (1978).

Lubinska, L., *Brain Res., 130,* 47–63 (1977).

Lubinska, L., *Brain Res., 233,* 277–240 (1982).

Ludvigson, M.A., and Sorenson, R.L., *Diabetes, 29,* 438–449 (1980).

Ludwin, S.K., in S.G. Waxman and J.M. Ritchie, Eds., *Advances in Neurology Vol. 31, Demyelinating Diseases,* Raven Press, New York, 1981, pp. 123–168.

McCaman, R.E., and Robins, E., *J. Neurochem., 5,* 18–31 (1959).

McDermott, J.R., and Wisniewski, H.M., *J. Neurol.*, *33*, 81–94 (1977).

McDonald, W.I., and Sears, T.A., *Brain Res.*, *93*, 583–598 (1970).

Madrid, R.E., Wisniewski, H.M., Iqbal, K., Pullarkat, R.K., and Lassmann, H., *J. Neurol. Sci.*, *50*, 399–411 (1981).

Maggio, B., Cumar, F.A., and Caputto, R., *Biochim. Biophys. Acta*, *650*, 69–87 (1981).

Matthews, M.R., and Raisman, G., *Proc. R. Soc. Lond. B*, *181*, 43–79 (1972).

Matsumoto, D.E., and Gould, R.M., *Soc. Neurosci.*, *9*, 50 (1983).

Matthieu, J.-M., Ginalski-Winkelmann, H., and Jacque, C., *Brain Res.*, *214*, 219–222 (1981).

Meiri, K.F., and McLean, W.G., *Brain Res.*, *238*, 77–85 (1982).

Mendell, J.R., Sahenk, Z., Warmolts, J.R., Marshall, J.K., and Thibert, P., *J. Neurol. Sci.*, *52*, 103–115 (1981).

Miani, N., *J. Neurochem.*, *9*, 537–541 (1962).

Mikoshiba, K., Nagaike, K., and Tsukada, Y., *J. Neurochem.*, *35*, 465–470 (1980).

Mithen, F.A., Agrawal, H.C., Eylar, E.H., Fishman, M.A., Blank, W., and Bunge, R.P., *Brain Res.*, *250*, 321–331 (1982).

Morell, P., Ed., *Myelin*, 2nd Ed., Plenum Press, New York, 1984.

Morell, P., Bornstein, M.B., and Raine, C.S., in G.J. Siegel, R.W. Albers, B.W. Agranoff, and R. Katzman, Eds., *Basic Neurochemistry*, 3rd Ed., Little, Brown and Co., Boston, 1981.

Nagara, H., Kobayashi, T., Suzuki, K., and Suzuki, K., *Brain Res.*, *244*, 289–294 (1982).

Nagata, Y., Mikoshiba, K., and Tsukada, Y., *Brain Res.*, *56*, 259–269 (1973).

Natarajan, V., and Schmid, H.H.O., in P.J. Dyck, P.K. Thomas, E.H. Lambert, and R. Bunge, Eds., *Peripheral Neuropathy*, 2nd Ed., W.B. Saunders Co., Philadelphia, 1984, pp. 531–561.

Natarajan, V., Dyck, P.J., and Schmid, H.H.O., *J. Neurochem.*, *36*, 413–419 (1981).

Natarajan, V., Yao, J.K., Dyck, P.J., and Schmid, H.H.O., *J. Neurochem.*, *38*, 1419–1428 (1982).

Nixon, R.A., *J. Neurochem.*, *7*, 237–244 (1976).

Nixon, R.A., Suva, M., and Wolf, M.K., *J. Neurochem.*, *27*, 245–251 (1976).

Norton, W.T., and Cammer, W., in P. Morell, Ed., *Myelin*, Plenum Press, New York, 1984a, pp. 161–199.

Norton, W.T., and Cammer, W., in P. Morell, Ed., *Myelin*, Plenum Press, New York, 1984b, pp. 369–403.

Norton, W.T., in A. Boese, Ed., *Search for the Cause of Multiple Sclerosis and Other Chronic Diseases of the Central Nervous System*, Verlag Chemie, Weinheim, 1980, pp. 64–75.

Norton, W.T., in G.J. Siegel, R.W. Albers, B.W. Agranoff, and R. Katzman, Eds., *Basic Neurochemistry*, Little, Brown and Co., Boston, 1981, pp. 63–92.

Ochs, S., *Axoplasmic Transport and Its Relation to Other Nerve Functions*, Wiley, New York, 1983.

Oderfeld-Nowak, B., and Niemierki, S., *J. Neurochem.*, *16*, 235–248 (1969).

Palmer, F.B., and Dawson, R.M.C., *Biochem. J.*, *111*, 637–645 (1969).

Palmano, K.P., Whiting, P.H., and Hawthorne, J.N., *Biochem. J.*, *167*, 229–235 (1977).

Patsalos, P.N., Bell, M.E., and Wiggins, R.C., *J. Cell Biol.*, *87*, 1–5 (1980).

Pentchev, P.G., and Barranger, J.A., *J. Lipid Res.*, *19*, 401–409 (1978).

Perry, G.W., and Wilson, D.L., *J. Neurochem., 37,* 1203–1217 (1981).

Pestronk, A., Drachman, D.B., and Griffin, J.W., *Expl. Neurol., 70,* 65–82 (1980).

Peterson, A., and Marler, J., *Neurosci. Lett., 38,* 163–168 (1983).

Peterson, R.G., Baughman, S., and Scheidler, D.M., *Neurochem. Res., 6,* 213–223 (1981).

Pevzner, L., in A. Lajtha, Ed. *Handbook of Neurochemistry,* 2nd Ed., Vol. 1, Plenum Press, New York, 1982, pp. 357–395.

Pleasure, D.E., Feldmann, B., and Prockop, D.J., *J. Neurochem., 20,* 81–90 (1973).

Poduslo, J.F., *J. Neurochem., 42,* 493–503 (1984).

Politis, M.J., Sternberger, N., Ederle, K., and Spencer, P.S., *J. Neurosci., 2,* 1252–1266 (1982).

Politis, M.J., Pellegrino, R.G., Oaklander, A.L., and Ritchie, J.M., *Brain Res., 273,* 392–395 (1983).

Porcellati, G., in A. Lajtha, Ed., *Handbook of Neurochemistry,* Vol. 2, Plenum Press, New York, 1972, pp. 393–422.

Privat, A., Jacque, C., Bourre, J.M., Dupouey, P., and Baumann, N., *Neurosci. Lett., 12,* 107–112 (1979).

Privat, A., Valat, J., and Fulcrand, J., *J. Neuropathol. Exp. Neurol., 40,* 46–60 (1981).

Prockop, L.D., and Pleasure, D.E., in S. Godensohn and S.H. Appel, Eds., *Scientific Approaches to Clinical Neurology,* Vol. 2, Lea & Febiger, Philadelphia, 1977, pp. 1437–1455.

Raff, M.C., Miller, R.H., and Noble, M., *Nature, 303,* 390–396 (1983).

Rapoport, S.I., *Blood Brain Barrier in Physiology and Medicine,* Raven Press, New York, 1976.

Rawlins, F.A., and Smith, M.E., *Neurobiol., 1,* 225–231 (1971).

Reigner, J., Matthieu, J.-M., Kraus-Ruppert, R., Lassmann, H., and Poduslo, J.F., *J. Neurochem., 36,* 1986–1995 (1981).

Renold, A.E., *Adv. Metab. Disord., 3,* 49–84 (1968).

Rerup, C.C., *Pharmacol. Rev., 22,* 485–518 (1970).

Richards, R.L., Aronson, J., Schoenbechler, M., Diggs, C.L., and Alving, C.R., *J. Immunol., 130,* 1390–1394 (1983).

Roach, A., Boylan, K., Horvath, S., Prusiner, S.B., and Hood, L.E., *Cell, 34,* 799–806 (1983).

Roelofsen, B., *Life Sci., 79,* 2235–2247 (1981).

Rosenbluth, J., *J. Comp. Neurol., 194,* 639–648 (1980a).

Rosenbluth, J., *J. Comp. Neurol., 193,* 729–739 (1980b).

Rosenbluth, J., *Brain Res., 208,* 283–297 (1981).

Rossiter, R.J., in J. Folch-Pi, Ed., *Chemical Pathology of the Nervous System,* Pergamon Press, New York, 1961, pp. 207–230.

Rossiter, R.J., McLeod, I.M., and Strickland, K.P., *Can. J. Biochem. Physiol., 35,* 945–951 (1957).

Rumsby, M.G., and Crang, A.J., in G. Poste and G.L. Nicolson, Eds., *The Synthesis, Assembly and Turnover of Cell Surface Components,* Vol. 4, Elsevier/North Holland Biomedical Press, Amsterdam, 1977, pp. 247–362.

Sahenk, Z., and Mendell, J.R., *Brain Res., 219,* 397–405 (1981).

Saida, T., Saida, K., Silberberg, D.H., and Brown, M.J., *Nature, 272,* 639–641 (1978).

Saida, T., Saida, K., Brown, M.J., and Silberberg, D.H., *J. Neurol. Exp. Neuropathol., 9*, 498–518 (1979a).

Saida, T., Saida, K., Dorfman, S.H., Silberberg, D.H., Sumner, A.J., Manning, M.C., Lisak, R.P., and Brown, M.J., *Science, 204*, 1103–1106 (1979b).

Saida, T., Saida, K., Silberberg, D.H., and Brown, M.J., *Annu. Neurol., 9*(Suppl.), 87–101 (1981).

Scaravilli, F., and Jacobs, J.M., *Nature, 290*, 56–58 (1981).

Scaravilli, F., and Jacobs, J.M., *Brain Res., 237*, 163–172 (1982).

Scaravilli, F., and Suzuki, K., *Nature, 305*, 713–715 (1983).

Schlaepfer, W.W., *Brain Res., 78*, 71–81 (1974a).

Schlaepfer, W.W., *Brain Res., 69*, 203–205 (1974b).

Schlaepfer, W.W., and Micko, S., *J. Cell Biol., 78*, 369–378 (1978).

Schroder, J.M., *Brain Res., 45*, 49–65 (1972).

Schroder, J.M., in P.J. Dyck, P.K. Thomas, and E.H. Lambert, Eds., *Peripheral Neuropathy*, W.B. Saunders, Philadelphia, 1975, pp. 337–362.

Schubert, T., and Friede, R.L., *J. Neuropathol. Exp. Neurol., 40*, 134–154 (1981).

Schwartz, M., Ernst, S.A., Siegel, G.J., and Agranoff, B.W., *J. Neurochem., 36*, 107–115 (1981).

Sears, T.A., Ed., *Neuronal-Glial Cell Interrelationships*, Springer-Verlag, Berlin, 1982.

Seemayer, T.A., Oligny, L.L., Tannenbaum, G.S., Goldman, H., and Colle, E., *Amer. J. Pathol., 101*, 485–488 (1980).

Shaikh, N.A., and Palmer, F.B., *J. Neurochem., 28*, 355–403 (1977).

Sheltawy, A., and Dawson, R.M.C., *Biochem. J., 111*, 147–155 (1969a).

Sheltawy, A., and Dawson, R.M.C., *Biochem. J., 111*, 157–165 (1969b).

Simmons, D.A., Winegrad, A.I., and Martin, D.B., *Science, 217*, 848–851 (1982).

Singer, M., and Steinberg, M.C., *Amer. J. Anat., 133*, 51–84 (1972).

Singer, S.J., and Nicolson, G.L., *Science, 175*, 720–731 (1972).

Sinicropi, D.V., and Kauffman, F.C., *J. Biol. Chem., 254*, 3011–3017 (1979).

Skene, J.H.P., *Cell, 37*, 697–700 (1984).

Skoff, R.P., in *Glial and Neuronal Cell Biology*, Alan R. Liss Inc., New York, 1981, pp. 93–103.

Smith, K.J., and Hall, S.M., *J. Neurol. Sci., 48*, 201–219 (1980).

Smith, K.J., Blakemore, W.F., Murray, J.A., and Patterson, R.C., *J. Neurol. Sci., 55*, 231–246 (1982).

Smith, M.E., *J. Neurochem., 16*, 83–92 (1969).

Smith, M.E., and Benjamins, J.A., in P. Morell, Ed., *Myelin*, 2nd Ed., Plenum Press, New York, 1984, pp. 441–487.

Smith, M.E., and Rauch, H.C., *J. Neurochem., 23*, 775–783 (1974).

Smith, M.E., Kocsis, J.D., and Waxman, S.G., *Brain Res., 270*, 37–44 (1983).

Smith, R.S., *J. Neurocytol., 9*, 39–65 (1980).

Soifer, D., Iqbal, K., Czosnek, H., DeMartini, J., Sturman, J.A., and Wisniewski, H.M., *J. Neurosci., 1*, 461–470 (1981).

Souyri, F., Chretien, M., and Droz, B., *Brain Res., 205*, 1–13 (1981).

Sparrow, J.R., and Kiernan, J.A., *Acta Neuropathol. (Berl.), 53*, 181–188 (1981).

Spencer, P.S., *Soc. Neurosci. Symp., 4,* 275–321 (1979).

Spencer, P.S., and Schaumberg, H.H., Eds., *Experimental and Clinical Neurotoxicology,* Williams and Wilkens Publ., Baltimore, 1980.

Spencer, P.S., Politis, M.J., Pellegrino, R.G., and Weinberg, H.J., in A. Gorio, H. Millesi, and S. Mingrino, Eds., *Symposium on Posttraumatic Peripheral Nerve Regeneration,* Raven Press, New York, 1981, pp. 911–929.

Stanbury, J.B., Wyngaarden, J.B., Fredrickson, D.S., Goldstein, J.L., and Brown, M.S., Eds., *The Metabolic Basis of Inherited Disease,* 5th Ed., McGraw-Hill, New York, 1983.

Steele, J.A., Poznansky, M.J., Eaton, D.C., and Brodwick, M.S., *J. Mem. Biol., 63,* 191–198 (1981).

Steinberg, D., in J.B. Stanbury, J.B. Wyngaarden, D.S. Frederickson, J.L. Goldstein, and M.S. Brown, Eds., *The Metabolic Basis of Inherited Disease,* 5th Ed., McGraw-Hill Book Co., New York, 1983, pp. 731–747.

Stewart, M.A., Passonneau, J.V., and Lowry, O.H., *J. Neurochem., 12,* 719–727 (1965).

Sumner, A.J., Saida, K., Saida, T., Silberberg, D.H., and Asbury, A.K., *Annu. Neurol., 11,* 469–477 (1982).

Sundaran, K.S., and Lev, M., *J. Neurochem., 42,* 577–581 (1984).

Suzuki, K., and Suzuki, Y., in J.B. Stanbury, J.B. Wyngaarden, D.S. Frederickson, J.L. Goldstein, and M.S. Brown, Eds., *The Metabolic Basis of Inherited Disease,* 5th Ed., McGraw-Hill Book Co., New York, 1983, pp. 857–880.

Takahashi, H., and Suzuki, K., *Acta Neuropathol., 62,* 298–308 (1984).

Takahashi, H., Igisu, H., and Suzuki, K., *Amer. J. Pathol., 112,* 147–154 (1983).

Takahashi, H., Igisu, H., and Suzuki, K., *Acta Neuropathol. (Berl.), 59,* 159–166 (1983b).

Tennekoon, G., Zarba, M., and Wolinsky, J., *J. Cell Biol., 97,* 1107–1112 (1983).

Tessler, A., Autilio-Gambetti, L., and Gambetti, P., *J. Cell Biol., 87,* 197–203 (1980).

Thomas, P.K., in R. Bellairs and E.G. Gray, Eds., *Essays on the Nervous System,* Clarendon Press, Oxford, 1974, pp. 44–70.

Thomas, P.K., and Eliasson, S.G., in P.J. Dyck, P.K. Thomas, E.H. Lambert, and R. Bunge, Eds., *Peripheral Neuropathy,* 2nd Ed., W.B. Saunders Co., Philadelphia, 1984, pp. 1773–1810.

Trotter, J., and Smith, M.E., in E.C. Alford, Jr., M.W. Kies and A.J. Suckling, Eds., *Experimental Allergic Encephalomyelitis. A Useful Model for Multiple Sclerosis,* Alan R. Liss, Inc., New York, 1984, pp. 55–60.

Tsai, P.Y., and Geyer, R.P., *Biochim. Biophys. Acta, 489,* 381–389 (1977).

Tsukita, S., and Ishikawa, H., *J. Cell Biol., 84,* 513–530 (1980).

Tytell, M., Black, M.M., Garner, J.A., and Lasek, R.J., *Science, 214,* 179–181 (1981).

Vaughn, J.E., and Peters, A., *J. Comp. Neurol., 133,* 269–288 (1968).

Vitadello, M., Couraud, J.Y., Hassig, R., Gorio, A., and DiGiamberardino, L., *Exp. Neurol., 82,* 143–147 (1983).

Vizoso, A.D., and Young, T.Z., *J. Anat., 82,* 110–134 (1948).

Vlassara, H., Brownlee, M., and Cerami, A., *Proc. Natl. Acad. Sci. USA, 78,* 5190–5192 (1981).

Vorbrodt, A.W., Lossinsky, A.S., and Wisniewski, H.M., *Brain Res., 243,* 225–234 (1982).

Waksman, B.H., and Reynolds, W.E., *Proc. Soc. Exp. Biol. Med., 175,* 282–294 (1984).

Waller, A.V., *Philos. Trans. Roy. Soc. Lond. (Biol.), 140,* 423–429 (1850).

Warden, C.H., and Friedkin, M., *Biochim. Biophys. Acta, 792,* 270–280 (1984).

Watson, W.E., *Brit. Med. Bull., 30,* 112–115 (1974).

Watson, W.E., *Cell Biology of Brain,* Chapman and Hall, London, 1976.

Waxman, S., *The Physiology and Pathobiology of Axons,* Raven Press, New York, 1978.

Waxman, S.G., and Ritchie, J.M., Eds., *Advances in Neurology,* Vol. 31, *Demyelinating Diseases,* Raven Press, New York, 1981.

Webster, G.R., *J. Neurochem., 21,* 873–876 (1973).

Weiss, D.G., Ed., *Axoplasmic Transport,* Springer-Verlag, Berlin, 1982.

Wender, M., Zgorzalewicz, B., and Wroblewsky, T., *Acta Neurol. Scand., 47,* 52–58 (1971).

Wender, M., Kozik, M., Adamczewska-Goncerzewicz, Z., and Goncerzewicz, A., *Acta Neuropathol. (Berl.), Supp. VII,* 36–39 (1981).

White, D.A., in R.M.C. Dawson and J.N. Hawthorne, Eds., *Form and Function of Phospholipids,* Elsevier/North Holland Biomedical Press, Amsterdam, 1973, pp. 441–482.

White, G.L., Schellhase, H.V., and Hawthorne, J.N., *J. Neurochem., 22,* 149–158 (1974).

Whiting, P.H., Palmano, K.P., and Hawthorne, J.N., *Biochem. J., 179,* 549–553 (1979).

Wilson, D.L., and Stone, G.L., *Annu. Rev. Biophys. Bioeng., 8,* 27–45 (1979).

Wisniewski, H.M., Madrid, R.E., Lassmann, H., Deshmukh, D.S., and Iqbal, K., in A. Boese, Ed., *Search for the Cause of Multiple Sclerosis and Other Chronic Diseases of the Central Nervous System,* Verlag Chemie, Weinheim, Germany, 1980a, pp. 89–95.

Wisniewski, H.M., Brosnan, C.F., and Bloom, B.R., in A.N. Davison and M.L. Cuzner, Eds., *Suppression of Experimental Allergic Encephalomyelitis and Multiple Sclerosis,* Academic Press, New York, 1980b, pp. 45–48.

Woelk, H., and Kanig, K., *J. Neurochem., 23,* 739–744 (1974).

Woelk, H., Kanig, K., and Peiler-Ichikawa, K., *J. Neurochem., 23,* 745–750 (1974).

Wood, J.G., and Dawson, R.M.C., *J. Neurochem., 22,* 631–635 (1974).

Wood, J.G., Jean, D.H., Whitaker, J.N., McLaughlin, B.J., and Albers, R.W., *J. Neurocytol., 6,* 571–581 (1977).

Yahara, S., Kawamura, N., Kishimoto, Y., Saida, T., and Tourtellotte, W., *J. Neurol. Sci., 54,* 303–315 (1982).

Yao, J.K., in P.J. Dyck, P.K. Thomas, E.H. Lambert, and R. Bunge, Eds., *Peripheral Neuropathy,* 2nd Ed. W. B. Saunders Co., Philadelphia, 1984, pp. 510–530.

Yao, J.K., and Dyck, P.J., *J. Neurochem., 37,* 156–163 (1981).

Yao, J.K., Natarajan, V., and Dyck, P.J., *J. Neurochem., 35,* 933–940 (1980).

Yates, A.J., and Thompson, D.K., *J. Neurochem., 30,* 1649–1651 (1978).

Index

Acetate, synthesis of, fatty acids in brain, 178–180
Acetoacetate, 180
Acetoacetyl-CoA synthetase, 180
N-Acetylaspartate, 179
Acetylcholine, 224, 310
Acetyl-CoA carboxylase, 179
Acyl, alkyl, and alk-l-enyl bond composition, 216–218
Acylation, 191–192
Acyl-CoA hydrolase, 115
Acyldihydroxyacetonephosphate, 58
Acyl group composition:
  brain phospholipids, 93–106
  peripheral nerve, 106–107
Acyltransferase, 115, 117, 122
Adrenergic receptors, 260–261
Alkyl- and alkenylglycerols, 11, 20
Alpha oxidation, fatty acids, 178
Alzheimer's disease, 307–308, 309, 310, 311
Amino acid neurotransmitters, 262–263
Analysis:
  conventional methods, 4–11
    deacylation and phosphate determination, 4–6
    molecular species, 10–11
    thin-layer chromatography, 6–10
  extraction procedures, 3–4
  free fatty acid in brain, 174–175
  high-performance liquid chromatography, 11–40
    class separation, 11–16
    mass spectrometry (MS), 22–40
    molecular species, 16–22
  introduction, 2–3
  purification, 4

Animal models:
  disorders of nervous system, 313–314
  neurological disorders, 321–367
    cell membranes, 323–324
    demyelination and hypomyelination, 348–361
    diabetic neuropathy, 361–366
    glial lipid metabolism, 326–327
    nervous system barriers, 324–325
    neuronal lipid metabolism, 325–326
    neurons and glia, 324–327
    Wallerian degeneration, 328–348
Arachidonate metabolism, enhanced phospholipid labeling, 285–287
Arachidonic acid, 119–120, 181, 189, 194, 220, 231
Astroglial cells, 89
Axonal transport, 140–153
  central nervous system, 141–149
  extra-axonal diffusion, 150–151
  historical, 140–141
  mechanisms of transport, 151–153
  peripheral nerve, 149–150
  phospholipid transport in regenerating nerve, 150
  retrograde transport, 151
Axon-myelin transfer, 153–161
  central nervous system, 154–155
  mechanism and function, 159–161
  peripheral nervous system, 155–159
AY9944, 314

Basal ganglia:
  biogenic amines and therapeutic interventions, 309–312
  clinical correlations, 307–308

Basal ganglia (*Continued*)
phospholipid composition of brain,
308–309
Base-exchange enzymes, 52
Benzoylated PI, PS, and PG, high-
performance liquid chromatography
separation, 17
Beta oxidation, fatty acids, 178
Biosynthesis, phospholipids in nervous system,
48–63
CDP-diacylglycerol, 60
phosphatidic acid, 58–60
phosphatidylcholine, 48–53
de novo synthesis, 48–51
interconversion or exchange, 51–53
phosphatidylethanolamine, 51–53
phosphatidylglycerol and
diphosphatidylglycerol, 60–62
phosphatidylinositol and
polyphosphoinositide, 62–63
phosphatidylserine, 51–53
plasmalogen and glycerol ether, 53–56
sphingomyelin, 56–58
Bis(monoacylglycero) phosphate, 301–303
Blood-brain and blood-nerve barriers,
324–325
Bovine brain sphingomyelin, CIMS of, 34
Brain phospholipids:
acyl group composition, 93–104
choline phosphoglycerides, 95–98
ethanolamine phosphoglycerides, 98–102
individual phospholipids, 94–95
inositol phosphoglycerides, 104
phosphatidic acid, 104
serine phosphoglycerides, 102–103
sphingomyelin, 103–104
total phospholipids, 93–94
composition, 82–93
capillary endothelial cells, 89–90
human brain, 82, 85–86
isolated cells and subcellular fractions, 89
miscellaneous subcellular fractions,
92–93
myelin, 90–92
neurons and astroglia, 89
primate, 86–87
rabbit, 84
rats, 82–84, 87–88
whole brain, 82
dietary effects, 107–115

EFA deficiency, 107–112
miscellaneous abnormalities, 114–115
perinatal undernutrition, 112–113
protein malnutrition, 113–114
introduction, 81
metabolism, 115–125
enxymes for biosynthesis, 115–117
fatty acids, 118–123
release of free fatty acids, 124–125
trans-unsaturated fatty acids, 123–124
turnover of myelin, 117–118
see also Fatty acids, in brain

Calcium gating hypothesis, 278–281
Capillary endothelial cells, 89–90
Catabolism, phospholipids in nervous system,
64–73
deacylating phospholipases, 64–67
degradation of plasmalogens and glycerol
ether, 67–68
phosphoinositide hydrolysis, 69–72
phospholipase D enzymes, 72–73
sphingomyelin degradation, 68–69
CDP-choline:*N*-acylsphingosine choline
phosphotransferase, 57
CDP-choline:1,2-diacylglycerol
cholinephosphotransferase, 50
CDP-cholinephosphate cytidyltransferase, 50
CDP-diacylglycerol synthesis, 60
CDP-ethanolamine, 51
CDP-ethanolamine:1,2 diacylglycerol
ethanolaminephosphotransferase, 51
CDP-nucleotide pathway, 224, 227
Cellular and subcellular localization, enhanced
phospholipid turnover, 271–277
Central nervous system:
axonal transport, 141–149
axon-myelin transfer, 154–155
degeneration, 345–348
Ceramide, 57, 69, 307
Cerebellum, plasmalogens of, 86
Cerebral cell cultures, metabolic regulation of
polar head groups, 222–227
Cerebrum, plasmalogens of, 86
Chemical ionization mass spectrometry
(CIMS), 23
Chloroquine, 314
Cholesterol esters, 338, 347
Choline, 48, 117, 223
Choline acetyltransferase, 224, 310

Choline phosphoglycerides, acyl group profiles, 95–98
Choline phosphokinase, 224
Choline plasmalogen, 227
Cholinergic receptors, 258–260
Ciliary ganglion of chicken, 155
Citrate, 179
Class separation, by HPLC, 11–16
Clonal neuronal lines, 210–212
Column chromatography, 4, 12
Corticotropin (1-24) tetracosapeptide, 263
C1300 neuroblastoma clone, 220
CTP:1,2-diacylglycerophosphate-cytidylyl transferase, 60
CTP:ethanolamine phosphate cytidyltransferase, 51
Cultured cells, neural origin, 201–239
    culture media, lipids, and cell growth, 212–214
    introduction, 202–204
    phospholipids and, 214–233
        cell growth and function, 228–233
        composition and metabolism, 214–228
    tissue and cell culture, 204–212
Culture media, neural cells, 212–214
Cycloserine, 360
Cytidine nucleotide pathway, 221

Deacylating phospholipases, 64–67
Deacylation, phosphate determination and, 4–6
Demyelinating disorders, 206
Demyelination, 348–355
De novo biosynthesis, 48–51
Δ-4-desaturase, 219–220, 221
Desaturation, brain fatty acids, 181–186
Developing and aging nervous system, 79–134
    brain, 82–104, 107–125
        acyl group composition, 93–104
        dietary effects, 107–115
        phospholipid metabolism, 115–125
    introduction, 81
    peripheral nerve, 106–107
    spinal cord, 104–106
Diabetic neuropathy, 361–366
Diacylglycerol, 10, 283
Diacylglycerol kinase, 59, 245, 247, 265, 313
Diacyl phosphoglycerides, 5, 20
Dietary effects, brain phospholipids, 107–115
    EFA deficiency, 107–112

miscellaneous abnormalities, 114–115
perinatal undernutrition, 112–113
protein malnutrition, 113–114
4,4-Diethylaminoethoxyhexestrol, 303, 314
Dihydroxyacetone phosphate, 191
Dimethylethanolamine phosphoglycerides, 228
Dipalmitoylglycerylphosphorylcholine, 14
Diphosphatidylglycerol (DPC), 7, 14, 138
Diphosphatidylglycerol synthesis, 60–62
Diphtheria toxin, 349, 351
Disorders of nervous system, 297–319
    animal models, 313–314
    introduction, 298–299
    neurological, 307–313
        basal ganglia, 307–312
        multiple sclerosis, 312–313
        other diseases, 313
    sphingomyelin lipidoses, 299–307
        Bis(monoacylglycero) phosphate storage, 301–303
        clinical heterogeneity, 299–300
        sphingomyelin, glycerophospholipids and sphingomyelinases, 303–307
Dissociated cell cultures, 207–210
    as aggregates in suspension, 209
    grown as monolayers, 207–209
    homotypic cultures, 209–210
Dissociated cerebral neurons, 214
Dissociated dorsal root ganglia cells, 214
Distal nerve, 330–339
    compositional changes, following injury, 332–333
Docosahexaenoic acid, 189, 217, 218, 219, 220
Dopaminergic receptors, 261–262

Elaidic acid (trans), 123–124
Elongation, brain fatty acids, 181–186
Enhanced phosphoinositide turnover, 241–295
    biochemical studies, 264–271
        general properties, 264
        hydrolysis, 266–269
        labeling, 264–266
        and prelabeling, 269–271
    functional significance, 277–287
        arachidonate metabolism, 285–287
        calcium gate, 278–281
        diacylglycerol, 283–284
        endogenous calcium ionophore, 281–282
        inositol phospholipid hydrolysis, 282–283

Enhanced phosphoinositide (*Continued*)
    inositol trisphosphate, 282
    plasma membrane, 284–285
  introduction, 243–253
    historical review, 243–244
    neural preparations and turnover, 253
    phosphatidate-phosphatidylinositol cycle, 244–247
    subcellular localization of enzymes, 247–253
  receptors, 253–263
    adrenergic, 260–261
    amino acid neurotransmitters, 262–263
    cholinergic, 258–260
    dopaminergic, 261–262
    histaminergic, 261
    nerve growth factor, 262
    peptidergic, 263
    serotonergic, 262
  turnover, cellular and subcellular localization, 271–277
    neuronal and glial, 271–272
    site, 274–277
    subcellular locus, 272–273
Enzymic pathways, phospholipid metabolism in nervous system, 45–78
  biosynthesis, 48–63
  catabolism, 64–78
  introduction, 46–48
Essential fatty acid (EFA), 213
Essential fatty acid (EFA) deficiency, 107–112
  in cells and brain subcellular membranes, 110–111
  linoleic acid, 107–109
  linolenic acid, 109–110
  metabolism of brain phospholipids, 112
  reversal, 111–112
Ethanolamine, 223
Ethanolamine phosphoglycerides, 11, 29–31, 117, 224, 225, 227
  acyl group composition, 98–102
Ethanolamine plasmalogen, 53–56, 219, 221, 229
Experimental allergic encephalomyelitis (EAE), 352–353
Experimental allergic neuritis (EAN), 352–353
Extra-axonal diffusion, 150–151
Extraction, free fatty acids, 175
Extraction procedures, 3–4

Fatty acids:
  in brain, 173–199
    introduction, 174–177
      free fatty acids, 175–177
      techniques for analysis, 174–175
    oxidation, 178
    release of free fatty acids, 186–191
      pathological response, 186–189
      regulation, 189–191
    synthesis, 178–186
      elongation and desaturation, 181–186
      from glucose and acetate, 178–180
      from ketone bodies, 180
    transport, 177–178
    utilization, 191–194
      acylation, 191–192
      prostaglandin formation, 192–194
  effects and alteration, neural cell phenotype, 230–233
  neural cells, 218–221
    metabolic studies, 221
    uptake and metabolism, 218–221
  see also Brain phospholipids
Fatty acid synthetase, 115
Fluorogenic spray reagents, 9
Free fatty acids (FFA), 124–125
  release of, 186–191
Friedrich's Ataxia, 312

Galactosylcerebrosidase, 358, 359
Galactosylsphingosine (psychosine), 360
Gas-liquid chromatography (GLC), 10
Gentamicin, 303, 314
Glia cells, 210–212
Glial lipid metabolism, 326–327
Glial preparations, polar head group composition and metabolism, 221–222
Glia-neuron interaction, 207
Glucose synthesis, fatty acids in brain, 178–180
Glutamate, 179
Glutamic, aspartic, and 4-aminobutyric acid (GABA), 262–263
Glycerol ether (alkyl-acyl) synthesis, 53
Glycerol ether phospholipids, degradation of, 67–68
sn-Glycerol-3-phosphate acyltransferase, 191
Glycerophosphate dehydrogenase, 58

Glycerophospholipids, 303–307
Glycerophosphoryl derivatives, 5
Golgi apparatus, 140, 153

High-performance liquid chromatography
(HPLC), 11–40
class separation, 11–16
–mass spectrometry (MS), 22–40
ethanolamine phosphoglycerides, 29–31
phosphatidylcholine, 24–29
phosphatidylinositol, 31–34
phosphatidylserine, 31
phospholipid mixtures, 34–40
sphingomyelin, 34
molecular species, 16–22
Histaminergic receptors, 261
Homotypic cultures, 209–210
Human brain, development and aging, 82,
85–86
Huntington's disease, 307, 309, 311
3-Hydroxybutyrate, 180
12-Hydroxyeicosatetraenoic acid, 192
Hypoglycemia, 188
Hypomyelination, 355–361

Infantile metachromatic leukodystrophy, 302
Inositol bisphosphate, 271
Inositol monophosphate, 263
Inositol phosphoglycerides, acyl group profile,
104
Inositol trisphosphate, 271, 282
Intracellular phospholipid transfer, 161–167
general properties, 162–163
historical, 161–162
mechanism and physiological role, 165–167
transfer proteins of nervous system,
163–165
Ion-exchange chromatography, 5
Ischemia, 175, 186, 188

3-Ketodihydrosphigosine, 56
Ketone bodies, synthesis of fatty acids, 180
Krabbe's disease, 358–359

L-dopa therapy, 309
Lecithin, 312
Lewy bodies, 308
Linoleic acid, 177, 183
deficiency, 107–109

Linolenic acid, 177, 183
deficiency, 109–110
Lipomodulin, 190–191
Lipoxygenase, 192
Lung phosphatidylcholine, molecular species,
28
Lysophopholipases, 67
Lysophosphatidic acid, 59–60
Lysophosphatidylcholine, 64, 67
Lysophosphatidylethanolamine, 64
Lysophosphatidylinosito 63, 64
Lysophospholipids, 5
Lysoplasmalogenase, 125

Medulla oblongata, of rat brain, 88
Membrane flow, 140
Metabolic turnover, phospholipid constituents
in mature brain, 203
Microchromatography, 7
Microwave irradiation, 175
Molecular species analysis, 10–11
by HPLC, 16–22
Monoacylglycerols, 59, 60
Monoacyl phosphoglycerides, 5
Monolayers, dissociated cells grown as,
207–209
Multiple sclerosis, 312–313
Myelin, 90–92, 138, 203, 207, 326–327, 347
phospholipid transfer proteins, 165
Myelinogenesis, 206, 213
Myotonic muscular dystrophy, 313

Nerve growth factor (NGF), 262
Nerve regeneration, 342–343
Nervous system barriers, 324–325
Nervous tissue culture, 204–212
clonal neuronal and glial cell lines, 210–212
dissociated, 207–210
organotypic explants, 204–207
Neural origin, cultured cells, 201–239
culture media, lipids and cell growth,
212–214
introduction, 202–204
phospholipids and, 214–244
acyl, alkyl, and alk-1-enyl bond, 216–218
cell growth and function, 228–233
cerebral cell cultures, 222–227
composition and metabolism, 214–228
effects of fatty acids, 230–233

Neural origin (*Continued*)
    fatty acids, 218–221
      isolated neuronal and glial preparations,
        221–222
      turnover following ligand-cell interaction,
        229–230
    tissue and cell culture, 204–212
      clonal neuronal and glial cell lines,
        210–212
      dissociated, 207–210
      organotypic explants, 204–207
Neuroblastoma tumor, 211
Neurological disorders, secondary
    involvement, 307–313
Neuronal lipid metabolism, 325–326
Neuronal preparations, polar head group
    composition and metabolism,
    221–222
Neurons and glia, phospholipid metabolism,
    324–327
Neurotensin, 263
Niemann-Pick disease, 299, 301, 303, 305, 313,
    323
Nonspecific phospholipid-transfer protein, 163
Norepinephrine, 310

Octanoic acid, 187
Octapeptide, 263
Oleic acid, 123, 177
Oligodendroglia, 326, 352
Organotypic explants, 204–207
Oxidation, long-chain fatty acid, 178
2-Oxoglutarate, 179

Palmitaldehyde, 69
Palmitic acid, 177, 181
Parkinson's disease, 307, 308, 309, 311
PC12 rat pheochromocytoma cells, 220, 231
Pentobarbital, 188
Peptidergic receptors, 263
Perinatal undernutrition, 112–113
Peripheral nerve:
    acyl groups, 106–107
    axonal transport, 149–150
    axon-myelin transfer, 155–159
Peroxidation, polyunsaturated fatty acids, 189
Peroxisomes, 323
Phosphate determination, deacylation and,
    4–6

Phosphatidate-phosphatidylinositol cycle,
    244–247
Phosphatidic acid (PA), 3, 82, 138, 227, 229
    acyl group profile, 104
Phosphatidic acid synthesis, 58–60
Phosphatidylcholine, 24–29, 52, 65, 72–73,
    216, 219, 222, 226, 227, 304, 310, 336
    de novo synthesis, 48–51
    synthesis by interconversion or exchange,
      51–53
Phosphatidylcholine-transfer protein, 163
Phosphatidyldimethylaminoethanol, 226
Phosphatidyldimethylethanolamine, 228
Phosphatidyl-*N, N*-dimethylethanolamine, 52
Phosphatidylethanolamine (PE), 3, 52, 65, 67,
    138, 216, 219, 220, 222, 224, 225,
    226, 229, 231, 310
    de novo biosynthesis, 48–51
    synthesis, 69
    interconversion or exchange, 51–53
Phosphatidylglycerol, 304
    synthesis, 60–62
Phosphatidylinositol (PI), 3, 31–34, 138, 221,
    227, 229, 310, 338
Phosphatidylinositolbisphosphate (PIP_2), 7
Phosphatidylinositol bisphosphate
    phosphodiesterase, 71, 72
Phosphatidylinositol-4,5-bisphosphate, 63, 364
    364
Phosphatidylinositol kinase, 63
Phosphatidylinositolphosphate, 7, 364
Phosphatidylinositol-4-phosphate
    (diphosphoinositide), 63
Phosphatidylinositol synthesis, 62–63
Phosphatidylinositol-transfer protein, 163
Phosphatidylserine (PS), 3, 31, 65, 310
    synthesis by interconversion or exchange,
      51–53
Phosphocholine, 223, 224
Phosphoethanolamine, 223, 224
Phosphoglycerides, 216
Phosphoinositide hydrolysis, 69–72
Phosphoinositides, 59
Phospholipase A, 349
Phospholipase A_1, 66–67, 68, 69–70,
    189–190, 354
Phospholipase A_2, 66, 69–70, 189–190, 354
Phospholipase C, 304, 313
Phospholipase D, 313

enzymes, 72–73
Phospholipid exchange proteins, 161
"Phospholipid-labeling effect," 244
Phospholipid mixtures, HPLC-MS of, 34–40
Phospholipids:
  analysis, 1–40
    conventional methods, 4–11
    extraction procedures, 3–4
    HPLC, 11–40
    purification, 4
  biosynthesis, 48–63
    CDP-diacylglycerol, 60
    phosphatidylcholine, 48–51, 51–53
    phosphatidylethanolamine, 51–53
    phosphatidylglycerol and
      diphosphatidylglycerol, 60–62
    phosphatidylinositol and
      polyphosphoinositide, 62–63
    phosphatidylserine, 51–53
    plasmalogen and glycerol ether, 53–56
    sphingomyelin, 56–58
  brain, see Brain phospholipids
  catabolism, 64–73
    deacylating phospholipases, 64–67
    degradation of plasmalogens and glycerol
      ether, 67–68
    phosphoinositide hydrolysis, 69–72
    phospholipase D enzymes, 72–73
    sphingomyelin degradation, 68–69
  cultured cells, neural origin, 201–239
    cell growth and function, 228–233
    composition and metabolism, 214–228
  developing and aging nervous system,
    79–134
    brain, 82–104, 107–125
    peripheral nerve, 106–107
    spinal cord, 104–106
  disorders of nervous system, 297–319
    animal models, 313–314
    neurological, 307–313
    sphingomyelin lipidoses, 299–307
  enhanced phosphoinositide turnover,
    241–295
    biochemical studies, 264–271
    functional significance, 277–287
    receptors, 253–263
    turnover, cellular and subcellular
      localization, 271–277
  fatty acids in brain, 173–199

  normal brain, 175–177
  oxidation, 178
  release, 186–191
  synthesis, 178–186
  techniques for analysis, 174–175
  transport, 177–178
  utilization, 191–194
  transport, exchange, and transfer, 135–172
    axonal transport, 140–153
    axon-myelin transfer, 153–161
    general considerations, 137–140
    intracellular phospholipid transfer,
      161–167
Phospholipid-synthesizing enzymes, 155
Phosphotransferase, 116
Pineal gland, 274
Plasmalogen (alkenyl-acyl) synthesis, 53–56
Plasmalogens, 15, 82, 84
  degradation, 67
Plasma membrane, 203, 285–286
Polyphosphoinositides, 8–9, 83–84, 338, 353,
  358, 363
Polyphosphoinositide synthesis, 62–63
Polyunsaturated fatty acids (PUFA), 217
  synthesis, 183–186
Primate brain, development and aging, 86–87
Prostaglandins, formation and release,
  192–194
Protein malnutrition, 113–114
Purification, phospholipid fraction, 4

Rabbit brain, development and aging, 84,
  88–89
Rat:
  brain:
    development and aging, 82–84, 87–88
    phospholipids, HPLC-MS analysis,
      37–39
    capillary endothelial cells, 102
Receptors, enhanced phosphoinositide
    turnover, 253–263
  adrenergic, 260–261
  amino acid neurotransmitters, 262–263
  cholinergic, 258–260
  dopaminergic, 261–262
  histaminergic, 261
  nerve growth factor, 262
  peptidergic, 263

Receptors (*Continued*)
  serotonergic, 262
Regenerating axons, myelination of, 343–345
Regenerating nerve, phospholipid transport, 150
Retrograde response, 339–342
Retrograde transport, 151
Reversed-phase HPLC, 16–17, 20

Schwann cells, 326, 331, 335, 338, 349–350, 352, 356, 358–359, 360
Serine, 223, 224
Serine phosphoglycerides, acyl group profiles, 102–103
Serotonergic receptors, 262
Serotonin, 262, 310
Sodium-potassium ATPase, 365
Sphingomyelin, 5, 13, 82, 84, 85, 89, 301, 302, 303–307, 308, 314
  acyl group profile, 103–104
  bovine brain, CIMS of, 34
  HPLC analysis, 18–20
  quantitative HPLC analysis, 16
  storage in brain, 300–301
Sphingomyelinase, 300, 303–307
Sphingomyelin degradation, 68–69
Sphingomyelin lipidoses, 299–307, 313–314
Sphingomyelin synthesis, 56–58
Sphingomyelin-transfer protein, 163
Sphingosine, 56–57
Sphingosine-l-phosphate, 69
Sphingosylphosphocholine, 57–58
Spinal cord, acyl group profiles, 104–106
Stearic acid, 118–119
Streptozotocin, 361
Sulfatides, 354
Superior cervical ganglion, 274
Synaptogenesis, 207, 213

Tardive Dyskinesia, 307, 308, 311, 312
Thin-layer chromatography (TLC), 5, 6–10
Thromboxane B_2, 192
Transbilayer movement, 139–140
Transfer proteins, nervous system, 163–165
  mechanism and physiological role, 165–167
Transport, exchange, and transfer of phospholipids, 135–172

axonal transport, 140–153
  central nervous system, 141–149
  extra-axonal diffusion, 150–151
  historical, 140–141
  mechanisms, 151–153
  peripheral nerve, 149–150
  phospholipid transport in regenerating nerve, 150
  retrograde transport, 151
axon-myelin transfer, 153–161
  central nervous system, 154–155
  mechanism and function, 159–161
  peripheral nervous system, 155–159
general considerations, 137–140
intracellular phospholipid transfer, 161–167
  general properties, 162–163
  historical, 161–162
  mechanism and physiological role, 165–167
  transfer proteins of nervous system, 163–165
introduction, 136–137
Transport, fatty acid in brain phospholipids, 177–178
Triacylglycerols, 192
Triparanol, 314
Triton WR1339, 303
Triton X100, 305
Turnover, meylin lipids, 117–118

Ultraviolet light, 11–12
Trans-Unsaturated fatty acids, 123–124

Vasopressin, 263
Vertical gaze ophthalmoplegias, 299, 300

Wallerian degeneration, 328–348
  central nervous system, 345–348
  distal nerve, 330–339
  myelination of regenerating axons, 343–345
  nerve regeneration, 342–343
  retrograde response, 339–342
Whole brain, development and aging, 82

Y79 retinoblastoma cells, 220

Zellweger syndrome, 323

Home Supply (Lumber)
160 Van Wickle Ave,
   Hawthorne,
   427-7400